Anxiety

For Churchill Livingstone:

Editorial director (Nursing and Allied Health): Mary Law
Project manager: Valerie Burgess
Project development editor: Valerie Bain
Design direction: Judith Wright
Project controller: Derek Robertson
Illustrator: Charles Simpson
Copy editor: Diane West
Indexer: Elizabeth Ball
Sales promotion executive: Hilary Brown

The Management of
Anxiety
A GUIDE FOR THERAPISTS

Diana Keable BSc (Hons), DipCOT

Head Occupational Therapist, Mental Health, Harrow and Hillingdon Health Care Trust, London

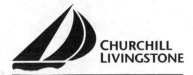

CHURCHILL
LIVINGSTONE

NEW YORK EDINBURGH LONDON MADRID MELBOURNE SAN FRANCISCO AND TOKYO 1997

CHURCHILL LIVINGSTONE
Medical Division of Pearson Professional Limited

Distributed in the United States of America by Churchill
Livingstone, 650 Avenue of the Americas, New York,
N.Y. 10011, and by associated companies, branches and
representatives throughout the world.

First Edition 1989
Second Edition 1997

ISBN 0 443 05527 0

British Library Cataloguing in Publication Data
A catalogue record for this book is available from the British
Library.

Library of Congress Cataloging in Publication Data
A catalog record for this book is available from the Library
of Congress.

Medical knowledge is constantly changing. As new
information becomes available, changes in treatment,
procedures, equipment and the use of drugs become
necessary. The editors, contributors and the publishers
have, as far as it is possible, taken care to ensure that the
information given in this text is accurate and up to date.
However, readers are strongly advised to confirm that
information, especially with regard to drug usage, complies
with the latest legislation and standards of practice.

Neither the publishers nor the author will be liable for any
loss or damage of any nature occasioned to or suffered by
any person acting or refraining from acting as a result of
reliance on the material contained in this publication.

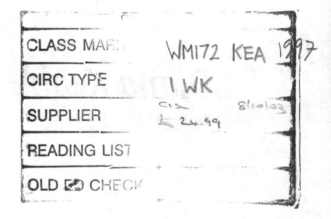
The
publisher's
policy is to use
**paper manufactured
from sustainable forests**

Produced through Longman Malaysia, PP

Contents

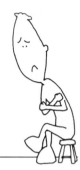

Contributors

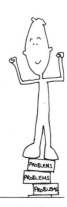

Kathryn Ashworth DipOT Henley Management Diploma
Head Occupational Therapist,
Bristol Royal Infirmary, Bristol
16 Section on 'Pain management'

Jenny Coleman DipCOT SROT
Head Occupational Therapist,
Napsbury Hospital and Community Mental
Health, Barnet Healthcare NHS Trust, London

Rosemary Johnson BSc
Occupational Therapist,
Bristol Royal Infirmary, Bristol
16 Section on 'Pain management'

Sue Hutchings BA MSc CertEd(FE) TDipCOT
Senior Lecturer, School of Occupational
Therapy,
Oxford Brookes University, Oxford
*13 From assessment to evaluation: procedures and
practicalities*

Alice Mackenzie BSc MSc DipCOT
Head Occupational Therapist,
Riverside Mental Health Trust, London
18 Working with older people

Peter O'Hanlon MBChB MRCPsych
Associate Specialist in the Psychiatry of Old Age,
Oxleas NHS Trust, Bexley Kent
*2 Section on 'Neurobiological mechanisms and drug
management in anxiety'*

Kate Radford MSc DipCOT
Research Occupational Therapist, Stroke
Research Unit,
Nottingham City Hospital NHS Trust,
Nottingham
16 Section on 'Cardiac rehabilitation'

Juliet Vinçom BSc (Hons)
T'ai Chi Teacher, Surrey
18 Working with older people

Gill Westland BA(Hons) DipCOT
Director, Cambridge Body Psychotherapy,
Cambridge
20 Understanding occupational stress and burnout

Preface

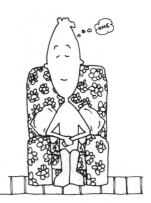

Since the publication of the first edition of this book, the body of knowledge relating to it has moved forward at an astonishing pace. The second edition, therefore, seeks to reflect some of these developments. In addition, while the first book was aimed almost exclusively at those working in the mental health field, this edition has tried to redress the balance by including a large section on using anxiety management techniques in the treatment of somatic conditions.

The more modern science discovers about stress responses the more it recognises that human beings are fully integrated psychophysiological units. Sadly, despite this, the notion that some kind of 'cut off' point exists between the mind and body – placed somewhat arbitrarily around the neck area – is, still, widespread. We, as clinicians, may inadvertently collude with this misplaced and deeply rooted construct among those we work with and for, perhaps because it seems so difficult to challenge. I hope that this book will provide clinicians from a wide range of settings with the theoretical knowledge and practical tools to support them in tackling this awesome task.

I hope that this explains why the second edition has been expanded to cover the use of anxiety management in the following additional clinical areas: the psychophysiological approach (including pain management and cardiac rehabilitation), older people, and community settings. This book also contains a chapter on occupational stress for clinicians, and the chapter on assessment and evaluation has been completely rewritten. A short section on the role of chemotherapy in anxiety has also been added. Finally, the book has been reorganised and more comprehensively illustrated to increase its appeal and accessibility.

The book has been enormously enhanced and broadened in its scope by those who contributed chapters, all experts in their respective fields. A great number of people have helped me to produce the book in small but significant ways. I hope they know that I know who they are! One outstanding example was David Farlie and his family, who patiently and expertly provided me with the technical support (and numerous cups of tea) necessary to process information produced by a variety of computer systems, each ranging from 'dinosaur' to 'state-of-the-art'.

To my professional colleagues for their interest and encouragement, and to my boss, Will Evans, for his flexibility, I am extremely grateful. Affectionate appreciation is also due to my two children for putting up with a very preoccupied Mum during the writing of this book, and to their Dad, for being there when I was on the planet 'stressor' attempting to practise what I preach.

1

Introduction

Diana Keable

STRESS AND MODERN SOCIETY

The concept of stress is now widely recognised. Although stress has always been an integral part of the human condition, it sometimes seems as if it was invented especially for the present time! Different periods in history have been associated with different kinds of stress. In times gone by, people were concerned primarily with survival — avoiding death by starvation, disease or violence. Sadly, this is still the case today in some beleaguered parts of the world. Yet the word 'stress' is commonly associated with western civilisation, in which the majority do not have to face severe hardship or the stark struggle merely to survive. How is it then that western societies are suffering from so much stress? After all, it could be argued that if we are protected from 'genuine' stress we may react by becoming neurotic!

Part of the answer lies in the very subtlety of modern pressures. These involve largely emotional factors such as uncertainty, insecurity, relationship problems, time pressure, fears of inadequacy and role conflicts. Today, the societal and moral structures that used to guide the decisions, actions and beliefs of the individual are undergoing massive upheaval. For example, less than 100 years ago in this country, just about everyone used to go to church each Sunday. Nowadays, it is only the minority who do so. The remaining majority have to decide how to structure their Sunday in alternative ways. The need to make even small decisions such as this can lead to stress. Sunday used to be regarded as a day of rest which gave people a kind of

1

'permission' to relax. Without this formalised opportunity to rest, many people are now unable to allow themselves to relax, being constantly goaded by the guilty feeling that they ought to be doing something 'useful'.

Similarly, the support afforded by the family structure is being eroded by the increasing breakdown of marital relationships. An insecure generation of young people is growing up in a world where permanent, caring relationships are the exception. Older people are forced to live alone in large anonymous cities or institutions. Violent crime appears to be increasing in a context of alienation within and between communities. Greater mobility has led to the mixing of different cultures with often incompatible needs and behaviours. Threatened minority groups are staking their individual claims within society and are, at best, met with misunderstanding and intolerance. Even men and women sometimes appear to be turning on each other in their attempts to carve out new roles or preserve old ones. Occupational and economic stresses also take their toll, either through the competitive, highly pressurised career or the spectre of unemployment. Add to all this upheaval, the accelerated pace of modern life where minutes, even seconds, matter. Today's world is a rapidly changing one in terms of technological development and high-speed information exchange systems, not least the all too efficient media, which constantly bombards us with distressing news and new challenges. Clearly, we are confronted with a system of stressors which the human being has not been prepared to withstand.

As mentioned before, it is the subtle nature of contemporary stressors which makes them so difficult to cope with effectively. Nature has provided us with a very limited repertoire of possible reactions to stress, i.e. the well-known 'fight or flight' responses. But, modern pressures can rarely be effectively dealt with by simply fighting them or running away. For example, in a stressful job interview, we cannot punch the interviewer on the nose, or run out of the room, and still expect to get the job! Patently, either of these actions would be highly inappropriate. However, this does not stop us from experiencing the same primitive internal responses which are preparing us for fight or flight. These feelings must be suppressed if we wish to achieve many of the goals of modern life. Unfortunately, there is a price to pay. Even if we are not exactly clear why modern society suffers so much from stress, we do know that it suffers badly. We know this because of the rising incidence of stress-related disease and death. The following examples of medical, psychological and social problems are held to be particularly related to stress:

- cardiovascular diseases, e.g. coronary arteriosclerosis
- gastrointestinal disease, e.g. ulcer
- respiratory disorders, e.g. asthma
- immunological disturbance, e.g. reduced resistance to infection
- dermatological disorders, e.g. psoriasis
- locomotor disorders, e.g. rheumatoid arthritis
- genitourinary disorders, e.g. impotence
- cancer
- pain, e.g. headache, back pain
- drug and alcohol abuse
- anxiety and depressive disorders
- psychosis
- fatigue, lethargy
- impaired task performance and cognitive function, e.g. poor memory and concentration
- behavioural disruption, e.g. impaired function in the work-place
- frequent minor illness
- suicide
- avoidance of social and occupational activities inside and outside the home.

Of course, the foregoing are only examples and do not entail a comprehensive list. Increasingly, the problems we suffer from are being related to stress in some way — but this is not always supported with the proper evidence. Much has been said about the stress of modern society. However, optimum levels of stress can energise and motivate individuals to improve performance, to the ultimate benefit of society as a whole. Berthold described anxiety as being the 'mother of the drive to know'.[1] Moderate stress also facilitates the shaping of behaviour during the process of growing up. Levitt[2] has described anxiety as a

'Janus-headed creature that can impel man to self-improvement, achievement, and competence, or can distort and impoverish his existence and that of this fellows'. Thus, the outlook need not be purely negative.

Since this book is primarily about anxiety, we will now begin to focus on this common disorder, which is inextricably linked with stress.

ANXIETY AND PSYCHIATRIC ILLNESS

What is anxiety? Before going any further, it is necessary to differentiate the terms we are using. We have already addressed the subject of stress. This is not the same as anxiety. Stress, or more properly, a stressor, is an external pressure which is brought to bear upon the individual. These stressors may bring about a variety of signs and symptoms which invariably include anxiety. Being anxious is often roughly equated to being 'in a state of stress'. Anxiety is a normal human response to stress. It may only be regarded as a disorder when it occurs in the absence of an appreciable degree, or kind, of threat or danger. In this lies the irony of anxiety. Although its original purpose was, and still is, to enhance survival and the learning of adaptive behaviour, excess anxiety impairs physical and cognitive performance.

Anxiety disorders are characterised by excessive physiological arousal, cognitive and behavioural disturbance. They are also associated with marked subjective distress and apprehension. The aversive nature of anxiety naturally motivates the sufferer to take action directed at reducing its intensity. This may take several forms: e.g. fight/flight behaviour, faint/freeze behaviour, evasive/protective manoeuvres, clinging behaviour and vocalisation of distress. Anxiety may be a diffuse, free-floating but persistent feeling of unease, i.e. generalised anxiety; or it may be a fear that is attached only to specific objects or situations i.e. phobia. It may also occur intermittently in an extremely acute form i.e. panic attacks. Anxiety may take the form of a 'state' which is a temporary feeling of subjective and physical ten-

sion. Alternatively, it may be described as a 'trait', in which it takes the form of a relatively permanent personality characteristic. People affected by trait anxiety have a tendency to experience more frequent and marked anxiety states in response to a wider range of stimuli than the general population. A short glossary of terms can be found at the end of this chapter.

The psychiatric classification of anxiety disorders

The classification of anxiety disorders has developed considerably over the last two decades. This has helped to inform the diagnostic process, and provided the basis for national and international research into these disorders. However, debate about whether a realistic classification system has finally been arrived at continues. The 1994 *Diagnostic and statistical manual of mental disorders* (DSM IV)[3] has provided the most recently up-dated classification of anxiety disorders:

- panic disorder without agoraphobia
- panic disorder with agoraphobia
- agoraphobia without panic disorder
- specific phobia
- social phobia
- obsessive compulsive disorder
- post-traumatic stress disorder
- acute stress disorder
- generalised anxiety disorder
- anxiety disorders due to a general medical condition
- substance-induced anxiety disorder
- anxiety disorder not otherwise specified.

The ICD-10[4] classification of mental and behavioural disorders gives a similarly lengthy list. However, the disorders are grouped differently and a few additional categories are included: e.g. somatoform anxiety, dissociative/ conversion disorders and other neurotic disorders. An alternative and much simpler classification, based on the cognitive–behavioural model, divides anxiety into five distinct categories:[5]

- generalised anxiety (acute and chronic)
- panic disorders

- simple phobias (single/multiple)
- agoraphobia
- evaluation anxiety, e.g. social/test anxiety.

The emphasis of the cognitive–behavioural treatment approach varies according to the category of anxiety being targeted.

WHAT CAUSES ANXIETY?

The aetiology of anxiety disorders is an enormous and highly complex subject to which a lengthy part of this book is devoted. Even so, this still provides only an introduction to the wide-ranging issues involved. What does seem certain is that anxiety disorders do not arise from one single cause. Rather, several contributory factors may be in operation at once, including:

- familial influences (including neurobiological and personality factors)
- early psychological trauma
- stressful life events
- faulty learning.

There has been some dissent about whether generalised anxiety disorder (GAD) actually qualifies as a separate category.[6] Whereas psychological models of panic and phobic disorders have been fairly well-established for some time, GAD is relatively new and less well understood.[7] GAD is thought to be fuelled by trait anxiety/neuroticism, and these elements are thought to have a heritability factor of 50%.[8,9] Studies have also shown that being older than 24 years of age, separated/widowed/divorced/unemployed, and a 'home-maker' are significant correlated with GAD. GAD is also frequently associated with other mental disorders.[6]

Relatively recent theoretical developments on the aetiology of anxiety disorders strongly suggest that in panic disorder, distinct neurobiological and psychological features are present.[5,10,11,12,13,14] In panic, these factors are thought to interact together via a feedback loop.[14] Accordingly, affected individuals anticipate the next panic attack with anxious apprehension, and are highly vigilant to bodily sensations which might signal an impending attack. This phenomenon, related to the learning model, has sometimes been termed the 'vicious circle' or 'spiral of anxiety'. Various neurological influences have been advanced to account for susceptibility to panic reaction in certain individuals:[5]

- chemoceptor oversensitivity triggering panic reaction in response to raised levels of sodium lactate or carbon dioxide
- asymmetric cerebral blood flow in the parahippocampal gyrus (subcortical area of the brain)
- high reactivity of the noradrenergic system of the brain
- underactivity of benzodiazepine receptors in the brain.

There is support for the proposition that any of these factors may be at work in causing a pathological oversensitivity to chemical changes associated with arousal.

Studies[15,16,17] of personality traits associated with phobic and panic disorders have also attempted to draw a profile of the characterological factors typically involved:

- imaginative
- self-deprecatory
- perfectionist
- excessively conscientious
- overly ambitious in setting standards/goals for themselves
- strong drive to please others
- highly sensitive to negative evaluation by others
- tendency to avoid conflict, disapproval or situations in which either may be elicited
- tendency to fearfulness and preoccupation with maintaining control or avoiding change
- maladaptive cognitive styles including a preponderence of negative and irrational thinking, including catastrophising, over-generalisation and jumping to conclusions.

THE EFFECTS OF ANXIETY

Anxiety disorders may have serious deleterious effects upon physical and mental health, functional ability and quality of life. Chronic anxiety may provide the trigger for physical disease to develop, or it may exacerbate an existing condition. Similarly, anxiety is a major component of the majority of psychiatric disorders, including psychosis. Stressful events are a common precipitating factor in acute psychotic episodes. Anxiety is the most disabling and distressing feature of many psychiatric conditions.

In the clinical setting, anxiety and depressive disorders are often indistinguishable. Also, the aetiological differentiation between anxiety and depression is still the subject of hot theoretical debate.[18,19,20] This difficulty is compounded by the closely interrelated neurological factors involved in depression and anxiety (neurobiological mechanisms are discussed in Section B of Chapter 2). However, Beck and Emery[13] have attempted to provide a practical guide to clinical differentiation between the two conditions.

Anxiety also has adverse effects on cognitive function, causing impairment of memory, task performance and concentration. These effects often occur when attention is diverted from the task and is taken up with apprehensive rumination about arousal symptoms, catastrophic imagery, self-preoccupation or preoccupation with attaining excessively high standards. Decision-making ability and occupational performance may be severely affected. Avoidance of ordinary behaviours such as shopping, travelling and participation in social functions is common. Anxiety also tends to interfere markedly with social and sexual functioning. The anxious individual may avoid people and be unable to maintain meaningful and healthy relationships. Conversely, overdependence on family and close friends may place additional, sometimes intolerable, burdens on relationships. Excessively anxious people may also tend to resort to illness behaviour as a way of coping with stress.

PREVALENCE

The size of the problem is considerable. In 1993, within the UK, estimates[21] of the number of those with a mental health disorder consulting NHS general practitioners totalled 4.2 million. This represented almost 10% of the overall consulta-

tion rate of 45.4 million in that year. The percentage share of days of certified incapacity due to mental illness (during 1992–93) was also remarkably high compared to other disorders. For male mental illness this was 16.1% — the third highest share, exceeded only by circulatory and musculoskeletal disorders. For female mental illness the percentage share was 26%, the second highest group, exceeded only by musculoskeletal disorders. These figures serve to highlight the widespread occupational disruption associated with mental illness in general.

Of all mental disorders, anxiety-related conditions are estimated to represent the second largest group, exceeded only by depressive disorders.[22,23] Epidemiological studies suggest that 15% of the general population suffer from either depression or anxiety over a period of one year.[24] Department of Health estimates[22] put the prevalence of anxiety disorders within the UK at 1.6–6% of the population. Thus, for every 500,000 people, 8,000–30,000 suffer from an anxiety-related disorder. Lifetime and 12-month prevalence studies[23] of psychiatric disorders in the USA show that of all anxiety disorders, social and simple (specific) phobias were the most prevalent.

TREATING ANXIETY WITH DRUGS — THE PROBLEMS

Just over a decade ago, benzodiazepines, or minor tranquillisers, were still being prescribed widely and relatively indiscriminately. At that time they were generally regarded as the treatment of choice for anxiety-related conditions. They were believed to be safe, effective and non-addictive. More recently, considerable alarm has been generated concerning the risks of dependency which is associated with the consumption of benzodiazepines. In 1982, between 18 and 20 million prescriptions were issued for tranquillisers in the UK.[25] Over the last decade, the psychiatric service has been faced with the daunting prospect of helping long-term consumers to withdraw from these drugs. This has been made all the more necessary in view of the growing recognition that minor tranquillisers only remain effectual for a relatively short period of time. After that brief period, habituation occurs and a greater dose is needed to control anxiety symptoms. Although thousands of people had been taking benzodiazepines for many years, they were no longer getting any benefit from them in terms of anxiety reduction. However, when withdrawal from benzodiazepines is attempted, a distressing recurrence of anxiety symptoms often occurs. The withdrawal symptoms may be more intense than the original symptoms for which the client started taking the drugs (see Section B of Chapter 2).[26,27,28,29] The Department of Health, in its Health of the Nation initiative in relation to mental illness,[22] emphasised that one of the principal themes for management action is to reduce dependence on benzodiazepines.

A COMPREHENSIVE APPROACH TO THE TREATMENT OF ANXIETY

We know that anxiety has severe effects on all aspects of human function, whether physical, cognitive or behavioural. Thus, a limited approach, such as that offered by chemotherapy, will rarely answer the purpose. Of course, therapists have been using a variety of relaxation training methods in treating anxiety for many years. However, although popular, and to some extent successful, single relaxation techniques generally focus on only one or two aspects of anxiety. Into this breach the newer comprehensive approaches to anxiety control have stepped, e.g. cognitive behaviour modification (CBM)[30] and anxiety management training.[31] These are not single techniques, but programmes or courses of training comprising a variety of different aspects of anxiety control. Firstly, they emphasise education about the physical, mental and behavioural effects of anxiety. Secondly, they involve training in a variety of different physical and cognitive skills which can be applied according to the different demands of the stressful situation confronting the client. Thirdly, as part of the programme, actual rehearsal and application of the new skills outside the treatment setting is emphasised. This ensures that skill learning is reinforced and applied to the situations in which

it is needed most. The programmes are usually carried out within a group context, which has both economic and learning advantages. Although there are several different comprehensive anxiety-reduction programmes, they have generally been given the umbrella term 'anxiety management'. It should also be noted that several studies have shown CBM to be more effective than chemotherapy in treating anxiety, particularly on a long-term basis.[32,33,34] Large sections of this book are devoted to the clinical application of CBM techniques.

THE ROLE OF THE THERAPIST/HEALTH CARE PROFESSIONAL IN DEALING WITH ANXIETY

In this introduction we have briefly looked at the pervasive and distressing effects of stress and anxiety. We now need to consider what therapists and other health care professionals may have to offer in dealing with these problems.

Many therapists have a valuable and practical contribution to make in the field of anxiety and stress control. In the author's opinion, therapists are in a unique position to use active anxiety reduction techniques to advantage in their work. This is partly because they are usually experienced in dealing with the functional problems associated with psychological disorders. That is, many therapists are used to looking at the way the disorder has affected the client as a whole person. The client is also seen in the context of his lifestyle, work and relationships.

Who is the 'therapist'?

Anxiety management methods are being used increasingly widely by a number of different professionals in a variety of health-related fields, including occupational therapists, community psychiatric nurses, other specialist nurses, social workers, physiotherapists and psychologists. The material in this book is meant to be of particular relevance to all these groups, and the term 'therapist', does not mean to exclude any professional who may be using the techniques.

However, the anxiety-reduction techniques covered here require that the professional adopts the role of a therapist in relation to his or her client. The term 'therapist' is, however, a very vague one, with wide-ranging and subjective connotations. In this context, then, it is taken to indicate a therapist whose role includes teaching, treatment and empathic listening. The therapist is using active treatment techniques which depend on the participation of the client. The therapist is working with the client, and this is necessarily a dynamic, cooperative relationship.

Who is the 'client/patient'?

The recipients of the interventions discussed in this book have been termed variously 'client' and 'patient'. These terms have been used interchangeably as deemed appropriate to the setting in which the intervention is generally delivered. However, it is recognised that there is still widespread disagreement about the political connotations attached to both terms.

WHAT THIS BOOK COVERS

When the first edition of this book was written, almost a decade ago, the concerns of mental health care professionals were its primary focus. The goal of the new edition has been to address the needs of a wider readership, acknowledging the strengthening links between mental and physical health care practice. Accordingly, a major area that has been expanded upon here is the psychophysiological approach. It is hoped that this material will be particularly useful to health care professionals working in medical and surgical settings. It is recognised that they are constantly faced with the challenge of anxiety, which may precipitate a wide range of disorders or hamper recovery. This edition has been laid out in three main parts:

1 Theoretical concepts
2 Treatment techniques
3 Clinical application

The theoretical concepts have been emphasised because, in order for treatment to be carried out with insight, an appreciation of the theoretical issues involved is indispensable. The subject area is extremely complex and wide-ranging; contributions have been made towards the theoretical understanding of anxiety from many different schools of thought.

The following chapters focus on treatment techniques. A description of various anxiety-reduction techniques is given, together with a plan for an eight-module anxiety management course. Further information in the form of 'client packs' can be found in the appendix at the end of the book. Ideas for supplementary activities which the therapist can use in anxiety-control training sessions are also suggested.

Part 3 contains several completely new chapters which illustrate some of the wider contexts in which anxiety management can be usefully applied, e.g. community settings, physical disorders, older people. Teaching resources and suggestions for dealing with common problems in the clinical application of the techniques are given. The topics of assessment, evaluation and research are also addressed with a particular focus on the need to demonstrate clinical outcomes. The book finishes with a new chapter devoted to the needs of health care professionals themselves — understanding and surviving occupational stress and burnout.

GLOSSARY

This is a short glossary of terms based on the DSM IV classification system.[3]

Acute stress disorder: Intense anxiety occurring in the immediate aftermath of an extremely traumatic event.

Agoraphobia: Intense anxiety and/or avoidance behaviour relating to certain places or situations, usually located outside the home environment, e.g. supermarkets. May or may not be accompanied by panic attacks.

Anxiety disorder due to a medical condition: Intense anxiety symptoms judged to be a direct physiological consequence of a general medical condition.

Generalised anxiety disorder: Pervasive,

persistent and excessive anxiety with no discrete focus, and of at least six months' duration.

Obsessive compulsive disorder: Obsessional thoughts which are experienced as intrusive and distressing, and/or compulsive behaviour, e.g. hand-washing rituals engaged in as a means of reducing the anxiety resulting from obsessional thoughts.

Panic attack: Intermittent episodes of sudden onset involving feelings of intense fearfulness/terror. They are accompanied by symptoms of acute physiological arousal, e.g. breathlessness, palpitations, trembling, chest pain, choking sensations and fears of losing control/going mad/imminent death.

Panic disorder: A disorder characterised by recurrent panic attacks. It may or may not be accompanied by agoraphobia.

Post-traumatic stress disorder: Intense anxiety and preoccupation with a previous traumatic event. This involves a feeling of re-living the event in the form of flashbacks and prompts the subject to avoid stimuli which reminds them of the trauma.

Social phobia: Intense anxiety associated with certain social/performance situations. Often associated with avoidance behaviour.

Specific/simple phobias: Intense anxiety brought about by exposure to a certain object/situation, e.g. spiders, lifts. Avoidance behaviour is usually a strong feature.

Substance-induced anxiety disorder: Intense anxiety symptoms judged to be a direct physiological consequence of drug/medication/toxin exposure.

REFERENCES

1 Berthold F 1963 Anxious longing. In: Hiltner S, Menniger K (eds) Constructive aspects of anxiety. Abingdon, New York

2 Levitt E E 1980 The psychology of anxiety, 2nd edn. Lawrence Erlbaum, Hillside, New Jersey, ch 11

3 American Psychiatric Association 1994 Diagnostic and statistical manual of mental disorders (DSM IV), 4th edn. American Psychiatric Association, Washington DC

4 World Health Organization 1992 The ICD-10 classification of mental and behavioural disorders — clinical descriptions and diagnostic guidelines, World Health Organization, Geneva

5 Michelson L, Ascher L M (eds) 1987 Anxiety and stress disorders — cognitive behavioural assessment and treatment. Guilford Press, New York

6 Wittchen H, Zhao S, Kessler R C, Eaton W W 1994 DSMIII-R Generalised anxiety in the national co-morbidity survey. Archives of General Psychiatry 51(5):355–364

7 Andrews G 1993 Panic and generalized anxiety disorders. In: Freeman H L, Kupfer D J (eds). Current opinion in psychiatry 6(2):191–194

8 Andrews G 1991 Anxiety, personality and anxiety disorders. International Review of Neurobiology 3:293–302

9 Oakley Browne M 1991 The epidemiology of anxiety disorders. International Review of Neurobiology 3:242–252

10 Gelder M G 1986 Panic attacks: new approaches to an old problem. British Journal of Psychiatry 149:346–352

11 Clark D M 1986 A cognitive approach to panic. Behaviour Research and Therapy 24(4):461–470

12 Thyer B A, Nesse R M, Curtis G C, Cameron O G 1986 Panic disorder: a test of the separation anxiety hypothesis. Behaviour Research and Therapy 24(2):209–211

13 Beck A T, Emery G 1985 Anxiety disorders and phobias. Basic Books, USA

14 Barlow D H 1992 Cognitive behaviour approaches to panic disorder and social phobia. Bulletin of the Meninger Clinic 56 (2 suppl.A):14–28

15 Zane M D, Milt H 1984 Your phobia: understanding your fears through contextual therapy. American Psychiatric Press, Washington DC

16 Angyal A 1965 Neurosis and treatment: a holistic theory. Wiley, New York

17 Hardy A B 1982 Phobic thinking; the cognitive influences on the behavior and effective treatment of the agoraphobic. In: Dupont R L (ed) Phobia: A comprehensive summary of modern treatments. Brunner/Mazel, New York

18 Stavrakaki C, Vargo B 1986 The relationship of anxiety and depression: a review of the literature. British Journal of Psychiatry 149:7–16

19 Lesse S 1982 The relationship of anxiety to depression. American Journal of Psychotherapy, XXXVI (3):332–349

20 Goldberg R J 1995 Diagnostic dilemmas presented by patients with anxiety and depression. The American Journal of Medicine 8:278–284

21 Office of Health Economics 1995 Compendium of health statistics, 9th edn. Office of Health Economics, London

22 Department of Health 1994 The health of the nation: key area handbook — mental illness, 2nd edn. HMSO, London

23 Kessler R C, McGonalgle K, Zhao S, et al 1994 Lifetime and 12-month prevalence of DSMIII-R psychiatric disorders in the US. Results from the national co-morbidity survey. Archives of General Psychiatry 51(1):8–19

24 Montgomery S A 1990 Anxiety and depression. Wrightson Biomedical Petersfield

25 The National Medical Advisory Committee 1994 The management of anxiety and insomnia. A report by the National Medical Advisory Committee. HMSO, Edinburgh

26 Haddon C 1984 Women and tranquilizers. Sheldon Press, London

27 Melville J 1984 The tranquilizer trap — and how to get out of it. Fontana, London

28 Stopforth B 1986 Outpatient benzodiazepine withdrawal and the occupational therapist. British Journal of Occupational Therapy 49(10):318–322

29 Tyrer P, Owen R, Dawling S 1983 Gradual withdrawal of diazepam after long-term therapy. Lancet 25:1402–1406

30 Meichenbaum D 1977 Cognitive behavioural modification. Plenum Press, New York

31 Suinn R M, Richardson F 1971 Anxiety management training: a nonspecific behaviour therapy program for anxiety control. Behavior Therapy 2:498–510

32 Lindsay W R, Gamsu C V, McLaughlin E, Hood E M, Espie C A 1987 A controlled trial of treatments for generalized anxiety. British Journal of Clinical Psychology 26:3–15

33 Clark D M, Salkovskis P M, Hackmann A, Middleton J, Anastasiades P, Gelder M 1994 A comparison of cognitive therapy, applied relaxation and imipramine in the treatment of panic disorder. British Journal of Psychiatry 164(6):759–769

34 Michelson L K, Marchione K 1991 Behavioral, cognitive and pharmacological treatments of panic disorder with agoraphobia: critique and synthesis. Journal of Consulting and Clinical Psychology 59(1):100–114

Theoretical concepts

It is difficult to single out theories which relate only to one aspect of anxiety since it can only be understood by taking several factors into account at once. Anxiety is a multifaceted creature in which physiological, emotional, behavioural and cognitive factors act interdependently. An attempt has been made to demonstrate the connections between the different aspects of anxiety throughout the text. However, for the sake of clarity, the subject is dealt with in five chapters, each focusing on a specific aspect of anxiety.

2

The physiology of anxiety

Diana Keable
(Physiological theories of anxiety)

Peter O'Hanlon
(Neurobiological mechanisms and drug management in anxiety)

PHYSIOLOGICAL THEORIES OF ANXIETY

HISTORICAL DEVELOPMENT

Many of the early thinkers and researchers in this field recognised the unique and powerful link between the emotional and physical aspects of anxiety. One of the first contributors to the development of psychophysiological theory was Descartes in 1648 who saw the mind and body as being separate entities. This dichotomy was termed 'dualism'. At that time, one of the major concerns was to determine the nature of the initiating centre of thought and feeling, and its anatomical location. He noted that the emotions could have direct effects on bodily responses. Central to his thinking was the influence of the environment in the initiation of emotion. He propounded the idea that the pineal body, which he called the 'seat of the soul', was the main mediating centre between the body, with its sensory and motor functions, and the soul, which experienced the emotions.

Thus, an external event which elicited emotion was transmitted from the sensory organs through nerve pathways to the pineal body, or soul. From thence, the emotions passed via the brain and nerves to the bodily organs to be translated into physical reactions and behaviour. Information about the physical activity was then transmitted back to the pineal body, serving to heighten the emotional state (Fig. 2.1).

We no longer credit the pineal body with

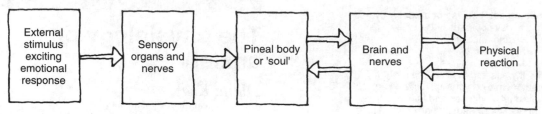

Figure 2.1   The Descartes model.

having such an important function as the soul. However, some of Descartes' ideas made a sound contribution to the developing understanding about the process of communication between physical, emotional and behavioural systems. This was, perhaps, the first example of a 'feedback loop' process, about which more will be said later on in this chapter. Little further headway was made until several centuries later. In the late 1880s, the James–Lange theory emerged which was described by two independent researchers.[1,2] This theory suggested that bodily changes could, in themselves, produce emotion, and that it was bodily reactions to stimuli that actually caused the effect. For example: 'we are angry because we strike', or 'we are afraid because we tremble' (Fig. 2.2).

This view was incompatible with the early theories of Descartes who put the initiating centre of anxiety in the 'soul'. However, the James–Lange notion still carries some weight today. Indeed, our perception of the bodily changes associated with our emotions, serves to intensify the state of feeling. The use of beta-blockade chemotherapy to reduce peripheral feedback in anxiety states is also relevant to this observation. By suppressing the uncomfortable physiological symptoms of anxiety, these drugs are able to reduce emotional

distress levels in some cases. Some anxious clients report that physical symptoms are the major obstacle preventing them from coping. For example: 'if only my hands would stop trembling, I could cope better in exams'.

By the 1920s, the science of neurophysiology had progressed considerably and the James–Lange theory was discredited by Cannon.[3] He argued that bodily reactions could not be responsible for initiating emotion, and suggested that the individual perceived the emotion and the physical reaction simultaneously. His experiments showed that animals still demonstrated the full range of emotion despite spinal cord lesions, which precluded the normal bodily reactions to stimuli. He also argued that bodily reactions are similar in different emotions; joy and fear, for example, are physiologically similar states. Additionally, he observed that emotional states could not be brought about by artificially inducing visceral changes, for example, by injecting adrenalin. His work was later supported and developed by Bard in 1928, and their collective work has become known as the Cannon–Bard theory.

The Cannon–Bard theory placed the main control centre initiating emotional reactions in the thalamus. The thalamus was thought to be responsible for receiving sensory information and communicating with the cortex and bodily organs to bring about behavioural responses (Fig. 2.3).

Cannon was also the first to describe the characteristic 'fight/flight' stress reaction and the part the sympathetic nervous system had to play in producing it.[4] These ideas were developed during the 1930s by Hans Selye. His important work on the human stress response represented a milestone in stress physiology.[5] Selye's work will be discussed in depth later in this chapter.

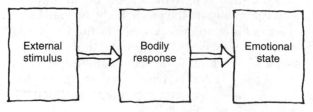

Figure 2.2   The James–Lange model.

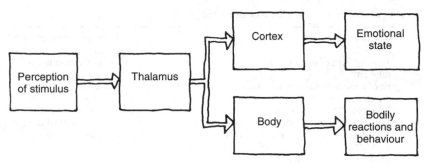

Figure 2.3 The Cannon–Bard model.

In 1937 Papez[6] described other brain sites which are associated with emotion, comprising the limbic system as it is now known. In contrast with the Cannon–Bard theory, he emphasised the role of the hypothalamus, rather than the thalamus, as the main control centre in the initiation of emotional responses. These findings have since been confirmed and developed further and will be elaborated upon later in this chapter.

So far we have seen how the developing sciences arrived at answers to very generalised questions about basic human emotional responses. The focus then began to diversify and various theories emerged about how individuals vary in the way they respond to stress. The part played by cognitive, environmental and personality factors in determining the human emotional response began to be examined.

In 1953, Ax[7] noted some differences in the way physiological arousal manifested itself in response to different emotions. He observed that while anger tended to increase diastolic blood pressure, fear increased muscle tension potentials. Similarly, Alexander[8] developed his 'specificity theory' which related certain emotions, personality types and conflicts to specific psychosomatic disorders and autonomic response patterns. The subject of psychosomatic disease and personality is highly pertinent to the study of anxiety and will be discussed further in Chapter 5.

Finally, recent evidence is beginning to highlight the bearing of genetic influences in the aetiology of anxiety disorders and other anxiety-related problems including panic disorder and various phobic conditions. Studies have shown that the prevalence of anxiety and related disorders is higher among the relatives of affected subjects than among control families. Marks[9] has suggested that this effect indicates a specific genetically determined autonomic predisposition.

Table 2.1 shows some of the key developments is psychophysiology.

THE BRAIN AND ANXIETY

The primitive lower brain, or subcortex, is responsible for initiating and controlling states of physiological arousal and for the involuntary homeostatic functions. The higher brain, or cortex, is responsible for perceiving and interpreting stressors, and initiating and coordinating voluntary action. The key lower brain structures have direct neural links with the cortex. Recent studies suggest that three main brain sites are responsible for regulating anxiety, i.e. the prefrontal area of the cortex, and the amygdala and hypothalamus in the subcortex (Fig. 2.4) (see Kalin, 1993, Further Reading).

The integrated process by which the main brain centres handle stress is initiated by the cortex when a stressor is first perceived by the individual. In particular, the prefrontal cortex is involved in the cognitive evaluation of the stressor. The subcortical structures are then called in to play. The amygdala, sited within the limbic system, is held to be responsible for generating the fear response. The hypothalamus has long been known to be a vital organ in regulating the stress response and is responsible for activating two other important agents, the autonomic and endocrine systems. The hypothalamus (discussed in more detail further on in this section)

Table 2.1   Some important milestones in the evolution of psychophysiology

Descartes 1648	The pineal body as the 'seat of the soul' The concept of mind-body dualism	Attempted to locate and explain system or organ responsible for the emotions, e.g. anxiety
James–Lange 1880s	Bodily reactions as the cause of emotions	
Cannon–Bard 1920s	The role of the thalamus The characteristic 'fight/flight' stress response Autonomic and endocrine responses	Defined the term 'stress', and the basic physiological processes involved
Papez 1937	The 'Papez' circuit — role of the limbic system and hypothalamus in the stress response	
Selye 1930s	'Stress'. The general adaptation syndrome: 'GAS'	
Ax 1953	Differences in physiological arousal patterns in response to different emotions	Developed theory of psychosomatic disease and the influence of personality
Alexander 1950s	Relationship of specific emotions to specific organic disorders and individualised response patterns	
Schacter and Singer 1962	Influence of cognition upon physiological arousal	Cognitive aspects of psychophysiology

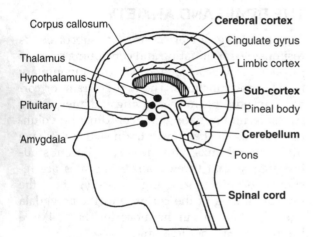

Figure 2.4   A diagrammatic cross-section of the brain.

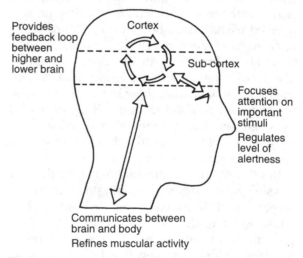

Figure 2.5   The reticular activating system.

mediates between these two systems and is also involved with the limbic cortex in regulating emotion and basic visceral functions.

The cingulate gyrus, sited below the upper part of the motor cortex has an inhibitory effect on emotional reactions. The cortex controls skeletal muscle potentials and brain wave frequencies. Under stress, beta wave frequencies can be observed to increase. Beta waves predominate in the brain as arousal increases; in the relaxed state theta and alpha waves are the more conspicuous.

The relationship between the cortex and subcortex is a complex and interesting one. These structures are not separate but communicate through feedback loops provided by the reticular activating system (RAS) (Fig. 2.5). Incoming information is sorted through this system, which focuses attention on relevant stimuli and rejects unnecessary input. The RAS also regulates levels of alertness and refines muscular activity. Additionally, the RAS transmits nervous impulses between the body and the cortex, providing a link between intellectual and neurophysiological activity. Stimuli arising from the autonomic system are also screened from the cortex.[10,11]

Of further relevance to the relationship between the higher and lower brain, in 1960, Simeons,[12] presented a 'cortical censorship communications' model. This involved the primitive 'fight/flight' responses and the higher brain functions. He posited the existence of a conflict between cortical and subcortical reactions. According to Simeons, the higher brain seeks to inhibit or 'euphemise' the primitive reactions of the lower brain. Thus we speak of indigestion when the appetite is blunted by fear, and of palpitations when the heart rate is felt to quicken.

Schacter[13] described the stress of modern society as having a persistent, ongoing quality. Physical activity serves to release accumulated tension. However, in modern society, a literal 'fight/flight' reaction is rarely appropriate. So, the subcortex continues to augment the arousal state while the cortex continues to restrain it. The result, he postulates, is a chronic tension cycle.

The hypothalamus

Stimulation of the hypothalamus produces integrated emotional and behavioural responses, both autonomic and skeletal.[14] Three main stress reactions have been observed on experimental stimulation of the hypothalamus in animals: alarm, flight and rage. Among other structures in the diencephalon, the hypothalamus assists in the control of body temperature and contains centres involved with hunger and pleasure. Its main function during stress is to activate and regulate the autonomic and endocrine systems.

The hypothalamus lies below the thalamus at the base of the forebrain. It has direct links with the pituitary gland, the limbic structures, the cortex and thalamus. Neuronal pathways from the hypothalamus also go to the brainstem and spinal cord. The hypothalamus and pituitary are also affected by various hormones from other endocrine glands which provide a regulatory feedback loop (Fig. 2.6).

The hypothalamus is connected to the pitu-

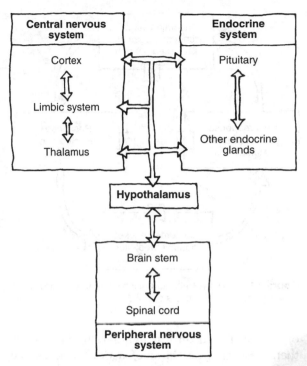

Figure 2.6   The hypothalamus and its links with the endocrine and nervous systems.

itary, or master gland, by two pathways. The first of these is via endocrine connections to the anterior (frontal) lobe; the second is via neuronal connections to the posterior lobe. Basically, the hypothalamus has two lobes concerned with the regulation of arousal. The anterolateral lobe inhibits sympathetic nervous system activity and the release of activating hormones from the pituitary; the posteromedial lobe has the opposite effect.

Papez's circuit

A recent hypothesis concerning the limbic system and its related structures, Papez's circuit, suggests that this region might act as a 'behavioural inhibition system'.[6,15] One function of this system is to predict the nature of stimuli to which the organism is about to be subjected. The actual incoming stimuli are then checked against this prediction, and labelled according to their level of importance, familiarity or aversiveness to the

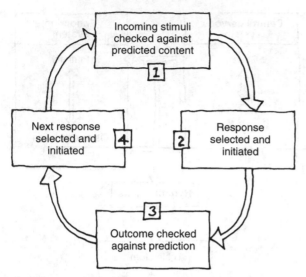

Figure 2.7   How the behavioural inhibition system governs ongoing behaviour (Papez's circuit).

organism. Based on this evaluation, the system then chooses what kind of action is necessary and initiates the required brain and bodily responses (Fig. 2.7). For example, imagine a person walking across a field. The sensation that will result from each step is predicted before it occurs. When a step has been taken, the actual sensation that occurred is compared and matched with the prediction. If the expected sensation occurs with each step the person continues to walk on. However, should the person catch a foot in a rabbit hole and stumble, a mis-match will occur. The system would then evaluate the new sensory event and alter the ongoing motor behaviour accordingly — such as increasing attention on the terrain and stopping while the foot is extracted.

In unexpected crisis situations, the system is involved in instigating the appropriate behavioural reaction such as the 'fight or flight' response. Anxiety symptoms are held to be the result of accelerated activity in the behavioural inhibition system. According to this hypothesis, people who are chronically anxious are said to have highly reactive behavioural inhibition systems.

The thymus and the immune system

Finally, the role of the brain in regulating the immune system is worthy of note, particularly with regard to the disruptive effects of stress. The hypothalamus appears to influence the thymus which, in turn, initiates and regulates immune system activity. The thymus is involved with the production of 'T' lymphocytes for antibody regulation. Some research on animals suggests that when the dorsal hypothalamic area is cut, thereby affecting the function of the thymus, a predisposition to disease occurs. The thymus appears to be stress responsive in humans also, and its function is disorganised by hormones produced during states of stress. It has been proposed that the normal function of the immune system in protecting the organism from disease is interrupted during stress.[16] This may reduce resistance to general infection as well as serious disease states such as cancer.[10]

THE AUTONOMIC NERVOUS SYSTEM AND ANXIETY

The autonomic nervous system (ANS) plays a crucial part in instigating and maintaining appropriate levels of physiological arousal. It has two main branches — the parasympathetic (PNS) and sympathetic (SNS) nervous systems. Broadly, the SNS is responsible for the 'stress' response and the PNS for the 'relaxation' response. Thus, during stress states, the SNS is dominant, preparing the individual for the 'fight or flight' response. Blood flow is redirected from the digestive organs to the fighting muscles and the heart rate increases. During relaxed states, the PNS is dominant, preparing the individual for digestion, recuperation and sleep. Apart from the digestive tract, there is a general slowing down of all bodily systems (Fig. 2.8).

Major SNS effects are:

- increased blood flow to skeletal muscles
- increased muscle tension
- increased breathing rate
- increased heart rate and blood pressure
- increased sweat output
- increased skin conductivity
- decreased gut motility
- decreased saliva output.

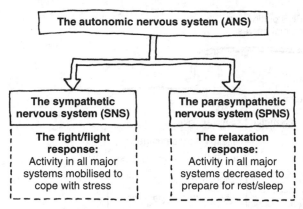

Figure 2.8   The dual function of the autonomic nervous system.

Major PNS effects are:

- decreased blood flow to skeletal muscles
- decreased muscle tension
- decreased breathing rate
- decreased heart rate and blood pressure
- decreased sweat output
- decreased skin conductivity
- increased gut motility
- increased saliva output.

The two branches of the ANS work partly in concert. Some sites and systems are under the sole control of the SNS, i.e. the sweat glands, lung muscles, blood glucose levels and the basal metabolic rate. Others, such as the ciliary muscles of the eye, are under the exclusive control of the PNS. Most organs, however, are innervated by both the PNS and SNS. In this way, the total system is homeostatically balanced allowing the individual to respond appropriately to his needs within the immediate environment.

Upper PNS nerve fibres issue from the brain stem and the lower PNS nerves from the sacral region. SNS nerves arise from the thoracic and upper lumbar vertebrae and synapse in the sympathetic chain of ganglia which extends from the cervical to the sacral region. In general, acetylcholine is the major neurotransmitter for the PNS, and noradrenalin for the SNS (Fig. 2.9).

Individual responses and the ANS

The foregoing description is only a general out-line of autonomic function. While the SNS is usually predominant during stress, some individuals may respond to stressors with PNS dominance, for example, causing a fall in heart rate, blood pressure and blood glucose. Cold sweating, dizziness, reduced respiratory action and fainting may occur in stress states.

At the individual level, no clear relationships exist between measures of temperament or personality traits and autonomic responding. Mixed patterns involving a clustering of SNS and PNS reactivity which are unique to each individual tend to occur, showing a stereotyped response to stress. This individualised reaction to stress does not simply consist of either SNS or PNS dominance, as Eppinger and Hess proposed in 1910 when they described the sympatheticotonic and parasympatheticotonic types.[17] This theory was criticised and discarded after Lacey[18] demonstrated in 1956 that individuals do not respond with simple PNS or SNS dominance under stress. The concept of autonomic specificity was proposed, describing individual patterns or 'reaction profiles'. In this way, individuals may react strongly on one physiological measure and very little on another. It was suggested that the nature of the reaction profile might be determined by the total life experience of the individual as well as genetically determined physiological factors.

However, several studies have been carried out relating physiological arousal patterns to various behaviour disorders. In anxiety neurosis, fairly consistent results have demonstrated sympathetic hyperactivity on all readings. Anxiety disorders have also been correlated with a pattern of raised heart-rate levels, frontalis muscle tension, forearm blood flow, skin conductance, respiration rates and blood pressure. In depression, a more mixed picture can be seen with SNS dominance on some systems and PNS dominance on others. But it is well known that depression is often associated with anxiety. In depression, heart rate and muscle action potentials are usually increased, with a fall in salivation rates, indicating SNS action. Electrodermal activity is reduced, however, suggesting PNS action.[19] These issues remain unresolved and it seems wise to conclude that generalisations relat-

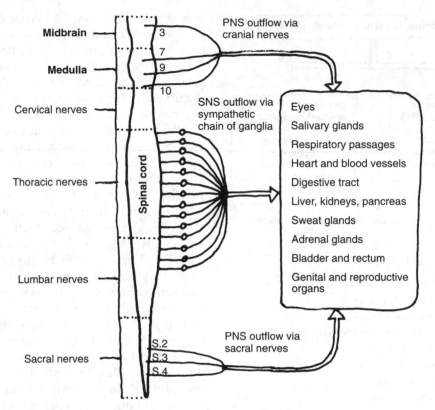

Figure 2.9 The autonomic nervous system — a schematic diagram.

ing the ANS responses to particular personality types or psychiatric disorders are misleading.

A further issue concerns the variations in the intensity of the SNS response between different individuals. Each individual has a base-line norm of autonomic arousal, or starting point. It has been shown that a high baseline norm will generally lead to a smaller reaction under stress, and a low baseline norm will lead to a larger reaction. This phenomenon is termed the 'law of initial values'.[20,21] It causes difficulties when attempting to measure the autonomic aspects of anxiety disorders accurately. For example, let us suppose that a researcher wants to know whether clinically anxious people have higher heart rates than controls in reaction to stress. The clinically anxious group may have a higher baseline heart rate to start with, although the readings taken after stress being applied may not be significantly greater than those of the control group. This is because the actual change between the baseline and final reading may be smaller in the anxious group, while the reaction of the control group to stress may actually be greater. Regarding autonomic responses, a ceiling effect tends to apply — fortunately, the heart rate does not go on increasing ad infinitum! If our researcher was unaware of the 'law of initial values' he might be misled by his results and conclude that there are no significant differences between the heart-rate reactions of anxious subjects and controls during stress.

Interestingly, a relationship between sympathetic activity and perception has been demonstrated. Calloway and Thompson[22] found that when sympathetic activity increases in response to a stressor, the constancy of size perception is decreased. This results in a diminished awareness of distant objects. It was concluded that a negative feedback loop between autonomic activity and perception exists, so that when an organism sees an approaching threat that cannot immediately be removed or reduced, the magnitude of the threat is decreased by the inhibition of size perception. Perhaps this phenomenon could be said to function as a kind of 'defence mechanism', although in psychophysiological terms.

THE ENDOCRINE SYSTEM AND ANXIETY

Working in close coordination with the ANS, the endocrine system has an important role in the total stress response. The endocrine system of glands comprises the pituitary or 'master gland', the thyroid, parathyroids, islets of Langerhans, adrenals and gonads. The system works through feedback loops. The hypothalamus regulates the pituitary which, in turn, regulates the remaining endocrine glands (Fig. 2.10).

During stress, the pituitary is stimulated by the hypothalamus to release several chemical 'messengers' to the slave glands directly into the bloodstream. These include vasopressin, adrenocorticotrophic hormone (ACTH), and thyrotropic hormone (TTH). Vasopressin contracts the arteries and causes blood pressure to rise. ACTH and TTH pass to the adrenal and thyroid glands which then work together to increase circulation and basal metabolic rates.

The adrenal glands

The two adrenal glands are composed of an outer layer — the cortex — and an inner layer — the medulla. Adrenalin and noradrenalin from the medulla and corticoids from the cortex are released directly into the bloodstream (Fig. 2.11).

Adrenalin stimulates the production of glucose from glycogen in the liver which is released into the bloodstream, increasing carbohydrate metabolism. Adrenalin also dilates the coronary and skeletal muscle arteries, increases heart rate, blood volume and body temperature. Gaseous exchange is facilitated by bronchial dilatation and shallow breathing results. Smooth (visceral) muscles tend to relax while the sphincters are constricted.

Noradrenalin constricts the peripheral arterioles and increases blood pressure. It has sometimes been suggested that adrenalin is the major hormone in states of fear while noradrenalin is predominant in anger. Glucocorticoids from the adrenal cortex tend to raise blood sugar levels and inhibit inflammation. Additionally, the mineralocorticoids cause retention of sodium and chloride, while potassium levels are reduced. The corticoids are associated with the immune response and prolonged presence of these pro- and anti-inflammatory hormones, as in chronic stress, may interfere with the function of the immune system. The corticosteroids also tend to dilate the bronchi so that gaseous exchange is

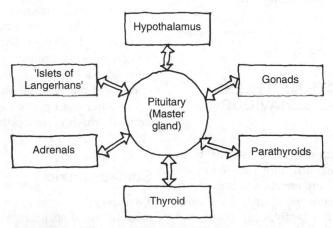

Figure 2.10 A diagrammatic model of the endocrine system.

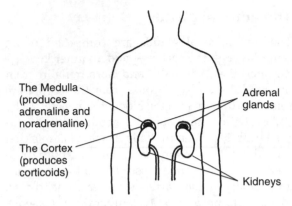

Figure 2.11 The adrenal glands.

enhanced while gut activity is inhibited. Renin production from the kidney is also increased thus raising the blood pressure. Blood volume, and consequently blood pressure, rises as interstitial fluid is withdrawn from the peripheral cells and tissue spaces.

The thyroid gland

At the same time, TTH acts on the thyroid gland causing the release of thyroxine. The rise in thyroxine levels under stress conditions results in increased sweating, muscle tremor, heart rate and exaggerated breathing. These effects are rapidly debilitating and very similar to those of adrenalin. Adrenalin tends to predominate in short-term stress whereas thyroxine is released in greater quantities in prolonged stress.[10,19] The pituitary is held to be particularly important in maintaining a sustained stress response, rather than in the initial 'emergency' phase.

FURTHER ASPECTS OF STRESS PHYSIOLOGY AND BEHAVIOUR

Activation theory

Current theories of emotion have so far been insufficient to account fully for the complex interrelationship between emotional behaviour and physiological stress reactions. However, Lindsley[23] proposed the 'activation' theory of arousal. According to this, the cortex is stimulated by ascending discharge from the subcortex which results in a continuum of arousal from deep sleep (characterised by delta waves) to states of rage or terror (characterised by beta waves). This arousal continuum operates irrespective of the type of emotion excited, yet enables the organism to react appropriately to stimuli. Excessive arousal, however, has been observed to disrupt performance.

The work of Schacter and Singer

Schacter and Singer's well known study[24] demonstrated that where physiological arousal is perceived, the subject will tend to label it in terms of the environmental cues available to him at that time. In a group of students, half were injected with saline, a neutral substance, and half with adrenalin to induce arousal. Half of each group were kept naive and not told about the content of the experiment. In one group a stooge (actor) incited euphoria and in the other, anger. The naive subjects who had received the adrenalin labelled their mood changes according to the stooge-induced cues. This important work raises interesting points about the states of arousal and anxiety. While anxious clients will invariably report their symptoms as being unpleasant, the symptoms of euphoria, or even ecstasy, may not be greatly dissimilar. Therefore, although anxiety clients invariably view their arousal symptoms as being disagreeable, this may be influenced considerably by the negative cognitive associations they hold concerning the symptoms. Certain people, described as sensation-seekers, actively and willingly expose themselves to potentially dangerous situations in which they will experience physiological arousal. The widely experienced and paradoxical state of 'falling in love' is yet another example of heightened physiological arousal which is generally experienced as desirable.

Somatic anxiety

Two decades ago, Tyrer argued that 'somatic' anxiety was distinguishable from ordinary anxiety by the way in which an individual perceived bodily feelings.[25] He posited that in true somatic anxiety a demonstrable link between symptoms and actual physiological events exists — the somatically anxious individual was shown to have an intensified awareness of bodily symptoms associated with increased arousal, and these were a correct reflection of autonomic function. This differed from ordinary psychic anxiety where mood was the primary factor and bodily feelings reported were not clearly related to what was actually occurring in physiological terms. In somatic anxiety, subjective feelings were held to be closely mediated by bodily changes.

These observations are reminiscent of the old James–Lange concepts[1,2] in which bodily feelings were held to be the instigator of emotions. This was discounted by Cannon[3,4] who had shown that animals with spinal cord lesions still demonstrated emotional behaviour. However, Hohmann[26] found that humans with spinal cord lesions reported reduced emotional intensity, and that this effect was at its most marked in high-level lesions.

The alexithymia construct

During the past decade our understanding of these apparently conflicting issues has been advanced considerably through the emergence of the alexithymia construct.[27,28] Put simply, alexithymic clients demonstrate a marked tendency to somatise their emotions. This is characterised by preoccupation with physical symptoms in conjunction with a distinct lack of psychological awareness. This important and highly relevant construct is discussed in Chapter 5.

In summary, although we may reject the notion that our emotions are dependent on bodily feelings, we must acknowledge the extraordinarily powerful and complex interactive links between the mind and body. In the understanding and control of anxiety disorders, therefore, the importance of bodily aspects cannot simply be ignored. Clinicians who attempt this will find their attempts confounded by the rising clamour of complaints about physical symptoms!

Bodily responses to different stimulation

Individuals vary in the way in which they respond bodily to different types of cognitive stimulation, but some general tendencies have been observed. For example, during mental problem-solving tasks SNS activity has been shown to increase. In experiments, the intensity of the SNS response has been correlated with the difficulty of the task. Also, tasks requiring intake of external stimuli have the effect of reducing the heart rate, while tasks requiring attention to internal states cause an increase in heart rate. Internal stimulation such as mood states are also reflected in individualised patterns of facial muscle activity. Additionally, in social situations, bodily responses are related to emotional reactions within those situations. Physiological arousal is increased where subjects like or dislike the people they are with, and reduced if the relationship is a neutral one. Regarding fear-producing stimuli, such as parachute-jumping, it has been shown that with practice people can learn to keep their physiological arousal levels from becoming excessive in order to continue coping with high fear levels.[19]

Many studies have attempted to demonstrate differences in the autonomic responses of people with anxiety disorders. Parameters measured have included electrodermal activity, heart rate, blood pressure, respiration rate and adrenalin, thyroxine and lactate levels. Some differentiation has been shown on heart rate and sweat-gland measurements and also in consistently low alpha brain wave activity in anxiety subjects. While results conflict, clearer distinctions appear in subjects under stimulation than in those at rest. This is due to the 'law of initial values' in which a ceiling effect causes controls to appear more responsive than anxiety subjects, since the latter already have a higher baseline norm of arousal. As has already been stated, those with a higher baseline norm will show a smaller reaction under stress. It cannot, therefore, be asserted that people with anxiety disorders are more reactive to stress. But anxiety subjects do consistently adjust to stressors more slowly than controls in experimental situations, and this suggests impaired habituation. In other words, highly anxious people take longer to acclimatise to stressful conditions.[20,21]

Perceptual studies have yielded interesting results relevant to these issues. The opposing dimensions of 'augmentation' and 'reduction' have been observed in which 'augmentors' tend to overestimate stimulation intensity, and 'reducers' to underestimate it. As a consequence, reducers appear to tolerate pain more easily. In studies of the physiological characteristics of anxiety, anxious subjects are more sensitive to pain and more likely to perceive stimuli as painful or emotionally threatening than controls.[29]

Conversely, another dimension has been described, that of repression-sensitisation. Some individuals, 'repressers', appear to repress threatening thoughts about their state of physiological arousal while others, 'sensitisers', tend to exaggerate them. Interestingly, repressers tend to show more physiological responsivity than sensitisers.[19] We have all observed people who deny that they are under stress, while it is obvious from the merest glance that they are indeed suffering from stress. This may show itself overtly in increased sweating, trembling or a tense posture.

The implications of all the foregoing observations for the treatment of anxiety are considerable. A wide range of possible response patterns to stress have been described. A flexible but focused approach to treatment is required in this field. Biofeedback is an example of a method of physical arousal control which is highly suitable for use in the treatment of specific physical stress responses. Through the use of this technique, anxious clients can learn to control specific maladaptive physiological responses. However, the process underlying biofeedback remains unclear. Biofeedback is described in Chapter 8 where relaxation training techniques are discussed.

THE WORK OF HANS SELYE

It was Selye who first used the term 'stress' in its relation to human psychophysiology.[5] The term is normally used in engineering to describe external pressure upon a mechanical structure, and it has been suggested that he really meant to use the word 'strain'. However, the use of the less common term was provident in that it suggested a new idea. Selye's theory described the 'general adaptation syndrome' or GAS, as it is generally abbreviated. GAS has three phases:

- alarm reaction (involving shock and countershock phases)
- resistance (adaptive response)
- exhaustion.

1 The alarm phase involves general mobilisation of all systems immediately upon presentation of the threat or stressor. The stressor can be either psychological or physiological in nature. There is a large and rapid increase in adrenocortical hormone levels during the alarm phase.

2 The resistance phase involves selection of the most appropriate organ or system to deal with the particular stressor. Adrenocortical hormone levels reduce once a specific system is delegated. Internal resources are then directed towards the support of this system, leaving others vulnerable. This may reduce the resistance of the organism to disease.

3 The exhaustion phase is reached when the specific system delegated becomes overloaded. At this point, the adrenocortical hormone levels increase again and the alarm phase is reinstigated. A different system may then be delegated to handle the continuing stress.

The three-phased GAS is useful in mobilising protective resources in emergency situations, but, if prolonged, may lower resistance. In providing energy for an adaptive reaction to stress, the GAS response suppresses immune reactions and inflammatory responses to invading pathogens. It is suggested that the 'weakest link' or most vulnerable part of the body breaks down first when under stress. Therefore, factors including heredity and prior disease may predispose an organism towards a specific somatic disorder. Thus, long-standing stress increases susceptibility to a wide range of infection and other disorders.

The local adaptation syndrome (LAS) mirrors

the action of GAS. When a local injury occurs, inflammation at that site to isolate invading organisms should result. However, this reaction can be disrupted by corticoid anti-inflammatory steroids which are present in the system as a result of stress. These syntoxic agents can suppress resistance to infection by allowing coexistence with a pathogen. In this way, a fairly minor wound may become septic, possibly resulting in the development of a serious infection.

In a converse manner, allergies, in which an inappropriate internal reaction to an innocuous substance occurs, may also be associated with stress. Allergic reactions involve high levels of inflammatory corticoids. Under normal circumstances these agents promote the destruction of pathogens, thus defending the body against disease. Under stressful conditions the allergic response may be aggravated. This causes the distressing symptoms of the allergy to increase while the body redoubles its efforts to attack a harmless substance as if it were a potentially damaging one.

Selye based his conclusions on experimental work which involved subjecting rats to prolonged stress. Drastic bodily changes, including irreversible organ damage, resulted. The rats showed enlargement of the adrenal cortex and atrophy of the thymus, spleen and lymph nodes. A severe reduction of eosinophil (white) cells and bleeding ulcers in the stomach and duodenum were also observed.

According to Selye, adrenocorticotrophic hormone (ACTH), plays an important role in GAS. In acute stress, adrenalin and noradrenalin from the adrenal medulla are most prominent. In chronic stress the corticoids are the primary agents. The kidney is also held to play an essential role in GAS. This organ is normally responsible for maintaining a suitable chemical and water balance in the blood and tissues. When corticoid levels are raised for a prolonged period, blood pressure may rise and damage the kidney — this may occur in chronic stress conditions. Damage to the arteries may also occur under these conditions. This is associated with a build up of cholesterol plaques and the development of atherosclerosis. The liver is normally respon-

sible for regulating corticoid levels in the blood, but when the organism is under stress, this organ is bypassed, allowing high levels to continue. Additionally, sustained stress can produce increased hydrochloric acid secretion in the stomach leading to the formation of ulcers. In short-term stress conditions, hydrochloric acid levels are usually decreased.[10] Selye added to his physiological observations some suggestions on ways of dealing with stress:

- remove unnecessary stressors from lifestyle
- do not allow neutral events to become stressors
- develop skill in dealing with stressful situations
- seek relaxation.

Selye described the objective of stress regulation as the achievement of an optimum level of stress (eustress), between the extremes of hyperstress (overload), distress and hypostress (boredom).[5]

He also suggested a code of ethics which might be instrumental in helping people to achieve this balance:

- follow your own natural predilections and stress levels
- practise 'altruistic egoism' (i.e. take care of yourself for the sake of those around you)
- earn thy neighbours' love.

The work of Selye has provided a comprehensive and solid foundation upon which the theory of stress physiology has developed. His work on the effects of chronic stress is still highly relevant to the clinical situation, and in the application of relaxation methods to clients suffering from anxiety disorders.[30] The concept of the fight/flight response has adequately described the mechanisms involved in acute stress and has also contributed to our understanding of panic attacks. For clients presenting a more insidious picture, Selye's theories may serve to clarify some of the more obscure symptomatology encountered. Educating anxious clients in basic stress physiology has great value in dispelling their often alarming fantasies about what might be happening inside the body. To do so is more likely to reassure worried clients than to encourage hypochondriasis. Commonly, clients attribute their anxiety symptoms to imagined fatal underlying disease. Lack of knowledge about the normal workings of the body prevails widely. Because physical symptoms often predominate in the clinical picture of anxiety, these symptoms are often the main focus of the client's complaints. Education about the links between the bodily and mental state can increase the client's insight and cooperation in treatment.

NEUROBIOLOGICAL MECHANISMS AND DRUG MANAGEMENT IN ANXIETY

NEUROTRANSMITTERS AND ANXIETY

Neurotransmitter molecules are the means by which nerve cells communicate with one another. With their own 'address' and 'message', the system is not unlike a cellular postal service. The lengthy list of transmitters includes a small number that play a significant role in anxiety and other major psychiatric disorders:

- noradrenalin
- adrenalin
- serotonin ~ 5 hydroxytryptamine (5-HT)
- GABA
- dopamine
- acetylcholine
- histamine.

Although nerve cells vary in shape and size a branching pattern is common to most types[31] (Fig. 2.12). The large number of branch endings, the dendrites, provide an extensive surface area for contact with other cells. As the dendrite tapers it comes to resemble a button-like structure known as the synaptic knob (Fig. 2.13).[32] It is here that the neurotransmitter is stored in vesicles and where it is released to cross over the synaptic cleft carrying its message to the neighbouring neurone. Receptor sites on the postsynaptic neurone are 'shaped' to fit the neurotransmitter ensuring that the 'message' reaches the right

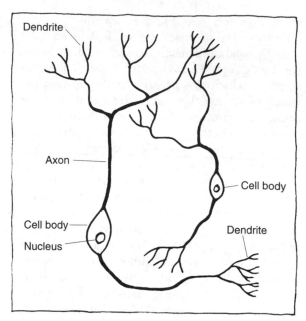

Figure 2.12 Nerve cells.

address. Once captured by the receptor the neurotransmitter will excite or inhibit the postsynaptic neurone — dampening down its activity or alternatively stirring it up. Dysfunction of neurotransmitter activity lies at the heart of most major psychiatric disorders. Depression seems likely to be due to underactivity whilst psychosis and anxiety may arise through excessive activity.

Treatments in common use influence neurotransmitter activity in a number of different ways. For example, some antidepressants will interfere with the reuptake mechanism that captures neurotransmitters from the synaptic cleft. Because the neurotransmitter is prevented from returning into the cell, it remains available within the cleft to engage with its receptors. In contrast, a betablocker will interfere with receptors in a way that prevents the neurotransmitter from making contact and passing on its message — a chemical blockade.

We still await an integrated model that can adequately explain the interplay between neurotransmitters and the phenomena that we associate with anxiety disorders. Such a goal may never be possible if the disorders we include under this umbrella are not as closely related or

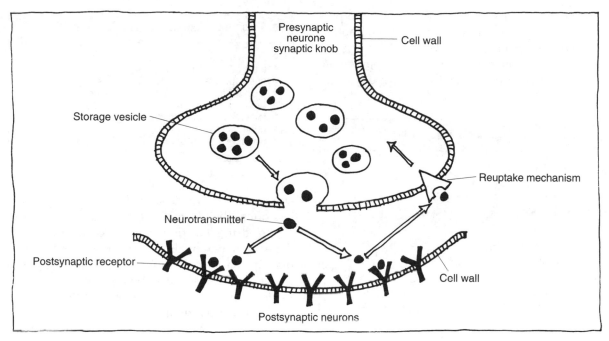

Figure 2.13   Synaptic cleft.

as unitary as our current classificatory systems imply. Irrespective of the uncertainties that remain, recent developments have lent support to the view that the noradrenergic and serotonergic systems, with their associated neurotransmitters noradrenalin and serotonin (5-HT), have a central role in the mechanisms underlying anxiety in the central nervous system (CNS). Learning how neurotransmitters modify the way an organism responds to stress has helped us to understand how established treatments have the effect that they do. In a similar vein, it has encouraged the development of treatments that are targeted in a way that maximises benefit and reduces the likelihood of unwanted effects.

The classificatory system DSM IV[33] recognises several forms of anxiety disorder including: generalised anxiety disorder, panic disorder with or without agoraphobia, other phobias and obsessive compulsive disorder. To complete the picture, account must be taken of the many other disorders in which anxiety can be an associated feature. Anxiety is such a common concomitant of depression that some have challenged the existence of these disorders as discrete entities.[34]

This blurring of boundaries is also reflected in the range of drugs that are commonly used to treat anxiety. For example, antidepressants can be effective in the management of panic, and for intractable forms of anxiety for which some antipsychotic drugs may also have a useful role. Similarly, the benzodiazepine Alprazolam has been described as having antidepressant properties in addition to its anxiolytic effect in both general anxiety and agoraphobic panic.

BENZODIAZEPINES

This important group of drugs enjoyed widespread usage following their introduction in the 1960s. Known primarily for their anxiolytic properties they have also been used as hypnotics, anticonvulsants and for muscle relaxation. Their mode of action is closely linked with the inhibitory neurotransmitter GABA which in turn is thought to have a modulating effect on both the serotonergic and noradrenergic systems. The group has evolved to include forms that differ in their duration of action (see Box 2.1).[35] Drugs with a short period of action (<12hrs) —

Temazepam, Oxazepam — are less likely to produce a hangover effect when used as hypnotics. In contrast, longer acting forms (> 24 hours) — Diazepam, Clobazam — are more appropriate when cover is required throughout the day.

Box 2.1 Duration of action of benzodiazepines

Short-acting:

- Temazepam
- Oxazepam

Medium-acting:

- Lorazepam
- Flunitrazepam

Long-acting:

- Diazepam
- Nitrazepam
- Chlordiazepoxide
- Clobazam
- Alprazolam

The benzodiazepines have a number of extremely valuable characteristics that help to explain their rapid growth in popularity (see Box 2.2). Their potency as anxiolytics and sedatives is combined with a speedy response and an impressive margin of safety, particularly when taken in excess.

Box 2.2 The advantages of benzodiazepines

- powerful anxiolytic
- sedative
- anti-convulsant
- speedy response
- safer in overdose

Drawbacks, including impaired concentration, unsteadiness, disinhibition and memory dysfunction have been eclipsed by the discovery of tolerance to the drug effect, dependency and a withdrawal syndrome (see Box 2.3).

Withdrawal is seen in almost half of those receiving treatment for more than six months. Symptoms may include features indistinguishable from anxiety. Seizures and perceptual

---

Box 2.3 The drawbacks of benzodiazepines

- drowsiness
- impaired concentration
- unsteadiness
- disinhibition
- memory dysfunction
- tolerance to the drug effect
- dependency
- withdrawal syndrome

---

abnormalities are described though they occur less often. Risk factors include the use of shorter acting drugs, a precipitous reduction and a dependent personality.[36] The point of recovery may be hard to distinguish as the symptoms merge into those seen before treatment commenced. Benzodiazepines have suffered a fall from grace as shifts in public opinion and medical practice have encouraged a more cautious attitude to their promotion — a change reinforced by a number of legislative developments around the world. Despite this, these drugs continue to be widely prescribed — particularly for elderly people.[37] Until the search for an alternative has borne fruit they are likely to remain the drugs of choice for acute distress.

BUSPIRONE

Originally developed as a potential antipsychotic, Buspirone was found to be an effective anxiolytic. Modulation of the serotonergic system through its affinity for the receptor $5HT^{31}$ is thought to be central to its mode of action.[38] Although the absence of sedation and muscle relaxation are useful features, it is the apparent freedom from dependence and withdrawal that has probably had the greatest impact on its use. Side effects include nausea, dizziness, headache and lightheadedness. In contrast to the benzodiazepines, a latency of two to three weeks limits its usefulness in acute distress.

BETA-BLOCKERS — PROPANOLOL

By reducing the autonomic symptoms of

anxiety, beta-blockers help to curtail the cycle of negative thoughts that can arise during an attack. Propanolol and other beta-blockers are particularly well suited to individuals whose symptoms are primarily somatic. Their mode of action arises through their affinity for the beta adrenergic receptors found in the heart, lungs, gut, skeletal muscle and bladder. Usage is limited by a number of important contraindications including: asthma, COAD, uncontrolled heart failure and heart block.

ANTIDEPRESSANTS

The family of antidepressants has grown since their introduction in the 1950s. Early forms have been refined in the hope of securing greater specificity with fewer side effects. The selective serotonin reuptake inhibitors (SSRIs), now established in common clinical practice, represent the latest phase in this continuing process.

Antidepressants are thought to exert their action by increasing the availability of neurotransmitters, either by preventing their reuptake into nerve cells or by interfering with the process of degradation. In the search for greater specificity, drugs with a preferential action on the serotonergic system have attracted much attention for both their clinical effect and their freedom from the more serious drawbacks associated with antidepressants.

Tricyclic, Monoamine oxidase inhibitor (MAOI) and SSRI drugs are all known to have an anxiolytic effect. Benefits of a more specific nature include a reduction in panic attacks following the use of Tricyclic and SSRI drugs and an improvement in phobic anxiety with an MAOI (Box 2.4). Tricyclics and SSRI drugs with increased serotonergic activity have been shown to modify the symptoms in Obsessive Compulsive Disorder. Tricyclic drugs have been dogged by a wide range of side-effects. Anticholinergic symptoms of dry mouth, constipation, urinary retention and blurred vision can be accompanied by drowsiness, postural hypotension and cardiac irregularities. MAOIs have until recently had the additional drawback of requiring the patient to follow a restrictive diet. SSRI drugs have a much improved profile but nevertheless can be associated with nausea and restlessness.

Box 2.4 Antidepressants

Tricyclics:
- Amitriptyline
- Dothiepin
- Clomipramine
- Imipramine
- Lofepramine

MAOI:
- Phenelzine
- Tranylcypromine
- Moclobemide

SSRI:
- Fluoxetine
- Sertraline
- Paroxetine

SSRI/SNAI:
- Venlafaxine

Antidepressants have an important and wide-ranging role to play in the management of anxiety. They can be invaluable for patients whose problems are persistent or recurrent and for whom the risks of using an alternative such as a benzodiazepine are too great.

ANTIPSYCHOTICS

Some antipsychotic drugs have been used in severe anxiety as an alternative to first-line treatments — Chlorpromazine and Thioridazine. The source of their sedative and anxiolytic properties is thought to be due to their affinity for histamine receptors. Short- and long-term side-effects mitigate against their continuous use as anxiolytics, though for some this may be a price worth paying for long-term symptom control.

REFERENCES

1 James W 1884 What is emotion? Mind 19:188
2 Lange C 1885 The emotions. In: Dunlap, K (ed) 1922 Translated by Haupt IA The emotions. Williams and Wilkins, Baltimore
3 Cannon W B 1927 The James–Lange theory of emotion. American Journal of Psychology 39:106–124
4 Cannon W B 1929 Bodily changes in pain, hunger, fear and rage, 2nd edn. Appleton, New York
5 Selye H 1956 The stress of life. McGraw–Hill, New York
6 Papez J W 1937 A proposed mechanism of emotion. Archives of Neurology and Psychiatry 38:725–743
7 Ax A F 1953 The physiological differentiation between fear and anger. Psychosomatic Medicine 15:433–442
8 Alexander F 1950 Psychosomatic medicine. Norton, New York
9 Marks I M 1986 Genetics of fear and anxiety disorders. British Journal of Psychiatry 149:406–418
10 Pelletier K R 1977 Mind as healer — mind as slayer. George Allen & Unwin, UK
11 Levitt E E 1980 The psychology of anxiety, 2nd edn. Lawrence Erlbaum, USA
12 Simeons A T W 1961 Man's presumptuous brain: an evolutionary interpretation of psychosomatic disease. Dutton, New York
13 Schacter S 1964 The interaction of cognitive and physiological determinants of emotional state. In: Berkowitz L (ed) Advances in experimental and social psychology. Academic Press, New York, Vol 1
14 Thompson R 1967 Foundations of physiological psychology. Harper and Row, UK
15 Gray J A 1982 The neuropsychology of anxiety. Clarendon Press, Oxford
16 Calabrese J R, Kling M A, Gold P W 1987 Alterations in immunocompetence during stress, bereavement and depression: focus on neuro-endocrine regulation. American Journal of Psychiatry 144(9):1123–1134
17 Eppinger H, Hess L 1910 Die Vagotonie. Berlin. Translated by Kraus W M and Jelliffe S E. Vagotonia: A clinical study in vegetative neurology. 1917 (2nd Rev.) Nervous and mental disease monograph series, No. 20. The Nervous and Mental Disease Publishing Company, New York
18 Lacey J I 1956 The evaluation of autonomic responses: toward a general solution. Annals of the New York Academy of Sciences 67:123–163
19 Grings W W, Dawson M E 1978 Emotions and bodily responses: a psycho-physiological approach. Academic Press
20 Lacey J I, Vanlehn R 1952 Differential emphasis in somatic response to stress. Psychosomatic Medicine 14:71–81

21 Terry R A 1953 Autonomic balance and temperament. Journal of Comparative Physiology and Psychology 46:454–460
22 Calloway E, Thompson S V 1953 Sympathetic activity and perception. An approach to the relationship between autonomic activity and personality. Psychosomatic Medicine 15:443–455
23 Lindsley D B 1951 Emotion. In: Stevens S S (ed) Handbook of experimental psychology. Wiley, pp 473–516
24 Schacter S, Singer E 1962 Cognitive, social and psychological determinants of emotional states. Psychological Review 69:379–399
25 Tyrer P 1976 The role of bodily feelings in anxiety. Institute of Psychiatry: Maudsley Monographs. University Press, Oxford
26 Hohmann G W 1962 Some effects of spinal cord lesions on experienced emotional feelings. Psychophysiology 3:143
27 Taylor G J, Bagby R M, Parker J D 1991 The alexithymia construct. A potential paradigm for psychosomatic medicine. Psychosomatics 32(2):153–164
28 Stuppy W P, Shipko S 1994 The dichotomy of alexithymia and panic disorder. In: International Journal of Psychosomatics (special annual issue) 41(1–4):30–33
29 Spielberger C D, Sarason I G, Kulcsar, Van Heck G L 1991 Anxiety, anger and curiosity. Stress and emotion series. Hemisphere Publishing Corporation, New York, Vol 14
30 Selye H 1976 Stress in health and disease. Butterworth, Massachusetts
31 Sukkar M Y, El-Munshid H A, Ardawi M S M 1993 Concise human physiology. Blackwell Scientific Publications
32 Gershon E S, Reider R O 1992 Major disorders of mind and brain. Scientific America September:89–93
33 American Psychiatric Association 1994 Diagnostic and statistical manual of mental disorders (DSM IV), 4th edn. American Psychiatric Association, Washington DC
34 Goldberg R J 1995 Diagnostic dilemmas presented by patients with anxiety and depression. The American Journal of Medicine 8:278–284
35 Gelder M, Gath D, Mayou R 1994 Concise Oxford textbook of psychiatry. Oxford University Press, Oxford
36 Tyrer P 1983 Gradual withdrawal of diazepam after long term therapy, Lancet 1(8339):1402–1406
37 Shorr R I, Robin D W 1994 Rational use of benzodiazepines in the elderly. Drugs and Aging 4(1):9–20
38 Tunnicliff G 1991 Molecular basis of Buspirone's anxiolytic action. Pharmacology & Toxicology 69:149–156

FURTHER READING

Forgays D G, Sosnowski T, Wizesniewski K 1992 Anxiety — recent developments in cognitive, psycho-physiological and health research. Hemisphere, Washington

Kalin N H 1993 The neurobiology of fear. Scientific American 268(5):94–101
Sims A, Snaith P 1988 Anxiety in clinical practice. John Wiley, Chichester

3

Behavioural and cognitive theories of anxiety

Diana Keable

THE DEVELOPMENT OF BEHAVIOURISM

The first major contributions to our knowledge of anxiety, based on the learning model, stemmed from Pavlov, Skinner and Watson in the early part of this century.[1,2,3] From their well known works emerged the 'stimulus–response' concept. According to this, certain stimuli, when associated with fear, could elicit an anxiety response. For example, if I get stuck in a lift on one or two occasions, I am very likely to develop a fear of lifts. Similarly, if a child is bitten by a ferocious dog, the child will respond with anxiety the next time he sees the dog. This response will occur even if the dog does not actually bite him again, because the child has learned to associate the dog (stimulus) with the fear (response) of being bitten.

Similarly, early researchers noted that behaviour aimed at reducing anxiety, could often minimise the danger that provoked it. Thus, the child who was bitten by a dog may learn the behaviour pattern of avoiding ferocious dogs in future. In this way, anxiety has a protective function and could become a learned response to a danger signal (conditioned stimulus) that was recognised to presage a harmful situation (unconditioned stimulus).[4] In our example, then, the actual fear of the dog is the conditioned stimulus for the avoidance behaviour.

However, classical conditioning theory has its limitations at the clinical level. For example, generalised anxiety appears to develop without repeated 'pairings' of a conditioned stimulus and unconditioned stimulus. Even in phobic anxiety, the original stimulus responsible for causing the fear to arise is often impossible to identify. Further, generalised anxiety is resistant to therapeutic attempts directed at 'unlearning' or the extinction of fear. It must be noted, however, that phobic disorders have tended to respond more successfully to learning-based treatment programmes such as systematic desensitisation. An example worth noting which relates to anxiety is that of superstitious or compulsive behaviour, such as ritual hand-washing or excessive checking. Obsessive–compulsive activities produce anxiety reduction in a similar way to phobic avoidance behaviour and are also very persistent; yet they do not usually relate to any reasonable or observable danger stimulus. Neurotic behaviour such as this, a largely human phenomenon, appears irrational because it is intended to reduce emotional discomfort rather than realistic physical danger. It can be seen that while the original learning theorists contributed greatly to our knowledge about anxiety, many questions still remain unresolved by the stimulus–response concept of anxiety.

THE WORK OF DOLLARD AND MILLER

Dollard and Miller[5] attempted to integrate psychoanalytic and behavioural theories. According to this approach, anxiety resulted from the vulnerability of a child to parental disapproval, rejection or trauma. Anxiety was not seen as being simply due to the pairing of a stressful event with a previously neutral one, as in the classical conditioning model. Neurotic anxiety was thought to be attached to cues associated with the arousal of, and attempt to gratify, important interpersonal needs. The function of internal conflict and defence mechanisms was emphasised. Dollard and Miller postulated that anxiety develops 'drive' properties and functions as a motivating force to gain relief or security in a similar way to primary drives, like hunger or pain avoidance. For example, the child's behaviour of avoiding the dog would be reinforced

through the resulting reward of anxiety reduction.[6] However, anxiety is seen as a secondary drive because, unlike a primary drive, it is not innate, it has been learned or acquired as a result of the individual's experiences. Secondary drives can become generalised and extend to a wide range of situations or objects associated in some way with the original fear stimulus. Following Dollard and Miller's line of reasoning, it is easy to see how excessive anxiety might develop. Firstly, if I am rewarded by relief from anxiety each time I successfully avoid using a lift, my fear of lifts and associated avoidance behaviour could get out of hand. Secondly, the fear of the child who was bitten by a ferocious dog might become extended to include all dogs, whether ferocious or not, and even people who speak in loud or angry tones.

Agreement between theorists has still to be achieved even within the strictly behavioural school of thought, e.g. 'Is anxiety a learned response or an acquired drive?' Two ways of looking at the question have been presented here. What is certain is the recognition that the learning models have added incalculably to our understanding of anxiety, how it comes about, is maintained and exacerbated.

Learning theory has also been of great practical use in the treatment of anxiety. In relaxation training, for example, learning theory is applied to techniques such as progressive relaxation, cue-controlled relaxation, systematic desensitisation and biofeedback. Generally, these methods attempt to teach subjects to recognise tension signals, or cues, and respond with relaxation-inducing behaviour. For example, systematic desensitisation and cue-controlled relaxation work through deconditioning by repeatedly pairing the fear stimulus with a competing relaxed response. In biofeedback, the principles of operant conditioning are utilised to enhance learned control over internal processes. Operant conditioning, as distinct from classical conditioning, involves an element of active, instrumental behaviour which is directed at achieving reinforcement or reward. Through operant learning, the required behaviour is reinforced each time it occurs and thus control is facilitated.

In summary, learning theory has suggested ways in which maladaptive and adaptive behaviour can be learned and reinforced. This has led to the development of systematic and structured programmes of relaxation training (RT) and anxiety management training (AMT), based on the premise that if anxiety can be learned, it can also be unlearned.

ANXIETY AND COGNITIVE PERFORMANCE

Before leaving the specific issue of learning, it is important to acknowledge how anxiety affects learning capacity itself. Sarason, Mandler and Craighill[7] showed that highly anxious subjects got poorer scores when given ego-involving (high-drive) instructions than when given neutral (low-drive) instructions. However, it is interesting to note that low-anxiety subjects did better when given high-drive instructions.

The inverted U concept, described by the Yerkes Dodson law, perhaps provides some insight into these results.[8] It proposes that there is an optimum drive level, according to the difficulty of the task, and that while drive level increases in anxiety, learning ability reduces. On complex learning tasks, highly anxious subjects resort to behaviours that are irrelevant to the task, thus reducing competence. Optimal performance is obtained in the middle ranges of anxiety (Fig. 3.1). Clients who continually sabotage their own performance by exposing themselves to excessive stress may benefit from learning to recognise their optimum stress tolerance levels.

Excessive anxiety seems to act as a kind of 'white noise' in the cognitive system. Sarason[9] describes the way in which anxious, negative self-preoccupation interferes with concentration, leaving the individual less able to process task-relevant information. Those attempting to teach relaxation techniques to anxious patients cannot have failed to observe this phenomenon. Test anxiety is another very common example and highlights the need for therapists to take into account the effects of extreme states of anxiety on learning capacity. A wide range of other thinking problems have been associated with anxiety, e.g.

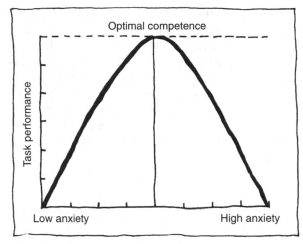

Figure 3.1   The inverted U concept.

excess vigilance and sensitivity to the possibility of threat, impaired judgement and objectivity.[10]

In converse fashion, however, fear of failure can act as a self-reinforcing motive system and actually increase achievement. Heckhausen[11] distinguishes between the 'hope of success' (HS) and 'fear of failure' (FF) motives. He posits that FF subjects often do better than HS subjects on difficult tasks and that some choose consistently higher risk goals than HS subjects. He states that when performance deficits do occur it is due to anxiety about the possibility of failure and not task difficulty.

ANXIETY, COGNITION AND COPING POTENTIAL

A further crucial issue relates to the effects of anxiety on cognitive and coping styles during stress. Each individual has a unique way of thinking and behaving when anxious or placed under stressful conditions. This can be described as the individual's coping style. We have all seen examples of extremes in coping style. On the one hand, the cool, collected person who never appears to get flustered no matter what; and on the other hand, the chronic worrier who appears to tear their hair out over quite trivial incidents. Occasionally, our assumptions are shattered when we observe the super-cool individual breaking down quite suddenly under accumulated strain; or by the worrier who copes admirably through an enormous personal crisis. Some coping styles are adaptive and enable the individual to respond positively to stress; others are maladaptive, serving to increase the stress on the individual. Equally, one coping style may be adaptive in a given situation but not in another. These are complex issues and what follows is an attempt to describe some of the factors at work in the coping process.

Lazarus,[12] an early proponent of the cognitive school, described how anxiety and coping are products of cognition. Firstly, initial appraisal of an event involves evaluation of whether it is either:

- irrelevant
- benign–positive
- stressful.

If the event is evaluated as being a stressful one, the individual then analyses whether it involves

- harm/loss that has already occurred
- harm/loss that is threatened
- a challenge that may be overcome.

Secondary appraisal then follows in the form of: 'what can I do about it?' If the individual has a firm sense of his ability to deal with the stressor, then appraisal of the threat tends to reduce its perceived intensity and leads to more effective coping. If this sense of self-efficacy is lacking, the perception of stress is intensified and adversely affects coping competence. As further information is received concerning the stressor, 'defensive re-appraisal' or 'cognitive manipulation' may occur, in order to reduce its stress-inducing characteristics. These responses may or may not lead to more effective coping. If the reappraisal and related response is a realistic one in the given situation, it is more likely to be successful.

Anticipatory anxiety is an important factor in the coping process and may have a variable influence on outcome. Although worry is generally assumed to have negative effects on performance, Janis[13] noted that the absence of prior 'work of worrying' led to inadequate coping with stress in certain persons. However, according to Rogers,[14] a psychologically defended person who resorts to denial of threat may be seen to cope better with stress than an open, sensitive person. Janis concluded that some 'work of worrying' before a stressful event is beneficial and serves to increase the level of tolerance to the threat. This must be distinguished from neurotic worrying, however, which is disproportionate and maladaptive in relation to the actual threat. Barlow[15] states that the 'distinguishing characteristic of individuals with panic disorder is the development of anxious apprehension about the next unexpected panic attack'.

Beck and Rush[16] describe how those with an anxiety neurosis tend to perceive a range of ordinary stimuli as potentially dangerous and may exaggerate unpleasant events (catastrophising tendencies). This danger-related thinking increases anxiety which leads to further irrational evaluations and misperceptions of situations. In several studies anxiety disorders have been shown to be associated with a persistent tendency to overestimate situational danger.[17,18,19]

The cognitive model of anxiety posits that anxious individuals invariably exaggerate the level of threat in a given situation and that this is associated with the following three reactions:

- increased autonomic arousal
- reduced ongoing behaviour
- selective scanning of environment for further threats.

Cognitively, this effect is compounded by 'negative automatic thoughts' and 'dysfunctional assumptions'.[20] Beck[10,21] reminds us that anxious thoughts and emotions are an integral part of a primitive survival mechanism, i.e. the 'fight or flight' syndrome, and therefore have an essentially protective function. However, in anxiety disorders, intrusive and aversive thoughts are a crucial feature and militate against successful coping.[22]

To summarise, 'coping' can be said to possess two functions. Firstly, as a practical problem-solving response, and secondly, as a way of managing emotions and thoughts adaptively in the face of stress.

Developed from cognitive and behavioural

models, the Cognitive Behavioural Modification (CBM) approach attempts to treat anxiety resulting from inadequate coping skills.[23] This involves the teaching of realistic, positive cognitive responses to stress which enhance coping ability; 'learned resourcefulness' as opposed to 'learned helplessness' is emphasised. While anxiety is accepted as a normal response to stress, neurotic anxiety results in maladaptive coping styles. In CBM, clients are given realistic education about the mental and physical concepts of anxiety to encourage more accurate appraisal of their symptoms. They are then given training in the realistic evaluation of stressful situations, and practice in responding with positive self-statements to facilitate coping. The debilitating effects of low self-esteem on cognitive function is recognised and realistic self-appraisal is encouraged. While acknowledging that severe anticipation anxiety may negatively affect coping style, the CBM approach exhorts patients/clients to prepare for, and cope with, the situations they dread in a practical and proactive manner.

ANXIETY AND COGNITIVE CONFLICT

Festinger[24] proposed a theory of cognitive dissonance which described the internal conflict and stress that results when an individual makes a descision or acts in a way that is 'out of character'. After such an event, the individual seeks to reduce the contradiction or discrepancy between his recent action or decision and his personal set of beliefs and opinions. He does this by altering or manipulating his cognitions in order to fit them in with the new decision or behaviour. Cognitive dissonance is held to be a powerful motivating force in producing attitudinal change, since people tend to seek to maintain cognitive consistency in order to avoid the anxiety associated with the dissonant state. Consistency is thought to be an especially important factor in relation to the integrity of the self-concept. Indeed, many people can be observed to try quite hard to maintain the consistency of their self-concept, even if it is a negative one. It has also been suggested that dissonance is more aversive when the self-concept is threatened. These issues

are relevant to the treatment of anxiety disorders. The self-concept of clients suffering from anxiety disorders is invariably negative. Considerable resistance is often observed when attempts are made to encourage anxious clients to re-evaluate their opinions of themselves more positively.

ANXIETY AND RATIONAL THINKING

First emerging in the mid-1950s, a treatment technique based on rational thinking was produced by Ellis: 'rational emotive therapy' (RET).[25] His work has since gained much ground following several research studies confirming the relationship between anxiety and negative or irrational thinking. For example, Himle, Thyer and Papsdorf[26] compared a general student sample with a clinically tested anxious one. They consistently found that certain irrational beliefs correlated with significant levels of test, state and trait anxiety.

In a further study, Thyer, Papsdorf and Kilgore[27] found that high levels of irrationality were associated with high levels of psychiatric symptomatology including state and trait anxiety. The work of Beck, Laude and Bohnert[28] also confirmed the premise that irrational cognitive processes are involved in anxiety neurosis. Using RET, Maxwell and Wilkerson[29] reported that, in a study of college students, they were able to reduce anxiety regarding achievement significantly, as well as increase emotional stability and self-confidence in dealing with everyday life challenges. The RET tenet holds that it is not external difficulties that create emotional states such as anxiety. Instead, the individual's own thoughts and beliefs about these difficulties produce the attendant negative emotions. Indeed, the individual's set of beliefs and attitudes towards a situation directs the way he reacts within it. If individuals inappropriately appraise a situation as potentially threatening, their behaviour is likely to be defensive or hostile as a result. This, in turn, tends to elicit an equally negative outcome, further reinforcing their irrational appraisal of the situation. While individuals cannot alter their feelings, they can re-evaluate and challenge the beliefs which underpin negative feelings. This allows more favourable beliefs and rational perceptions of events to be held.

However, Safran's[30] study suggested that while negative self-statements are associated with negative feelings and maladaptive behaviour, well-adjusted individuals do not necessarily use an inordinate number of positive self-statements. In fact, such a strategy might indicate a defensive coping style, involving an unrealistic distortion of events.

Finally, Smith, Ingram and Brehm[31] investigated socially anxious subjects and concluded that they were more excessively concerned with how others perceived them than with their own negative evaluations of themselves. Invariably, such responses are examples of irrational thinking, irrespective of their focus. The issue of rationality is brought to bear on client's cognitive responses as part of anxiety management programmes. Clients are taught to challenge the irrational beliefs which maintain and justify their anxiety. After all, neurotic anxiety is by definition not attributable to sources of real danger, and as such, is irrational. Clients are therefore shown how to re-appraise their fears realistically and this ability can function as a powerful coping skill.

THE WORK OF SELIGMAN

Helplessness

Anxiety is closely related to depression, and in the clinical situation the symptoms are often surprisingly difficult to differentiate. In the early 1970s, Seligman[32] produced important theories on the causes of the lack of autonomy seen in clients suffering from depression and anxiety. This feature he termed 'helplessness'. The basic theory posited that when organisms experience events in which certain results take place, irrespective of how they respond, learning occurs:

- behaviourally, this learning inhibits subsequent responses to control the outcome
- cognitively, it produces the belief that responses are ineffective
- emotionally, the outcome is traumatic involving anxiety and ultimately depression.

If, after having failed a few exams, I avoid sitting exams again, I might conclude that I should give up trying because I am too stupid to pass any exam. Once individuals believe that they have no control over their environment, it subsequently becomes difficult to learn that responding succeeds. The characteristic lack of volition, or helplessness, seen in clients with neurotic disorders is all too familiar with clinicians in the field. It is unfortunate that clients affected in this way are so often judged with the non-specific, umbrella term — 'unmotivated'.

Seligman based much of his theory on experimental work with animals. For example, after administering 'uncontrollable' or random shock to dogs, they were put in a shuttle box with a double-sided chamber. The random shocks resumed, but this time, by leaping over the barrier the dogs could turn off the shock. The uncontrollably shocked dogs made few attempts to escape compared to controls. The former displayed all the features of 'helplessness', characterised by apathy and passivity. Other experiments followed involving pairs of dogs 'yoked' uncontrollably to each other. The yoked dogs could not control their escape and demonstrated signs of 'helplessness' whether badly shocked or not. Maier[33] also got similar results — subjects responded with passivity and made no attempt to turn off the shock. Seligman's findings led him to criticise the renowned 'executive monkey' experiment.[34] In this study, four pairs of monkeys were yoked together but only one monkey of each pair (the executive) could avoid shock by pressing a bar. Seligman argues that Weiss, who repeated the experiment in a triadic design, found that the yoked (helpless) monkeys developed more ulcers and showed more stress than the 'executives' who had the most control.[35,36,37]

Seligman also pointed out the bearing of physiological forces in helplessness and noted that noradrenalin depletion had been found in animals with experimentally-induced 'helplessness'. Noradrenalin is a neurotransmitter substance present in the brain. Seligman suggested that the reduction in noradrenalin levels may be a causative factor in 'helplessness'. In support of this theory, he cites the work of Thomas,[38] who

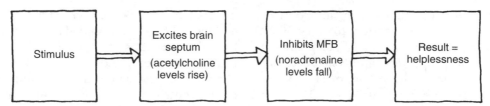

Figure 3.2   A physiological model of helplessness.

proposed an explanation of the possible process at work inside the brain. He posited that excitation of the brain septum, which inhibits the median forebrain bundle or adrenergic neurone tract (MFB), could cause 'helplessness' (Fig. 3.2). The MFB, when stimulated, gives rise to pleasure and positive reward sensations. Noradrenalin is its primary neurotransmitter. Thus, when the nearby septum, which is cholinergic, is stimulated, this action may inhibit the MFB and thus reduce noradrenalin levels.

What then, causes the septum to be stimulated with resulting noradrenalin depletion? This is not yet clear, but Weiss, in a series of animal experiments, showed that noradrenalin depletion occurs when uncontrollable shock is administered.[36,37,39,40,41] Accordingly, he suggests that uncontrollable shock is responsible for producing the physiological effects associated with 'helplessness'.

Seligman proposed that, separately, and in conjunction, physiological and cognitive changes can produce 'helplessness'. Seligman tested his 'helplessness' hypothesis on a variety of species including cats, fish, apes, rats and dogs. However some of his work has been criticised since too few studies have been carried out using human subjects on relevant problem areas. Of particular importance to anxiety and phobias, Seligman also proposed two other theories describing 'preparedness' and human 'safety-signal' conditioning.

Preparedness and safety-signal conditioning

Let us take 'preparedness' first. It can be seen that phobias frequently appear to relate to a selective set of objects, such as snakes, spiders or public places.[42] These fears are extremely difficult to treat and can be acquired in one exposure. He postulated that certain objects become the focus of phobias more readily than others, because they are important danger signals for man as a result of evolution and natural selection. Thus some objects or situations are highly 'prepared' to become objects of fear.

Regarding 'safety-signal' conditioning, Seligman stated that the presence of a safety-signal reduces anxiety because it increases predictability and consequently control. If, in an experimental situation, an animal is given warning of shock such as a light or buzzer, this acts as a safety-signal. In this condition, the animal can 'relax' until the light or buzzer warns of the coming shock. Seligman has given several examples of safety-signals used to deal with human anxieties, such as sirens for air-raid warnings. The use of the sirens allowed people to continue their everyday life unperturbed all the time the sirens remained silent. The lack of such safety-signals is held to produce great stress and ultimately 'helplessness'.[32]

Interestingly, however, McNally and Reiss demonstrated experimentally that a snake could be established as a safety-signal just as readily as a flower.[43] According to the preparedness theory, they argue, this should not have been possible — the snake being 'contra-prepared' to become a safety-signal.

ANXIETY AND PERSONAL CONTROL

A further theory, that of 'locus of control', is related to the 'helplessness' hypothesis. Rotter suggested that individuals differ in the degree to which they perceive the environment as being under their control.[44] Those with an 'internal' locus of control see events as being under their own control, whereas those with an 'external' locus see events as being due to 'luck, fate, chance or powerful others'. Johnson and Sarason investigated this proposition and concluded that negative life changes have the most adverse effects on those with external locus.[45] This was also correlated with higher levels of depression and anxiety. Hiroto confirmed that college students with external loci of control reacted more 'helplessly' to stress or change.[46] Sandler and Lakey's study supported these findings and observed that even where 'externals' received more social support, the stress reduction effect of this was only found in 'internals'.[47]

It has been suggested that 'internals' hold the conviction that they are able to manage their environment successfully and use practical, rational thinking strategies to achieve their ends. This results in increased motivation. Anderson investigated locus of control in 90 entrepreneurs over a period of two and a half years following a major disaster.[48] 'Internals' were found to perceive less stress, use more task-related coping behaviours, and less emotionally based behaviours than 'externals'. Indeed, it appears that those who are confident in their own ability to overcome difficulties rarely suffer from anxiety disorders. One of the most common disabling problems reported by anxious clients is that of poor self-esteem and related lack of confidence in their ability to deal with life's exigencies.

Seligman and others have indicated the important role of subjective control over aversive events in determining the level of stress manifested. For example, Geer, Davison and Gatchel showed that perception of control reduces autonomic reactivity to stressful stimulation such as shock.[49] In their study, half the subjects were told, incorrectly, that they could reduce shock by improving their reaction times, while the other half were not. The 'perceived control' subjects showed reduced galvanic skin response reactivity to shock. Similarly, a more recent study[50] demonstrated the powerful influence of control perception in subjects with panic disorder. All subjects were told (again, incorrectly) that they would be able to use a carbon dioxide inhaler to reduce panic when a light in the room was illu-

minated. Subjects were divided into two groups and the light was illuminated for one group only, thus giving an illusion of control. The illusion-of-control group reported significantly fewer panic attacks and associated anxiety symptoms than the no-control group. These results suggest that we merely have to believe in our own ability to control aversive events in order to reduce their degree of unpleasantness.

However, Averill stated that these conclusions may not always be warranted and that whether personal control increases or reduces stress also depends on the nature of the response and its context.[51] Reduction of uncertainty may be more effective than personal control in reducing stress. In some studies, on occasions where the opportunity for a control response was given, stress was increased.[37] In certain conditions then, signalled shock can reduce stress and this sensitisation acts in a similar fashion to the 'work of worry' concept proposed by Janis.[13] This concept describes a cognitive process by which individuals can prepare themselves to withstand a stressful event. This is held to be more effective than the use of psychological defences akin to denial.

Three types of personal 'control' have been posited:

- cognitive (interpretation of events)
- behavioural (action upon environment)
- decisional (possessing a choice of responses).

These three are related to stress in a complex fashion, sometimes increasing stress and sometimes reducing it.[51]

IMPLICATIONS FOR THE TREATMENT OF ANXIETY

Clinicians will be aware of the difficulties experienced by some clients in accepting and effectively utilising self-control techniques such as relaxation training. Some clients appear to find non-self-control treatments, e.g. drug treatment, considerably more credible. This is despite the inadequacy and drawbacks of drugs as a long-term solution to anxiety-related problems. In many cases, neurotic anxiety automatically carries with it the features of loss of control, helplessness and lack of reliance on personal resources. Additionally, poor self-esteem invariably goes hand in hand with anxiety — the two features being inextricably related in inverse proportions. For such a client, drug treatment may seem a more attractive option because it can be seen as an external, and therefore more powerful, agent than the client himself. Further, drug treatment does not require personal effort to make the treatment work, unlike relaxation training. It will be remembered that the helplessness syndrome inhibits behavioural responses to control outcome. In self-control-based treatments such as relaxation training, the therapist is asking the client to develop personal control resources which he does not believe he possesses. Little wonder, therefore, that such clients may not find relaxation training as credible as a drug regime.

The anxiety management models have recognised these factors, and their treatment regimes are designed accordingly. Heavy emphasis is placed upon the client acquiring autonomous control over symptomatology. Dependence on the therapist is avoided at the outset by having clients practise skills independently, both within the session and through homework assignments. Clients are also expected to undertake anxiety-arousing behavioural tasks and positively reinforce themselves when these have been achieved. Helplessness and an internal locus of control may be deeply rooted factors in an anxious individual. However, Seligman asserts that change is possible.[32] In experimental situations he literally dragged the uncontrollably shocked animals away from the shock compartment, despite their resistance. After repeatedly forcing the animals to protect themselves from shock in this way, he observed that they began to recover normal responsiveness. Of course, it is difficult to conceive of a treatment procedure like this for humans! Nevertheless, the anxiety management approaches are didactic and systematic, encouraging the learning of new and more independent ways of coping. Repeated rehearsal and reinforcement for success is also emphasised. Clinically it can often be observed that once a client manages to make even a small achievement, the vicious circle of dependence, apathy, low self-esteem and further anxiety, is broken.

REFERENCES

1 Pavlov I P 1938 Translated and edited by G V Anrep. Conditioned reflexes. Oxford University Press, Oxford: Humphrey Milford: 1927
2 Skinner B F 1938 The behaviour of organisms. Appleton-Century-Crofts, New York
3 Watson J B 1924 Psychology from the standpoint of a behaviourist. Lippincott, Philadelphia
4 Mowrer O H 1939 A stimulus–response analysis of anxiety and its role as a reinforcing agent. Psychological Review 46:553–565
5 Dollard J, Miller N E 1950 Personality and Psychotherapy. McGraw-Hill, New York
6 Miller N E 1948 Studies of fear as an acquirable drive. Journal of Experimental Psychology 38:89–101
7 Sarason S B, Mandler G, Craighill P G 1952 The effect of differential instructions on anxiety and learning. Journal of Abnormal and Social Psychology 47:561–565
8 Yerkes R M, Dodson J D 1908 The relation of strength of stimulus to rapidity of habit formation. Journal of Comparative Neurological Psychology 18:459–482
9 Sarason E G 1975 Anxiety and self-preoccupation. In: Sarason I G, Spielberger C D (eds) Stress and anxiety. Hemisphere, New York, Vol 2
10 Beck A T, Emery G 1985 Anxiety disorders and phobias. Basic Books, USA
11 Heckhausen H 1975 Fear of failure as a self-reinforcing motive system. In: Sarason I G, Spielberger C D (eds) Stress and anxiety. Hemisphere, New York, Vol 2
12 Lazarus R S 1966 Psychological stress and the coping process. McGraw-Hill, New York
13 Janis I L 1958 Psychological stress. Wiley, New York
14 Rogers C R 1951 Client-centred therapy. Riverside Press, Massachusetts
15 Barlow D H 1992 Cognitive behavioral approaches to panic disorder and social phobia. Bulletin of the Meninger Clinic 56 (2, suppl.A):14–28
16 Beck A, Rush A 1975 In: Sarason I G, Spielberger C D (eds) Stress and anxiety. Hemisphere, New York, Vol 2
17 Foa E B 1988 What cognitions differentiate panic disorder from other anxiety disorders? In: Hand I, Wittchen H (eds) Panic and phobias. Springer, New York, Vol 2
18 Lucock M P, Salkovskis P M 1988 Cognitive factors in social anxiety and its treatment. Behaviour Research and Therapy 26:297–302
19 Martin M, Williams R M, Clark D M 1991 Does anxiety lead to selective processing of threat-related information? Behaviour Research and Therapy 29(2):147–160
20 Hawton K, Salkowskis P M, Kirk J, Clark D M (eds) 1989 Cognitive behaviour therapy for psychiatric problems — a practical guide. Oxford University Press, Oxford

21 Beck A T 1976 Cognitive therapy and the emotional disorders. International Universities Press, New York

22 Wells A, Davies M I 1994 The thought control questionnaire: a measure of individual differences in the control of unwanted thoughts. Behaviour Research and Therapy 32(8):871–878

23 Meichenbaum D 1977 Cognitive behavioural modification. Plenum Press, New York

24 Festinger L 1957 A theory of cognitive dissonance. Peterson Row, Illinois

25 Ellis A 1962 Reason and emotion in psychotherapy. Lyle Stewart, New York

26 Himle D, Thyer B A, Papsdorf J D 1982 Relationships between rational beliefs and anxiety. Cognitive Therapy and Research 6:219–223

27 Thyer B A, Papsdorf J D, Kilgore S A 1983 Relationships between irrational thinking and psychiatric symptomatology. Journal of Psychology 113(1):31–34

28 Beck A T, Laude R, Bohnert M 1974 Ideational components of anxiety neurosis. Archives of General Psychiatry 31:319–325

29 Maxwell J W, Wilkerson J 1982 Anxiety reduction through group instruction in rational therapy. Journal of Psychology 112:135–140

30 Safran J D 1982 The functional asymmetry of negative and positive self-statements. British Journal of Clinical Psychology 21:223–224

31 Smith T W, Ingram R E, Brehm S S 1983 Social anxiety, anxious self-preoccupation and recall of self-relevant information. Journal of Personality and Social Psychology 44(6):1276–1283

32 Seligman M E P 1975 Helplessness. W H Freeman, USA

33 Maier S F 1970 Failure to escape traumatic shock: Incompatible skeletal motor responses or learned helplessness? Learning and Motivation 1:157–170

34 Brady J V 1958 Ulcers in 'executive' monkeys. Scientific American 199:95–100

35 Weiss J M 1968 Effects of coping response on stress. Journal of Comparative and Physiological Psychology 65:251–260

36 Weiss J M 1970 Somatic effects of predictable and unpredictable shock. Psychosomatic Medicine 32:397–409

37 Weiss J M 1971 a,b,c Journal of Comparative and Physiological Psychology (77):1–30
   a Effects of coping behaviour in different warning signal conditions on stress pathology in rats. pp 1–13
   b Effects of punishing the coping response (conflict) on stress pathology in rats. pp 14–21
   c Effects of coping behaviour with and without a feedback signal on stress pathology in rats. pp 22–30

38 Thomas E, Balter A 1974 Learned helplessness: amelioration of symptoms by cholinergic blockade of the septum. In: Seligman M E P 1975 Helplessness. W H Freeman, USA, pp 28,70,73,170

39 Miller N E, Weiss J M 1969 Effects of somatic or visceral responses to punishment. In: Campbell B A, Church R M (eds) Punishment and aversion behaviour. Appleton-Century-Crofts, New York, pp 343–372

40 Weiss J M, Stone E A, Harrell N 1970 Coping behaviour and norepinephrine in rats. Journal of Comparative and Physiological Psychology 72:153–160

41 Weiss J M, Glazer H, Pohoreckyh 1974 Coping behaviour and neurochemical changes in rats. Paper presented at the Kittay Scientific Foundation conference. New York

42 Seligman M E P 1971 Phobias and preparedness. Behaviour Therapy 2:307–320

43 McNally R J, Reiss S 1982 The preparedness theory of phobias and human safety-signal conditioning. Behaviour Research and Therapy 20:153–159

44 Rotter J B 1966 Generalised expectancies for internal vs external control of reinforcements. Psychological Monographs 80(609)

45 Johnson J H, Sarason I G 1978 Life stress, depression and anxiety: internal-external control as a moderator variable. Journal of Psychosomatic Research 22:205–208

46 Hiroto D S 1974 Locus of control and learned helplessness. Journal of Experimental Psychology 102:187–193

47 Sandler I N, Lakey B 1982 Locus of control as a stress moderator: the role of control perceptions and social support. American Journal of Community Psychology 102:187–193

48 Anderson C R 1977 Locus of control, coping behaviours and performance in a stress setting: a longitudinal study. Journal of Applied Psychology 62:446–451

49 Geer J H, Davison G C, Gatchel R I 1970 Reduction of stress in humans through non-veridical perceived control of aversive stimulation. Journal of Personality and Social Psychology 16:731–738

50 Sanderson W C, Rapee R M, Barlow D H 1989 The influence of and illusion of control on panic attacks induced via inhalation of 5.5% carbon dioxide-enriched air. Archives of General Psychiatry 46:157–162

51 Averill J R 1973 Personal control over aversive stimulation and its relationship to stress. Psychological Bulletin 80:286–303

FURTHER READING

Forgays D G, Sosnowski T, Wizesniewski K (eds) 1992 Anxiety — recent developments in cognitive, psychophysiological and health research. Hemisphere Publishing Corporation, Washington

with applying a realistic approach to decision-making or problem-solving tasks. The ego ethos is: 'In order to avoid adverse consequences, I must wait a while for what I want'.

Superego

The superego is popularly synonymous with the human 'conscience' and is associated with feelings of guilt. It is not present at birth, but develops in the growing child as a result of the internalisation of parental values and judgements. The child is punished when it transgresses against parental dictates. The superego arises in response to the need to avoid further punishment and control the id. Parental and social values are gradually absorbed into the superego so that the mature individual perceives these values as part of his own moral code. The superego ethos is: 'It is wrong to have/do that, if I seek it I must suffer severe punishment'.

The dynamics of anxiety

Freud described a dynamic internal struggle at work between the differing impulses of the id, ego and superego. These three parts are distinct, but interact with each other in the maintenance of psychological equilibrium. As the human organism develops, anxiety may result from conflict between the three facets of the personality. For example, libidinal impulses from the id may press for discharge but are met with the threat of punishment, such as castration anxiety, from the superego. Similarly, the ego may perceive the severity of the superego as 'danger' and respond with signal anxiety. Ultimately, the original impulses themselves become the stimulus which release signal anxiety. Thus, if an impulse arises from the id, the gratification of which had previously been punished, the superego now punishes the individual merely for having the impulse itself. Signal anxiety results, which immobilises the power of the id and leads to repression of the impulses. A reduction in anxiety results. The tendency to employ psychological defence mechanisms, such as repression, is reinforced by the need to maintain the reduction in anxiety. Thus, if the individual in our previous example is to avoid anxiety, he must find a way of banishing his wish for the forbidden object from consciousness.

Categories of anxiety

Freud broke down his concept of anxiety into three types: reality, moral and neurotic anxiety. All three are involved with the ego's response to actual, or potential, helplessness when threatened with overwhelming psychic 'danger'. The function of the ego is that of mediation between the instinctual demands to ensure that some gratification is achieved, while still preserving its own integrity. If such an outcome becomes impossible, pathological anxiety results.

1. In reality anxiety, the ego's aim is to expedite gratification of the instincts without making the organism vulnerable to danger, e.g. 'I must have/do this, but I must avoid coming to physical harm in the process'. If the ego is uncertain how to achieve this aim, fear-related anxiety results.

2. In moral anxiety, the ego's aim is to preserve its sense of its own goodness while at the same time placating the instincts. If the ego attempts to achieve this in a way which fails to meet the moral demands of the superego, shame or guilt result, e.g. 'If I am good and worthy, I cannot allow myself to have/do this'. If the ego cannot satisfy the aims of both id and superego, guilt-related anxiety results.

3. In neurotic anxiety, the ego's aim is to protect its own identity and structure while an uncharacteristic and powerful instinctive drive threatens to overwhelm it, e.g. 'I long to have/do this, but I cannot allow myself to perceive that I am the one who has/does this'. If the ego cannot satisfy these conflicting aims, neurotic anxiety results.[2,3]

In order to control anxiety and maintain the stability of the individual in the face of such conflicts, the ego employs various defence mechanisms. Freud's initial work on defence mechanisms was developed by later contributors in the field, including his daughter, Anna Freud, whose work is described next. Further examples of defence mechanisms will also be given at the end of this section.

ANNA FREUD

Anna Freud elaborated upon her father's theories about human instincts and drives, and the psychodynamic concept of the id, ego and superego. In particular, she is noted for her work on defence mechanisms.[4] Her basic premise was that the ego defends not only against the drives but also against the emotions associated with the drives. In adult neurosis the superego prevents the ego from coming to terms with the drives. Thus, the first motive for using defence strategies is superego anxiety. The purpose of the defences is to protect the ego from being overwhelmed by the demands of the id instincts.

Anna Freud described ten psychological defences: regression, repression, reaction formation, isolation, undoing, projection, introjection, turning against self and reversal. The tenth defence mechanism, sublimation, or displacement of instinctual wishes, is described as the only normal defence. Some common examples of defence mechanisms are given here.

Projection — the attribution of one's own feelings to another person. For example, a client may be unaware that he is angry with his therapist and instead blames the therapist, claiming that it is really she who is angry with him. This may be because his own angry emotions cause too much anxiety to permit acknowledgement and are defended against by projecting them onto the therapist.

Reaction formation — characterised by behaviour which is diametrically opposed to that which the individual truly wishes to engage in. For example, a client may have a deep-seated wish to behave in a powerful, aggressive manner, but instead goes to inordinate lengths to be meek and submissive. In this case, the submissive behaviour is used to defend against the forbidden impulse to dominate.

Isolation — having a thought without the accompanying emotion. For example, a client may express sad thoughts without showing the related emotion. In this case, the client may be defending against the true impact of the sadness due to anxiety that it might overwhelm him.

Repression — blocking an impulse from consciousness so that the individual is totally unaware of its presence.

Introjection — attributing the personal characteristics of another person to oneself. This occurs when the individual fears they have lost the other person, or their love, e.g. through bereavement. This is a way of denying the loss. In the neurotic adult, superego anxiety prevents acceptance of the id instincts and prohibits sexual and aggressive feelings. This leads to the setting up of ideal standards which are incompatible with psychological health. The adult neurotic ego fears the instincts because it fears the superego. Consequently, the aim of neurosis is to elude superego punishment. Defences are used to reduce anxiety arising from the ego's fear of being completely overwhelmed or destroyed by the power of the instincts. Thus, the role of the defences is to preserve the psychological organisation and stability of the individual.

Further motives for the use of defences may include conflict between incompatible impulses, e.g. heterosexuality and homosexuality or activity and passivity. This conflict arises due to the adult ego's need for integration and consistency between its impulses. The ego has a more marked tendency to defend against instincts which are associated with painful emotions than pleasurable ones.[5,6]

THE NEO-FREUDIANS

Between 1930 and 1950 the neo-Freudians emerged, bringing a more sociocultural slant to Freudianism. Exponents included Sullivan[7], Horney[8], Fromm[9] and Erikson[10]. According to the neo-Freudians, primary anxiety appears as the infant begins to perceive itself as being separate from its mother. This awareness involves the frustration of the infant's dependency needs, and provokes anxiety.

For instance, Sullivan saw human life as being the process of striving towards interpersonal acceptance as a human being. He described anxiety as the experience, and expression, of tension associated with disruptions in an individual's significant interpersonal relationships. Accordingly, anxiety occurs when disapproval from significant others is expected or expressed — the 'forbidding gesture'. Such a gesture would threaten the structure of the individual's internal world — the world of being an interpersonally acceptable human being. Sullivan also introduced the 'self-system' concept, which supplemented the prevailing understanding of psychic defence strategies. The self-system is described as a defensive psychic measure used to protect the individual from disagreeable or disruptive anxiety. Such defences involve various manoeuvres to control awareness so as to eliminate an event or impulse from consciousness, or alter its meaning, e.g. 'selective inattention', 'substitution' or 'dissociation'. These manoeuvres are aimed at reducing anxiety by distorting reality.

The neo Freudians were concerned with the effects of the socialisation process upon the growing child. Society, through parental influences, enforces restrictions upon the expression of instinctual impulses e.g. anger. The threat of parental disapproval or punishment, such as withdrawal of affection, forces the child to find a means of containing his unacceptable impulses. The child learns to use psychic defences to achieve this. In adulthood, anxiety may continue to arise whenever an unacceptable impulse, such as anger, is felt. This is because the forbidden impulses are an unconscious reminder of parental disapproval. The individual must continually adjust his defensive system in order to reduce anxiety. Under conditions of stress, pressure on the defensive system is increased. This may lead to the shoring up of old defences, or the erection of new ones, in order to preserve psychological integrity. A vicious cycle may result which predisposes the individual to develop severe psychological illness.

THE POST-FREUDIANS

The major exponents of this school include Klein, Fairbairn and Winnicott. The post-Freudians based their work upon much of Freud's original terminology and conceptual framework.[11,12] Their main contribution was to clarify the crucial role of infant development in the genesis of adult neurosis as well as developing and improving relevant treatment approaches.

The work of Klein

Klein, as a student of Sigmund and Anna Freud, contributed to the development of play therapy which she used in her work with children. This worked in a similar way to free association in classical psychoanalysis. Klein emphasised a reconstructive approach to therapy, focusing on events occurring at an earlier stage in development. Klein noted that in play, as in analysis, typical sequences occurred. For example, it has been observed that in the initial stages of analysis there is often a warm relationship and a productive flow of free association. This tends to run dry after a few weeks as more threatening material is encountered.

Klein posited that at the moment of birth, the experience of the infant is that of chaos, fraught with anxiety. The infant is only able to perceive disjointed impressions of the world and itself, so the environment is understood in terms of separate 'bits and pieces'. This includes the mother, who is perceived as a series of good and bad things or events (part-objects), rather than a whole person. The infant has no means of structuring the chaos since it has no language, is unable to differentiate between reality and fantasy, and has no understanding of time. The only solution available to the infant is to dissociate from its own physical pains such as hunger. The infant therefore perceives the bad part-objects (e.g. bad breast) arising from the environment as the cause of the pain. If then, the mother's breast, or good part-object, is presented, the infant perceives it as a rescuer and relaxes. In early development the cycle of hunger (bad breast) and feeding (good breast) is often repeated, thus when the bad breast scenario presents, this becomes a signal for the good breast. If the good breast is not a regular rescuer, the infant employs psychic defences as a way of dealing with its distress. This may become manifest in the adult neurotic as persecutory anxiety, and may involve the 'splitting' of good and bad part-objects, idealisation, projection and introjection. Adult neurosis is characterised by such defensive reactions, thus making stable relationships difficult to achieve.

Finally, Klein emphasised the importance of the death instinct in the genesis of anxiety. Accordingly, the ego splits itself and projects its own death instinct onto the breast. This causes the breast to be seen as 'bad' and leads ultimately to paranoia. Thus, the infant sees the bad breast (containing its own death instinct) as a persecutor, which seeks the infant's destruction.[13,14,15]

The Kleinian theory of development

The paranoid–schizoid position Klein described this phase as occupying the first 4–5 months of life. Termed the paranoid–schizoid position, this stage involves the perception of the breast as persecutory, resulting in withdrawal from it. The resulting conflict is compounded by the inability of the infant to perceive either itself or its mother as whole, discrete entities. It is also unable to perceive itself as being separate from its mother. The infant compensates for this by splitting its own ego into good and bad part-objects. This results in paranoid anxiety.

The depressive position This phase relates to the subsequent 6–8 months of life and involves the infant's recognition of its own separateness from the mother and from the breast. The infant realises that it contains both good and bad, and becomes aware of its own feelings of hate and guilt towards the mother. A state of ambivalence results, as the infant also becomes aware that its mother is a whole person, and the source of both the good and bad breast. In other words, she is both frustrator and provider. The infant fears that its anger towards the bad breast may have also destroyed the good breast. The only solution to the conflict is that of reparation for the destructive impulses towards her. This strategy allows the infant to re-incorporate and idealise the good breast. The acceptance of the ambivalent state, in which objects are seen as incorporating good and bad aspects, is a psychologically healthy attitude which facilitates the development of realism and maturity.

Fairbairn and Winnicott

The individual works of Fairbairn and Winnicott are complementary to the Kleinian concepts, although with different emphasis and terminology. Fairbairn, for instance, was concerned with the oral stage, as originally described by Freud. As a result of Fairbairn's work the early oral stage has been termed: 'love made hungry'. He stated that if the helpless infant were to be severely frustrated during this phase, schizoid withdrawal might result. Substantial deprivation at this stage is deeply damaging as the infant's unfulfilled needs grow to frightening proportions which can no longer be met. A sense of emptiness and hunger threaten to overwhelm the infant, and this is made still worse when the good breast is presented because the infant's needs have become insatiable, rather like a bottomless pit. The only solution is to reject the unreliable good breast entirely. Thus, in later relationships, a repressed wish to consume the love object would result in a difficulty in expressing feelings at all. For example, deeply disturbed individuals may appear to be devoid of emotion. Their unconscious fear may be that if a nurturing gesture were to break through their unconscious defences, the floodgates would open, overwhelming them with unsatisfied needs. In the late oral stage, termed 'love made angry', the infant responds with angry fantasies towards the love object if its wishes are frustrated. If the infant were to be continually frustrated, guilt and fear that the accumulated anger might destroy the love object would result. Severe frustration during this stage may lead to the development of separation anxiety. The whole oral stage lasts from 0 to 10 months.[16]

Winnicott affirmed the object–relations theories described above. He emphasised the importance of an early facilitating environment for healthy psychological development. His view was that an insufficiently nurturing mother cannot support the vulnerable infant ego, resulting in schizoid withdrawal.[14,17,18] His work has made a remarkable impact due to its insightful and empathic approach to the challenges of parenting, often characterised by the term: 'good-enough mother'.

Glossary of some post-Freudian terminology

Anxiety: is the ego's reaction to the death instinct. In order to defend against its own death instinct, the immature ego deflects it. This may result in either of the following reactions:

1. Paranoid anxiety occurs when the death instinct is projected onto external objects which are then experienced as persecutors. The infant is fearful that the persecutor may destroy the ideal object, e.g. good breast, as well as itself. Paranoid anxiety relates to the paranoid–schizoid position.

2. Depressive anxiety occurs when the infant fears that its own anger may destroy the ideal object. It relates to the depressive position when the infant experiences both its separateness from the object, or mother, and its own conflicting feelings of love and hate for the object, which contains both good and bad.

Bad object: is a part-object, e.g. bad breast, which has been split off in the paranoid–schizoid phase of development. The infant's own destructive impulses and anger are projected into the bad object, and all bad experiences are seen as arising from it.

Idealisation: is a schizoid defence mechanism, involving splitting and denial. The unwanted parts of the object, e.g. bad breast, are denied and rejected through the process of splitting, so that these parts become bad. The remaining parts then become associated with all the infant's good experiences and are thus idealised.

Ideal object: is a part-object, e.g. good breast, which has been split off and idealised by the infant while in the paranoid–schizoid phase of development.

Reparation: is the attempt to restore a loved object which the infant fears its hostile impulses may have harmed. This occurs in the depressive position and is associated with a constructive reaction to guilt and fear of having lost the ideal object.

Splitting: in the earliest phase of development, splitting occurs between the good and bad self, and the good and bad object. For example, the mother is not seen as a discrete entity, containing both good and bad, instead she is split and is perceived as two mothers — a good and a bad one.

The use of the foregoing psychological defences is held to continue into adulthood, and although they no longer directly involve infantile concerns, they are related symbolically to the unresolved conflicts of childhood.

SEPARATION ANXIETY: VARIOUS THEORIES

Towards the end of his life, Freud began to emphasise the significance of loss and separation from the maternal figure, and began to revise his earlier theories accordingly. Freud's original instinctual model posited that the mother is only sought in order to relieve tension due to the physiological drives of the infant. His concept of signal anxiety implied that the infant demonstrates anxiety as a distress signal to bring about the mother's return, and that this develops through the learning process. He also regarded anxiety about a known danger as realistic, and anxiety about an unknown danger as neurotic. However, large numbers of children show fear of the dark and strangers. According to this line of reasoning, the question was raised as to whether all children are neurotic. Additionally, children may show distress if the mother is absent, even when their physiological needs are being met.

A major contributor to the psychological concept of separation anxiety was Bowlby.[19] He pointed out that many common childhood fears have an evolutionary basis in human infants and are associated with survival. His formulation stated that where a young child has made an attachment to a mother figure and separation occurs, great distress results. Such early separation has the potential to cause severe psychological damage. We will return to Bowlby's important ideas in more detail in the next section.

Apart from Freud and Bowlby, several others have contributed their ideas to the theory of separation anxiety. Klein stated that separation anxiety stems from the infant's belief that his hostile impulses have destroyed her. This belief is due to projection of the infant's death instinct and his angry feelings towards the mother, whose absence serves to punish him. According to Klein, objective anxiety occurs as a result of the infant's dependence on the mother for the satisfaction of needs. In neurotic anxiety, however, the infant fears that the mother has been destroyed by his sadistic impulses and will never return. Somewhat similarly, Anna Freud described separation anxiety as being characteristic of an early phase of object relations when mother–child biological unity is frustrated. Winnicott stated that the earliest anxiety is caused by being 'insecurely held' or by inadequate and inconsistent support by the mother. In each of the foregoing viewpoints, the importance of actual mother–child separation in the genesis of anxiety is acknowledged in the theoretical framework. From a more sociological standpoint, Sullivan placed greater emphasis on disapproval and lack of affection from the mother in the aetiology of anxiety.[20]

THE CONTRIBUTION OF BOWLBY

Bowlby emphasised that separation, which obviates the rupture of the child's attachment to the mother, is the primary factor in early anxiety. Bowlby challenged the notions of the post-Freudians by stating that anxiety reactions to the loss of the love object can be observed months before the human infant could be credited with an awareness of losing the object's love. Similarly, Bowlby disputed Freud's instinct theories regarding separation anxiety by stating that the child's tie to the mother does not depend on learning that she is a need-gratifier, but precedes the infant's capacity for such learning. He claimed that the nature of the child's early attachment resembles 'imprinting', an ethological notion. Bowlby posited that separation anxiety is an evolved protest mechanism. This mechanism can be seen in animals who are assumed to lack the necessary cognitive equipment to learn that separation implies the impending frustration of their physiological needs.

According to Bowlby, the first time separation occurs intense fear is aroused, but if the child senses the prospect of further separation, a deeply rooted pattern of anxiety results. He outlined three phases to be observed when a young child experiences separation:

1. Vigorous protestation as the child tries to recover the lost mother — initial phase of separation anxiety.
2. Despair, but continuing vigilance for her return — grief and mourning phase.
3. Detachment as the child appears to withdraw and lose interest in the mother — defensive phase.

Bowlby's findings were collated from the observations in a number of studies of children separated from their mothers, notably due to hospitalisation or placement in residential nurseries. Of the characteristic responses listed above, the first two relate to 'anxious attachment'. In anxious attachment, the child is searching for his mother and still has hopes of finding her. If this does not occur, his distress deepens and he begins to lose hope. If the mother reappears, the child may react with excessively clinging, possessive and demanding behaviour towards his mother. The attendant insecurity of the anxious attachment phase may permanently predispose the child to be over-dependent on others in later life. In the third phase, that of withdrawal, the child has given up hope that his mother will return and appears not to care any more. If she does reappear at this stage, he may reject her. If the withdrawal stage is reached, the child may suffer severe psychological damage, and in some cases, where the separation is prolonged, permanent emotional detachment.

Bowlby reports several studies demonstrating that people with poor self-esteem and other psychological problems tend to have been reared in unstable environments. Firstly, without secure attachment in their formative years, adults may become chronically anxious about the availability of others when needed. Links between this proposition and the development and function of adult agoraphobia have also been made by others.[21,22] For example, the symptoms in some agoraphobic clients may have the effect of curtailing the freedom of movement of significant others, e.g. family members. In such a case, then, the agoraphobia may be a psychological strategy to reduce the anxiety produced by the absence of certain family members.

Secondly, Bowlby cited studies of empirical evidence showing that disrupted mother–child relations may ultimately cause certain forms of psychopathy. In extreme cases, where no attachment is achieved by age three, an antisocial personality disorder may result. Such an individual has 'given up' on relationships, whereas the adult with anxious attachment, albeit distressed and insecure, still desires love and hopes to make a worthwhile relationship.[23,24]

THE RELEVANCE OF THE PSYCHOANALYTIC THEORIES TO ANXIETY MANAGEMENT TRAINING

In the adult, a tendency to revert to infantile conflicts and reactions may result if a mature relationship is attempted. The post-Freudian concept of 'love made hungry' described by Fairbairn may be proffered to explain how muscular tension can be used as a defence against feelings, such as pleasure, which the individual may find too disturbing to deal with. For example, a few clients receiving relaxation training can be observed to react with unexplained and deep distress just at the point when they begin to relax. This suggests that muscular tension itself may act as a psychological defence in some cases and is used to hold back the onslaught of unmet needs. To illustrate this point further, Jacobsen and Edinger have described two case histories in which clients developed side-effects to relaxation training which seemed related to underlying dynamic issues.[25] In one case, the adverse reaction was thought to be due to a sense of being overpowered, which provoked a panic reaction associated with an unresolved homosexual conflict. In the second case, the anxiety symptoms themselves appeared to be of crucial necessity to the client's adjustment. They were periodically produced as a coping strategy for dealing with difficulties which the client seemed unable to face directly. It is interesting to note that both clients were World War II veterans with post-traumatic stress disorders and long histories of psychiatric problems.

Consideration of psychoanalytic concepts may also help to illuminate some of the underlying dynamic reasons for a client's difficulty in responding to treatment, especially the self-control-orientated approaches described here. For instance, the theories concerning separation anxiety and anxious attachment may help the therapist to understand the needs of clients who consistently behave dependently and maladaptively as if to elicit protective responses in others. Direct attempts to encourage such clients to use their own resources frequently flounder.

Somewhat differently, Michelson and Ascher[22] describe how hyperprotective parental styles may contribute to anxious insecurity and an inordinate need to control self, environment and events. They highlight the pitfalls of communicating excessive concern with the dangers in the world and the difficulties of dealing with them. Constant emphasis on the child's inability to deal with difficulties causes the child to feel particularly exposed to life's dangers. This may be part of an unconscious parental strategy to keep the child with them. Where parental threats of desertion and other emotive family scenes occur, feelings of insecurity outside the home are compounded. A conflicted self-image may result in the anxiously attached individual: while they do possess a sense of being loved and valued, they see themselves as being too weak to cope in the outside world. Rigid attitudes may be developed, particularly towards themselves, underpinned by a desperate need for control. This formulation is associated with obsessive/compulsive features.

In some cases, where early psychological trauma has been severe, relaxation training may be contraindicated, or at best, a waste of therapeutic time. An alternative treatment approach may be required. On the positive side, practical relaxation training and anxiety management programmes have proved to be of considerable help to quite deeply disturbed individuals if appropriately applied. However, while relaxation training and anxiety management have been used to good effect with psychotic clients, these techniques are not recommended for use during a florid phase of the illness, by any school of thought.

In conclusion, while one of the major benefits of relaxation training appears, on the surface, to be its lack of side-effects, more research appears to be required to confirm the truth of this assumption. Although anxiety management and relaxation training are essentially behavioural techniques, it may be useful to be aware of psychodynamic issues in the screening and treatment of anxious clients referred for anxiety management and relaxation training.

DEFENCE MECHANISMS VERSUS COPING STRATEGIES

Anxiety is involved to some extent in the formulation of all major neurotic and psychotic disorders. It is posited that the neurotic person suffers from the effects of accumulated unresolved childhood conflicts still requiring expression. The stresses of modern life therefore pose an extra burden and serve to compound adult relationships with difficulties. Various psychological defences are used to preserve stability and neutralise the painful effects of anxiety. For example, the obsessional defends against anxiety concerned with chaos by inordinate attempts to control everyday life. The agoraphobic deals with anxiety through flight towards the home, while the schizoid flees from reality. The hysterical defence is used by the 'defeated' individual who feels forced to resort to oblique or deceptive emotional manipulation to achieve his or her ends. Such strategies also serve to provide a 'safe', if indirect, outlet for hostility.[26]

Defence mechanisms are used to combat anxiety, and are therefore psychologically homeostatic. They may be considered to be adaptive or maladaptive according to individual circumstances. What characterises a defence mechanism from a coping mechanism is its tendency to be a rigid, automatic response to a specific stimulus. The effect of a defence mechanism is also generally to distort reality. Coping mechanisms are commonly more flexible, creative and objective responses.

Dollard and Miller are noted for their efforts to investigate psychoanalytic theory scientifically.[27] Their work on anxiety and conflict helped to refine knowledge about defence mechanisms. They stated that while all individuals have defences, these are only maladaptive in the neurotic individual. Some pertinent examples of defence mechanisms in common use as ways of coping with stress are given below.

Compulsivity: This has been described as the 'anti-childhood-incompetence-syndrome' and is used as a defence against anxiety concerned with punishment. It is characterised by excessive activity directed at controlling the environment, e.g. excessive checking behaviour or overly frequent hand-washing. In craftsmen it can be adaptive and lead to admirably high standards of perfection.

Counterphobia: This is a drive to overcome anxiety by facing it head on. This can only be described as pathological when it appears in an exaggerated form or if it ignores the actual danger imposed by the phobic object. Indeed, exhortations to 'face the fear' are a major feature of modern anxiety management regimes.

Regression: In regression the individual reverts to an earlier stage of development in an attempt to reduce anxiety. Thus, less responsibility is invited and dependency is increased. Normal individuals often regress while under stress and this may be expressed through habits such as nail-biting.

Ordinary behaviours such as drug or alcohol use, eating, smoking, laughing, crying, swearing, sleeping, talking, sublimation, fantasy, hyperactivity and displacement activities such as fidgeting are also widely used to reduce tension. These activities may have a function in helping to stabilise existing psychological defences. When defences fail, new ones are brought into action and old ones are strengthened and extended.[28,29,30]

REFERENCES

1 Freud S 1936 The problem of anxiety. Norton, New York
2 Freud S 1926 Inhibitions, symptoms and anxiety. Standard Edition, 20:77–174
3 Levitt E E 1982 The psychology of anxiety, 2nd edn. Lawrence Erlbaum, USA, ch 3
4 Freud A 1968 The ego and the mechanisms of defence. The Hogarth Press, London
5 Freud A 1965 Normality and pathology in childhood. Penguin Books, London
6 Freud A 1937 The ego and the mechanisms of defence. The Hogarth Press, London
7 Sullivan H S 1938 Introduction to the study of interpersonal relations. Psychiatry I:121–134
8 Horney K 1945 Our inner conflicts: a constructive theory of neurosis. Norton, New York
9 Fromm E 1944 Individual and social origins of neurosis. American Sociological Review IX(4)
10 Erikson E 1950 Childhood and society. Norton, New York, pp 219–234
11 Segal H 1975 Introduction to the work of Melanie Klein. The Hogarth Press, London
12 Guntrip H 1983 Schizoid phenomena, object relations and the self. The Hogarth Press, London
13 Meltzer D 1978 The Kleinian development. Clunie Press, Perthshire
14 Klein M 1932 Psychoanalysis of children. The Hogarth Press, London
15 Klein M 1948 Contributions to psychoanalysis. The Hogarth Press, London, pp 1921–1945
16 Fairbairn W R D 1952 Psychoanalytic studies of the personality. Tavistock, London
17 Winnicott D W 1960 The theory of the parent–infant relationship. The Hogarth Press, London
18 Winnicott D W 1972 The maturational process and the facilitating environment. The Hogarth Press, London
19 Bowlby J 1973 Attachment and loss. Vol II: separation, anxiety and anger. The Hogarth Press, London
20 Jones B A 1983 Healing factors of psychiatry in light of attachment theory. American Journal of Psychotherapy 37(2):235–244
21 Klein D F 1981 Anxiety reconceptualized. In: Klein D F, Rabkin (eds) Anxiety: new research and changing concepts. Raven Press, New York
22 Michelson L, Ascher L M (eds) 1987 Anxiety and stress disorders — cognitive–behavioural assessment and treatment. Guilford Press, New York
23 Bowlby J 1961a Separation anxiety: a critical review of the literature. Journal of Child Psychology and Psychiatry 1:251–269
24 Bowlby J 1961b Processes of mourning. International Journal of Psycho-Analysis 42:317–340
25 Jacobsen R, Edinger J D 1982 Side effects of relaxation treatment. American Journal of Psychiatry 139(7):952–953
26 Rycroft C 1968 Anxiety and neurosis. Pelican, UK
27 Dollard J, Miller N E 1950 Personaltiy and psychotherapy. McGraw-Hill, New York
28 Levitt E E 1982 The psychology of anxiety, 2nd edn. Lawrence Erlbaum, USA, ch 4
29 Dobson C B 1982 The hidden adversary. MTP Press, UK, ch 4
30 Heilbrun A B, Pepe V 1985 Awareness of cognitive defences and stress management. British Journal of Medical Psychology 58:9–17

5

Psychophysiological models of anxiety

Diana Keable

PSYCHOSOMATIC DISEASE

Psychosomatic diseases have been defined as: 'clinical conditions which are considered to be a compromise solution, in bodily terms, of emotional conflict, without initial irreversible structural changes in the organs concerned'.[1] The term 'psychosomatic disease' is often applied somewhat inclusively in the literature. However, in the interests of clarity, it should be differentiated from 'illness anxiety' (hypochondriasis), in that observable physical symptoms or organic pathology exists, e.g. hypertension, insomnia, skin conditions, irritable bowel syndrome and gastric ulcer. In illness anxiety (to be covered in greater detail later in this chapter) the problems are primarily of perceived, rather than actual, symptomatology, or of hypersensitivity to normal bodily sensations. Psychosomatic disease should also be distinguished from hysterical conversion syndrome in which anxiety is 'converted' into physical symptoms such as paraplegia or, famously, 'shell-shock'. Finally, it must be remembered that a mixed picture can also be seen in which the basis of symptoms is variable or uncertain.[2]

That a relationship exists between the emotions and bodily health is now beyond argument. Contrary to long-held beliefs, visceral responses may be modified by positive and negative conditioning, e.g. biofeedback. So integrated is the relationship between emotional and physiological reactions that lie detectors have been at least partially successful. Attempts have been made to detect deception through the measurement of skin resistance, respiratory and cardiovascular responses. These observations have widely recorded characteristic 'blips' when the subject is giving information that they know to be false. This is despite the fact that each individual's psychophysiological profile is unique.

THE DEVELOPMENT OF PSYCHOSOMATIC MEDICINE

Some of the earlier work in this field attempted to relate specific attitudes, psychological disorders and personality types to specific disease patterns. However, many contributors at that time tended to oversimplify. For example, Graham[3] related 18 physical disorders to specific psychological attitudes. Accordingly, an individual suffering with acne would possess the attitude of feeling 'picked on' and wanting to be left alone. Vomiting was associated with the feeling that some wrong had occurred for which the individual felt guilty and wished to expunge. Hypertension involved a constant feeling of impending threat and a need for continual vigilance. Alexander's specificity theory proposed that when increased arousal due to stress becomes chronic, organic pathology such as ulcer ultimately occurs.[4] He further postulated that the basic emotion causing increased SNS arousal is anger, while feelings of dependence cause increased PNS arousal (SNS and PNS are discussed in Chapter 2). These reactions were related to specific disease patterns, i.e. separation conflict being associated with asthma. This theory has been criticised widely in subsequent studies that indicate no such specific relationships. However, Robbins later put forward evidence to support the theory that hostility and dependency are significant factors in certain psychosomatic diseases.[5]

Other early research studies attempted to indicate that specific personality types are associated with specific disease patterns. For example, cancer was related to the 'too good to be true', martyr-like and repressed personality. Difficulties in relationships and loss during childhood were related with a tendency to develop cancer.[6]

Rheumatoid arthritis was related to a constellation of personality traits comprising qualities of self-sacrifice, self-consciousness, shyness, excessive inhibition and repressed anger; similar traits were also found in colitis patients.[7,8] Finally, migraine sufferers were said to be generally tense, nervous individuals who displayed high standards and martyr-like qualities.[9]

Later research was successful in highlighting the relationship between myocardial infarction and the 'Type A' personality. The Type A personality displays marked elements of hostility, time-urgency, and excessively ambitious and competitive behaviour. In contrast, Type B behaviour lacks these characteristics and belongs to more relaxed, phlegmatic personalities.[10] Epidemiological studies have demonstrated Type A behaviour to be a risk factor for coronary heart disease. RT and AMT programmes have been used to reduce this risk in Type A clients.[11,12,13,14]

It is now accepted that we cannot make the generalisation, for example, that people with asthma necessarily suffer from a separation conflict. Nor can it be assumed that all those with separation anxiety conflicts will respond to stress with PNS dominant reactions because of dependency feelings. It is acknowledged, however, that individuals show specific response patterns to stress and this has been termed 'organ specificity'. In other words, each individual has their own unique way of responding to stress, certain organs or systems tending to be more responsive than others. For example, one person may suffer predominantly from tension headaches, whereas another person may experience gastrointestinal difficulties or blood pressure problems when under stress. This reminds us of Selye who suggested that it is the most vulnerable organ or system in each individual that tends to break down under stress.[15,16] If we accept this line of reasoning, then each individual is already predisposed to develop certain psychosomatic diseases before stress is applied. This may have attractive implications for preventative medicine, but it should be noted that stress cannot be seen as a constant. Particular stressors interrelate in a variable fashion with each particular individual.

The stress-resistant or 'hardy' personality

It has been shown that the stress-resistant or 'hardy' personality type is associated with lower rates of illness linked with stressful life events. Kobasa[17] disagrees with the early conclusions of Holmes and Rahe,[18] i.e. that we are passive victims of life events. He states that: 'persons can rise to the challenges of their environment and turn stressful life events into possibilities or opportunities for personal growth and benefit.' He asserts that three existential concepts are necessary for this to be achieved:

- commitment — personal investment, involvement and belief in the value of one's activities, whether within the family, work or community environment
- control — believing that one can influence the course of events and acting accordingly
- challenges — perceiving change as an opportunity and a normal part of life rather than a threat; the ability to tolerate ambiguity and respond flexibly to life's challenges.

The foregoing comprise the three components held to be essential elements of the 'hardy' personality. In similar vein, Flannery[19] lists the five main features of the 'stress-resistant' personality:

- personal control
- task involvement
- adaptive lifestyle based on diet, stimulant reduction/hard exercise/relaxation
- active seeking of social support
- mood well-being.

He contrasts these features with those of 'learned helplessness', first described by Seligman,[20] and exhibited in clinical depression. He recommends the application of the first four features listed above as coping strategies in lowering the incidence of physical and psychological illness.

Cognitive style

Fisher and Reason[21] concluded that cognitive style is crucial in ameliorating the effects of stressful events on health. They pointed out that highly resourceful individuals are singular in their ability to reduce the interfering effects of their own stress reactions on ongoing behaviour. Thus, while some degree of worrying can be productive in preparing for contingencies, it may drive states of anxiety and depression, thus increasing the risk of illness in the long term. Where cognitive capacity is taken up by ruminative activity, this may lead to cognitive failure/absent-mindedness and reduce ability to deal with other aspects of life. This compounds stress levels as new problems arise in consequence and a vicious circle is set up with attendant damage to self-esteem and confidence. Fisher and Reason conclude that thinking too much can damage your health, but acknowledge that trying not to think about problems does not help either. This indicates that positive cognitive strategies are vital to successful coping.

THE AETIOLOGY OF PSYCHOSOMATIC ILLNESS

With regard to the aetiology of psychosomatic disease in general, various hypotheses have been proposed.

1. It is thought that the limbic system plays a major role in the development of psychosomatic disease in certain people. This mechanism involves the redirection of emotions into bodily organs via ANS action.[1]

2. In psychoanalytic terms, it has been proposed that early unresolved conflicts may become somatised, resulting in psychosomatic disease. The individual subconsciously brings this about as a solution to unbearable feelings of ambivalence which are 'split off' and projected on to the bodily organ affected.[1]

3. A 'necessary conditions' hypothesis has been postulated.[22] This states that three variables must be present for psychosomatic disease to occur:

- individual response stereotypy
- inadequate homeostatic restraints
- exposure to activating situations.

Accordingly, if the individual's most vulnerable

organ or system fails to adapt successfully to stressful conditions, psychosomatic disease results. Selye[15,16] stated that, during stress, harmonious biological states of equilibrium may be overridden, leaving the organism vulnerable to disease. Again, periods of relaxation may be beneficial in providing a homeostatic restraint when an individual is exposed to ongoing stressful conditions. Relaxation may give the vulnerable organ-system a chance to adapt and recover, whereas unrelieved arousal will inevitably lead to breakdown under the escalating pressure.

4. It has been recognised that anxiety and stressful life events are important aetiological factors in psychosomatic illness.[15,16] Further, physiological changes can ensue following life stress and, again, individual patterns of response to stress differ widely. No consistent evidence that anxiety increases susceptibility to one particular disease exists. Rather, it may increase general susceptibility to illness and impede healing thereafter.

THE HYPERVENTILATION SYNDROME

One interesting phenomenon worthy of close study by therapists involved in relaxation training is that of chronic hyperventilation. Whether it can be classified as a psychosomatic disease is debatable, but the syndrome is commonly associated with anxiety. Symptoms may involve dizziness, disturbances of consciousness and vision, visceral pain, muscular spasm, cold extremities, headache, paraesthesia, numbness and even blackout and tetany in extreme cases. Symptoms may also mimic cardiac ischaemia or tachycardia. Hyperventilation activates the SNS, and this is evident in clinical signs such as tachycardia, sweating palms and axillae, and dilated pupils. Emotional lability will also often accompany acute episodes.

Hyperventilation is characterised by rapid thoracic respirations in the forward and upward direction. Little lateral or diaphragmatic chest movement can be observed and periodic sighing respirations may be noted. The acute physiological effect of hyperventilation is to expel carbon dioxide in excessive quantities, thus reducing the partial pressure of carbon dioxide in the arterial blood. The consequent reduction in carbonic acid leads to a state of respiratory alkalosis. In turn, this results in cerebral vasoconstriction and hypoxia, also affecting peripheral nerve function. This process gives rise to the diverse array of symptoms which are commonly reported by hyperventilating subjects. Hyperventilation has been implicated as the main causal factor in many instances of chest pain where no organic pathology has been found.[23]

Attempts to correlate the psychological characteristics associated with hyperventilation have shown obsessional, perfectionist traits with a tendency to suppress feelings. Lum,[24,25] who has contributed much to our knowledge of hyperventilation, believes that the syndrome is the result of a learned habit of incorrect breathing rather than neurosis. He postulates that chronic hyperventilation ultimately leads to the development of anxiety neurosis. Lum asserts that the high cure rate of subjects treated by breathing reeducation alone supports his hypothesis.[26]

ILLNESS BEHAVIOUR

Mechanic has made valuable contributions to our knowledge about the concept of illness behaviour.[27,28] He produced a review of the social and psychological factors relating to hypochondriasis and the presentation of bodily complaints at clinics.[29] The review looked at what makes people decide they are 'ill', at what point they decide to seek medical attention, and what social and emotional issues relate to their decision. He made several useful observations in relation to these issues:

1. People tend to pay particular attention to bodily sensations when they depart from more familiar feelings. This is an important factor in leading to the decision to ask for medical attention.

2. When bodily sensations occur at the same time as increases in personal stress levels, then these sensations are more likely to be interpreted as illness than the normal course of events.

3. Psychologically vulnerable persons tend to express their emotional distress through bodily illness.

4. Hypochondria may be associated with low self-esteem. Those with high self-esteem may feel more capable of dealing with stress.

5. In hypochondria, symptoms presented are commonly those that occur when under stress and these tend to be vague and diffuse.

Several studies have shown that approximately one third of patients attending gastrological clinics do not actually have organic disorders.[30,31] One study reported that 22 patients with chronic abdominal pain had seen a total of 76 consultants.[32] The only measure showing consistent abnormality in this group was the Hamilton Rating Scale for Depression in which 14 out of 22 were rated as clinically depressed. A recent review of this subject[23] concluded that nonorganic abdominal pain is associated with psychiatric disorder, and that its onset was associated with stressful life events. These findings highlight the size of the problem, and the attendant economic implications.[33]

An aetiological model is reproduced in Figure 5.1 to demonstrate how illness anxiety may develop.[23] Most notable is the concept that the patient's interpretation (attribution) of their physical sensations/symptoms is the key factor. A cluster of factors tends to be present in order for such disorders to present in medical clinics:

- perception of severe somatic symptoms e.g. pain
- psychiatric disorder/psychosocial factors e.g. stressful life event, vulnerable personality
- fear of serious illness
- external health locus of control.[23]

The tendency to refer such clients for psychological treatment only as a last resort is still a lamentable fact. Although liaison psychiatry, a growing specialism, has done much to correct this tendency, a great deal of work remains to be done in increasing awareness of how to tackle these problems. It has been emphasised[2,23] that it is vital to refer early in order to avoid problems becoming chronic. The manner and timing of

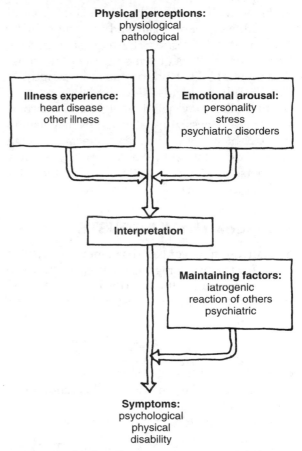

Figure 5.1 An aetiological model for non-cardiac atypical chest pain.[23] Reproduced here by kind permission of the Royal College of Psychiatrists.

referral can affect the client's ultimate willingness to accept psychological treatment. Wasting months or years on a series of irrelevant medical investigations is distressing for the client and only serves to consolidate the belief that their symptoms are due to some mysterious and malignant physical disease.

Salkovskis[34] has also identified four maintaining factors in illness anxiety:

- increased physiological arousal
- focus of attention on arbitrary physical signs
- avoidant behaviours
- reassurance-seeking.

A further crucial point to be considered in relation to illness anxiety is that of health locus of control (HLC). One study found that college students with internal health loci of control reported fewer clinic visits and were more likely to assert themselves, e.g. by requesting specific medications.[35] It has been suggested that those with internal HLC tend to cope more adaptively with health problems. Occasionally, however, external HLC may be advantageous. In chronic or terminal illness, for instance, this may lead to less self-blame and greater cooperation with health care providers.[35] See under the 'Anxiety and personal control' section of Chapter 3 for further discussion of locus of control.

THE ALEXITHYMIA CONSTRUCT

A relatively new concept has emerged over the past decade concerning the relationship between personality and health.[36,37] This has been termed 'alexithymia' to denote a cluster of characteristics including:

- difficulty in identifying and describing emotions
- difficulty in differentiating between the experience of emotions and bodily sensations of arousal
- limited ability to visualise; paucity of fantasy-related activity
- an externally oriented cognitive style that

tends to be literal and devoid of emotional content.

It has been proposed that due to the lack of an inner life of feelings and fantasies, alexithymic individuals become preoccupied with the minutiae of their physical symptoms. Alexithymia has been described as a 'lack of psychological mindedness'.[37] Paradoxically, although there is often a muted sensitivity to pain, such individuals often complain at length of physical symptoms in the absence of organic pathology. A central feature of the therapeutic approach to patients with alexithymia is to increase awareness of their emotional reactions.

Treatment strategies for both illness anxiety and alexithymia are aimed at changing beliefs and behaviour which maintain the problem. Experience has shown that few patients are reassured either by negative test results or by being told there is nothing wrong with them.[23] Better management in this area is vital and some therapeutic principles will be discussed later in this book (Ch. 16). Few clinicians will escape encountering clients who demonstrate the features discussed here, no matter which field they choose to practise in. Such clients frequently present the greatest challenge to the clinician's therapeutic expertise.

REFERENCES

1 Maxwell H 1978 Psychosomatic medicine, 2nd edn. Macmillan, London, ch 2

2 Hawton K, Salkovskis P M, Kirk J, Clark D M (eds) 1989 Cognitive behaviour therapy for psychiatric problems — a practical guide. Oxford University Press, Oxford

3 Graham D T, Stern J A, Winokur G 1960 The concept of a different specific set of physiological changes in each emotion. Psychiatric Research Reports 12:8–15

4 Alexander F 1950 Psychosomatic medicine. Norton, New York

5 Robbins P R 1969 Personality and psychosomatic illness: a selective review of research. Genetic Psychology Monographs 80:51–90

6 Kissen D M 1966 The value of a psychosomatic approach to cancer. Annals of the New York Academy of Sciences 125:777–779

7 Moos R H, Solomon G F 1965 Psychologic comparisons between women with rheumatoid arthritis and their non-arthritic sisters: (I) Personality test and interview rating data. Psychosomatic Medicine 27:135–149

8 Engel G L 1955 Studies in ulcerative colitis: The nature of the psychological process. American Journal of Medicine 19:231

9 Pelletier K R 1977 Mind as healer — mind as slayer. George Allen & Unwin, London

10 Beech H R, Burns L E, Sheffield B F 1982 A behavioural approach to the management of stress. John Wiley, Chichester

11 Friedman M, Rosenman R H 1974 Type A behaviour and your heart. Alfred A. Knopf, New York

12 Hart K E 1984 Anxiety management training and anger control for type A individuals. Journal of Behavioral Therapy and Experimental Psychiatry 15(2):133–139

13 Suinn R M, Bloom L J 1978 Anxiety management training for pattern A behavior. Journal of Behavioral Medicine 1:25–35

14 Roskies E, Kearney H, Spevack M, Surkis A, Cohen C, Gilman S 1979 Generalizability and durability of treatment effects in an intervention program for coronary-prone (Type A) managers. Journal of Behavioral Medicine 2:195–207

15 Selye H 1956 The stress of life. McGraw-Hill, New York

16 Selye H 1976 Stress in health and disease. Butterworth, Massachusetts

17 Kobasa S C 1982 The hardy personality: toward a social psychology of stress and health. In: Sanders G S, Suls J (eds) Social psychology of health and illness. L. Erlbaum Associates, New Jersey

18 Holmes T H, Rahe R H 1967 The social readjustment rating scale. Journal of Psychosomatic Research 11:213–218

19 Flannery R B 1987 From victim to survivor: a stress management approach in the treatment of learned helplessness. In: Van der Kolk B A Psychological trauma. American Psychiatric Press. Washington, USA

20 Seligman M E P 1975 Helplessness. Freeman, San Francisco

21 Fisher S, Reason J (eds) 1988 Handbook of life stress, cognition and health. John Wiley, Chichester

22 Sternback 1978 In: Grings WW and Dawson M E Emotions and bodily responses. Academic Press, ch 10

23 Mayou R 1992 Patients' fears of illness. In: Creed F, Mayou R, Hopkin A 1992 Medical symptoms not explained by organic disease. Mayou R 1992 Patients' fears of illness. In: The Royal College of Psychiatrists and the Royal College of Physicians of London, London

24 Lum L C 1976 The syndrome of habitual chronic hyperventilation. In: Hill O (ed) Modern trends in psychosomatic medicine. Butterworth, London, ch 11

25 Lum L C 1981 Hyperventilation and anxiety state. Journal of the Royal Society of Medicine 74:1–4

26 Tweeddale P M, Rowbottom I, McHardy G J 1994 Breathing retraining: effect on anxiety and depression scores in behavioural breathlessness. Journal of Psychosomatic Research 38(1):11–21

27 Mechanic D 1962 The concept of illness behaviour. J. Chron. Dis 15:189–194

28 Mechanic D 1986 The concept of illness behaviour: culture, situation and personal predisposition. Psychological Medicine 16:1–7

29 Mechanic D 1972 Social psychologic factors affecting the presentation of bodily complaints. The New England Journal of Medicine 286(21):1132–1139

30 Harvey R F, Salih S Y, Read A E 1983 Organic and functional disorders in 2000 gastroenterology outpatients. Lancet 1:632–634

31 Holmes K M, Salter R H, Cole R P, et al 1987 A profile of district gastroenterology. Journal of the Royal College of Physicians 21:111–114

32 Kingham J G C, Dawson A M 1985 Origins of chronic right upper quadrant pain. Gut 26:783–788

33 Sims A, Snaith P 1988 Anxiety in clinical practice. John Wiley, Chichester

34 Salkovskis P 1992 The cognitive–behavioural approach. In: Creed F, Mayou R, Hopkin A 1992 Medical symptoms not explained by organic disease. The Royal College of Psychiatrists and the Royal College of Physicians of London, London

35 Wallston K A, Wallston B S 1982 Who is responsible for your health? The construct of health locus of control. In: Sanders G S, Suls J (eds) Social psychology of health and illness. L. Erlbaum Associates, New Jersey

36 Taylor G J, Bagby R M, Parker J D A 1991 The alexithymia construct — a potential paradigm for psychosomatic medicine. Psychosomatics 32(2):153–164

37 Stuppy W P, Shipko S 1994 The dichotomy of alexithymia and panic disorder. In: International Journal of Psychosomatics (special annual issue) 41(1–4):30–33

6

Integrative and alternative models of anxiety

Diana Keable

LIFE EVENTS AND STRESS

Life events play a large part in determining stress levels and include those which are expected and unexpected. In the face of stressful events and change, the individual's capacity to employ adaptive methods of coping with stress is of crucial importance to physical and psychological health.

In 1948 Adolf Meyer first emphasised the importance of sociological life changes by the construction of a life chart. This organised medical data into the form of a dynamic biography.[1] Meyer regarded his patients as unique individuals, their illnesses being part of an idiosyncratic physical and mental response to their social situation and life events. He saw the need to understand the patient as a whole person to be a vital factor in preventing illnesses which, as a result of their total life history, each individual may be predisposed (Fig. 6.1).

Holmes and Rahe[2] correlated life events with illness onset and tested their hypothesis in a major work involving more than 5000 subjects. Their study showed that the frequency of stressful life events or changes tended to increase prior to disease onset. Thus, the more life events or changes that occur in a given period, the greater the likelihood of developing organic illness. Holmes and Rahe later postulated that these events lowered bodily resistance and that this was due to maladaptive coping attempts on the part of the individual. It was concluded that change, as opposed to aversiveness, was more stressful. Surprisingly, even ordinary changes

Year	Medical history	SEX-LIFE	THYROID	THYMUS	DIGESTION AND LIVER	RESPIRATION	REFLEXES	CEREBRUM	HEART	Life events	Age
1955	Birth – girl									First child	1
56										Learns to walk and talk	2
57	Whooping cough										3
58										Baby brother born	4
59										– reverts to thumb-sucking behaviour	5
60	Hospital admission – acute meningitis							▓			6
61										Develops school phobia	7
62											8
63										School phobia resolves	9
64											10
65											11
66											12
67	Commenced menstruation	▓									13
68		▓								First boyfriend	14
69		▓									15
70	Develops migraine headaches	▓						▓		Final exams	16
71		▓								Leaves school. First job	17
72		▓									18
73		▓								Receives promotion	19
74		▓						▓		Leaves parental home	20
75		▓						▓		Changes job	21
76	Develops appendicitis	▓			▓						22
77		▓			▓						23
78	Surgical removal	▓									24
79		▓								Marries	25
80	First pregnancy	▓									26
81	Delivered (Caesarian section)	▓								Son born	27
82		▓									28
83	Post-natal depression	▓									29
84	Depression resolves	▓								Returns to work	30

Figure 6.1 An example of a life chart based on Adolf Meyer's approach.

from a stable state qualified as being stressful. Holmes and Rahe produced a scale, 'The social readjustment rating scale', comprising 43 items. These items are mainly common events, including some that would normally be thought agreeable such as marriage or exceptional achievement. Other items include bereavement, divorce, holidays, Christmas, moving house, hire purchase loans, minor violation of law and changes in routine. All items were ranked by large numbers of subjects to arrive at the values attached to them regarding their stress content. Not surprisingly, bereavement was placed at the top of the list. Other fairly commonly occurring events also appear near the top of the hierarchy. Holmes and Rahe found that the resulting rating scale could be used to predict the onset of illness or health change.[2,3]

More recently, the direct causal link between life events and physical illness has been disputed. Murphy and Brown[4] found that the onset of organic illness was mediated by an intervening psychiatric disturbance occurring within a period of six months. Yet another study supported the theory that life events are an important factor in precipitating generalised anxiety.[5] These issues have been hotly debated over the last decade. This has resulted in a much clearer, although more complex picture than that originally proposed by Holmes and Rahe. Accordingly, the impact of life events must be considered in relation to individual circumstances and personality factors.[6] Life events must be understood in terms of their personal meaning to the individual. For example, those who either exaggerate a threat or deny anxiety unrealistically may be more prone to breakdown following stressful life events than those who admit to moderate anxiety. However, some defences against anxiety, i.e. compulsivity and counterbehaviour, can be constructive if moderate. 'Stress resistant' or 'hardy' personalities are held to cope with stressful life events more adaptively.[7,8] The components held to be associated with these personality constructs are discussed more fully in the previous chapter. Anxious clients often fail to identify sources of stress within their lifestyles, far less reduce them. The recognition that ordinary events can be highly stressful may facilitate acceptance of symptoms which some see as unjustified reactions in the absence of genuine stress. Additionally, many anxious clients consistently avoid making necessary changes because change itself is so stressful. Learning new ways of coping with change and its challenges in a more healthy and effective way is an important element of treatment. This is particularly so given that many

stressful life events cannot be avoided. It is notable that AMT programmes incorporate therapeutic material designed to reinforce such stress-resistant strategies. Again, in this way, anxiety management techniques may have a prophylactic role in enabling people to develop healthy coping mechanisms for dealing with stressful life events.

POST-TRAUMATIC STRESS DISORDER

Before leaving the subject of life events, it is necessary to consider the impact of severe trauma or overwhelming life experiences, e.g. major disasters, wars, rape and torture. This diagnostic category has become the focus of much interest in recent years, but was not introduced as a separate category of anxiety until 1980 when it first appeared in the *Diagnostic and statistical manual of mental disorders* (DSM III).[9] Post-traumatic stress disorder (PTSD) occurs in response to a major traumatic episode. This may involve devastating degrees of loss, physical harm, pain and fear, along with exposure to horrific events totally outside the individual's normal experience. The main symptoms are:

- intrusive and recurrent memories (flashbacks) and dreams of the traumatic episode
- impulsive re-enactment of situations reminiscent of the episode
- hyperreactivity, including aggressive outbursts and exaggerated startle response
- cognitive disturbances e.g. concentration
- sleep disruption
- avoidant behaviour, especially of activities reminiscent of the traumatic episode
- survivor guilt
- intermittent phases of numbed effect characterised by diminished interest and involvement in significant activities, and emotional and social detachment.

Onset may be immediate or delayed, appearing several months or even years after the trauma occurred. A state of fixation may result if the individual fails to come to terms with the trauma, resulting in profound personality changes:

- inability to utilise social support
- chronic recurrent depression
- psychosomatic symptomatology
- blocked affect / emotional numbing
- alexithymia.

The ability to control anxiety and aggression is disrupted, leading to extreme irritability which alternates with emotional withdrawal. This is compounded by feelings of helplessness, loss of control and vulnerability to further stress. There is a tendency to dissociate the trauma leading to loss of psychological integration. Affected individuals have described a feeling of being 'inhuman', with an impoverished inner life devoid of emotion, empathy and fantasy. This is frequently complicated by alcohol and drug addiction.[10]

Individuals vary in the extent to which they are vulnerable to damage by severe trauma and this is governed by a number of factors:

- the personal meaning of the trauma for the individual
- trauma severity — few can escape psychological impairment from very severe stresses such as torture
- genetic predisposition — stress resistance is partly an inherited trait
- developmental phase at which the trauma occurs — children are more vulnerable to long-term effects
- social support — can ameliorate the effects of trauma
- previous trauma experiences leave the individual more vulnerable to new traumatic episodes
- previous personality — psychologically vulnerable individuals are also less able to cope with trauma.

Treatment of PTSD involves a process of eliciting and working through the painful memories, thus enabling the individual to regain their sense of control and psychological wholeness. Resolution is achieved when the individual accepts the reality of the traumatic event and integrates it positively within the context of their current lifestyle outlook.[10,11,12,13]

SOCIOLOGICAL ASPECTS OF STRESS

Changes in society

Western societal structure has undergone great upheaval in recent times, and this has particularly affected occupational and sexual roles. Cultural conflicts have also been evident as mixed-race societies become more prevalent, concomitant with increased mobility across geographical boundaries. This has often involved different cultures in a bitter struggle to preserve their racial identities, or lose them, at great cost, in the attempt to integrate. Conflicts concerning the status of different cultures in society are all too common, tending to escalate in societies where resources are limited and some cultures may receive less than their fair share.

Roles and relationships

The stability of modern family life has become eroded with the increasing divorce rate and the attendant distress usually suffered by children from broken homes. The psychological significance of the family unit in the expression of mental illness is well known; but the supportive extended family, an important stress buffer for young couples with children as well as the elderly and their carers, is disappearing. It should be noted, however, that the picture regarding social support and stress is a complex one. It has been suggested that the presence of social support may sometimes interfere with the exercise of stress resistance or 'hardiness' in the face of stress.[7] Thus, when challenged with work-related stress, some individuals may be tempted to return to the bosom of a caring family rather than continue to tackle the problems.

Also, roles within the family are now more subtle, complex and demanding. Married women are commonly forced to attempt the triple role of home-manager, mother and breadwinner. For men, competition to secure suitable employment and pressure to adapt to new roles in the home are great.

Social stress and role conflict

The foregoing factors have contributed to a general increase in social stress. Status integration theorists propose that the level of social stress in a population is related to the stability and durability of its social relationships. Clearly, the security of family relationships is becoming increasingly threatened. In order to be both stable and durable, social relationships also depend on a significant degree of role conformity. In modern society roles are rapidly changing and are not so clearly defined as in previous times, resulting in a lack of role conformity. The terms 'mother', 'wife', 'father', 'husband', and even 'man' and 'woman', are undergoing rapid review concerning the expectations attached to these roles. Added to this, the degree of role conformity is reduced if conflicts between different roles exist, and if the status attached to these roles is incompatible. Role conflicts are now common in both sexes, caused by pressure to take on several, often incompatible, roles at once. This leads to a state of ambivalence and pressure to choose between the requirements of different roles. For example, the working mother is often torn by the conflicting demands of picking her children up from school or staying later at work to sort out a crisis which has arisen. Which is most important? Clearly, an agonising choice presented daily to many women, giving rise to a great deal of stress and often guilt.

In summary, sufficient levels of status-integration and role conformity are thought to be crucial in the maintenance of societal equilibrium.[14] The prevalence of these stabilising factors within our society is now lower than ever before. It is hardly surprising, therefore, that high levels of social stress are apparent.

Society and self

On a more individual level, threats to self-esteem are a crucial factor in bringing about social distress. This may include circumstances where expectations of self or society fail to be met. Self-esteem is derived from socialisation with significant others, including peers, during development. When a discrepancy between the real self and the ideal self is perceived, great anxiety is caused. This increases as the growing child becomes aware of societal and parental values and norms, measures himself against them, and finds himself wanting.[15]

Social anxiety is a common phenomenon, held to be a consequence of feelings of insecurity and sensitivity to the remarks of others.[11] In some cases this is a pervasive theme affecting many aspects of the individual's lifestyle; in others, it focuses on specific types of interaction, e.g. speaking/eating in public. Fear of negative evaluation by others is a central theme. One recent study[16] found that highly socially anxious subjects have a greater tendency to perceive negative implications in the emotional expressions of others (i.e. facial and auditory).

Sensory deprivation and social isolation are also responsible for creating anxiety in many individuals. These factors are increasingly prevalent, compounded by the breakdown of the family unit in modern western society, leading to great numbers of individuals living alone in industrial cities, or in institutions. For example, many disadvantaged groups live in institutions where they are starved of the ordinary intimate human contact and communication normally shared in families. Sensory deprivation is inevitable unless positive steps are taken to ameliorate this lack of stimulation in institutions and in the community. Elderly and psychologically vulnerable people are particularly prone to such stress, and much clinical work with these groups is aimed at resocialisation, and increasing cognitive and sensory stimulation.[17]

Occupational factors

Much has been said and written concerning the work-related stresses of our time. These may relate to the mind-numbing effects of repetitive work or to the daunting challenges borne by those who work long hours in highly responsible positions. The complex issues concerning work-related stress and, more importantly, how to cope with it, are discussed further in Chapter 20.

In a society where time pressures and their attendant stressful qualities are paramount, recreational outlets have also changed dramatically and many are now more pressurised in nature. Relaxing, restorative pursuits such as craft-work, walking or reading are replaced by competitive sports, or on the other extreme, by passive television viewing. The need for relaxation training on a wide scale is beginning to emerge as society develops in this vein.

A knowledge of how sociological factors relate to the stresses of modern living is useful to the clinician. This is particularly so in AMT which attempts to teach clients effective ways of coping with social anxiety. Many of the factors described above as triggers of social stress can be observed at work in the anxious client. Role conflicts, lack of self-esteem, inadequate social skills and social isolation are typical features of anxiety disorders.

ANXIETY, EXISTENTIALISM, AND THE HUMANISTIC SCHOOL OF THOUGHT

Existential theories are concerned with the question of the meaning of anxiety for human life. In Kierkegaard's view, man is anxious in the face of his finite freedom.[18] He is forced to choose between a set of limited alternatives without having the advantage of knowing the attendant consequences beforehand. Further, he knows that he will be held responsible for the choice he makes by those around him. Thus, man is anxious about the meaning of his life and about making choices that will ensure meaningfulness for his life. Failure to achieve this results in anxiety and despair.

Laing is a well-known exponent of existentialism, having rejected traditional psychiatric theory based on the medical model.[19] He emphasised the importance of having a strong sense of one's true self. We lose the sense of our real identity through the use of defence mechanisms, such as distortion and denial, in order to secure protection from emotional trauma. In this way, we cease to know ourselves as we really are, and as a result, we become alienated from ourselves and others.

Similarly, the humanistic approach involves a number of different but related perspectives which emphasise the personal experience and development of the individual. For example, Rollo May stated that neurotic anxiety develops when an individual is unable to deal with normal anxiety at a time of crisis in his growth as a person.[20] Anxiety results when a threat to personal values occurs. May posits that anxiety is necessary to develop personal values into mature ones which transcend the immediate situation. Mature values are those which involve the past and future, the immediate group, the community and, ultimately, humanity as a whole.

A central issue in the humanistic approach is that of personal motivation to achieve one's full potential as a person, or self-actualisation. Maslow developed a hierarchy of needs comprising deficiency motives and growth motives.[21] He stated that it is only when basic needs such as warmth, food, safety and self-esteem have been met that the individual is able to attend to higher motives and seek self-actualisation. Rogers, on the other hand, believes that we are all motivated towards self-actualisation and personal enhancement.[22] Anxiety occurs when we are diverted from this goal because we lack a favourable nurturing environment in which to grow and develop. The quest for the true self becomes disrupted and the real person is obscured by neurotic behaviour and the use of psychological defence strategies. Rogers' work in developing the client-centred counselling approach is well known and the techniques are widely used in modern psychological therapy.

Cracknell has described the background of the humanistic and existential theories in greater detail for therapists involved in the short-term psychiatric setting.[23]

KELLY'S PERSONAL CONSTRUCT THEORY

According to Kelly's theory of personal constructs, man knows the world by the constructions he places upon it and is bound by these possibilities for understanding events within his world.[24] Thus, man builds a representational model of the world in order to make sense of it, and to enable him to plan his behaviour in relation to it. This model is termed 'the construct system'. The constructs are also used to enable the individual to predict future events. The following are examples of constructs:

- friendly–aloof
- respect–despise
- fear–frighten.

These constructs comprise a negative and a positive dimension, but cannot merely be described as concepts. Each individual has his own set of constructs and deploys these to give meaning to his world and to prepare for change. According to Kelly, psychological suffering is the result of having rigid and inappropriate constructs about the world which preclude personal growth. For instance, an anxious person may be unable to relax because they construe this as laziness and indulgence. Thus they feel duty-bound to engage in continual activity and striving in order to avoid guilt. Such a person is trapped in a negative cycle, repeatedly testing out the same inappropriate and unhelpful construct system. Kelly's ideas resonate somewhat with those of Ellis[25] who described 'irrational belief' systems associated with neurosis.

Kelly used the psychotherapeutic relationship as a partnership in which therapist and client are engaged in exploring and scientifically testing out the client's constructs and trying to reconstrue them in a more appropriate and workable manner. Kelly defined various emotions such as anxiety, threat, fear, aggression and hostility. He described anxiety as a sense of awareness that one's constructs are inadequate to deal with change. Kelly also made useful contributions at the clinical level. In particular, he designed grids to enable clinicians to test attitudinal patterns in psychological diagnosis and research.

CONCLUSION

While some of the foregoing theories have only the loosest relationship to the teaching of anxiety management, the reminder that individuals are concerned with wider issues is a welcome one to the therapist. The therapist considers the anxious client as a whole person. As such, he is not seen as a creature composed merely of physiological–subjective responses. That he is concerned with others, has complex value systems, spiritual beliefs, intellectual and creative concerns as well as an individualised set of perceptions about the world must be acknowledged and understood. In order to be maximally effective, therapeutic approaches must take the whole person into account — in anxiety, as in all other aspects of psychological suffering.

REFERENCES

1 Lief A (ed) 1948 The commonsense psychiatry of Dr. Adolf Meyer. McGraw-Hill, New York
2 Holmes T H, Rahe R H 1967 The social readjustment rating scale. Journal of Psychosomatic Research 11:213–218
3 Morse D R, Lawrence-Furst M 1979 Stress for success. Van Nostrand Reinhold, USA
4 Murphy E, Brown G W 1980 Life events, psychiatric disturbance and physical illness. British Journal of Psychiatry 136:326–338
5 Blazer D, Hughes D, George L K 1987 Stressful life events and the onset of a generalized anxiety syndrome. American Journal of Psychiatry 144(9):1178–1183
6 Fisher S, Reason J (eds) 1988 Handbook of life stress, cognition and health. John Wiley, Chichester
7 Kobasa S C 1982 The hardy personality: toward a social psychology of stress and health. In: Sanders G S, Suls J

(eds) Social psychology of health and illness. L. Erlbaum Associates, New Jersey
8 Flannery R B 1987 From victim to survivor: a stress management approach in the treatment of learned helplessness. In: Van der Kolk B A Psychological trauma. American Psychiatric Press, Washington, USA
9 American Psychiatric Association 1980 Diagnostic and statistical manual of mental disorders (DSM III), 3rd edn. Washington, USA
10 Van der Kolk B A 1987 Psychological trauma. American Psychiatric Press, Washington, USA
11 Sims A, Snaith P 1988 Anxiety in clinical practice. John Wiley, Chichester
12 Foy D W, Donahoe C P, Carroll E M, Gallers J, Reno R 1987 Post-traumatic stress disorder. In: Ascher L M (ed) Anxiety and stress disorders — congnitive–behavioural assessment and treatment. Guilford Press, New York

13 Roberts G W 1995 Trauma following major disasters: the role of the occupational therapist. British Journal of Occupational Therapy 58(5):204–208

14 Fischer W F 1970 Theories of anxiety. Harper and Row, New York

15 Dobson C B 1982 Stress and the self-concept. In: The hidden adversary. MTP Press, UK, ch 3

16 Winton E C, Clark D M, Edelmann R J 1995 Social anxiety, fear of negative evaluation and the detection of negative emotion in others. Behaviour Research and Therapy 33(2):193–196

17 Orford J 1976 The social psychology of mental disorder. Penguin Books, Middlesex

18 Kierkegaard S 1941 The sickness unto death. Princeton University Press, USA

19 Laing R 1982 The voice of experience. Penguin, Middlesex

20 May R 1977 The meaning of anxiety, revised edn. Norton, New York

21 Maslow A H 1954 Motivation and personality. Harper and Row, New York

22 Rogers C R 1951 Client-centred therapy. Riverside Press, Massachusetts

23 Cracknell E 1984 Humanistic psychology. In: Wilson M (ed) Occupational therapy in short-term psychiatry. Churchill Livingstone, Edinburgh, ch 4

24 Kelly G A 1955 The psychology of personal constructs. Vol 1: A theory of personality. Norton, New York

25 Ellis A Reason and emotion in psychotherapy. Lyle Stewart, New York

SUMMARY OF PART 1

Considerable ground has been covered in order to provide an eclectic overview of the vast array of relevant theoretical approaches to anxiety. A complex picture has emerged in which behavioural, cognitive, physiological, social and psychodynamic issues contribute to a comprehensive knowledge of anxiety.

However, it is far from clear how they can be linked in a coherent manner. To what extent are the different theories discrete and incompatible entities? To what extent do they possess the potential to integrate meaningfully, or at least to coexist with some measure of comfort? These questions confront the enquirer with an awesome, if not impossible task.

To the extent that anxiety is a multifaceted syndrome involving many different variables, an eclectic study of its nature has the potential to be enlightening. Further, the treatment regimes focused upon in this book, i.e. methods related to anxiety management, involve a recognition of the wider picture of anxiety within their construction. This is unlike the purely physiological approach which attempts to ameliorate anxiety symptoms with drug treatment alone; or the psychodynamic approach which ignores the physiological components of anxiety. The AMT-related approaches to anxiety have attempted to encompass many of the different tenets outlined here. In the opinion of the writer this has served to great advantage in the clinical treatment of anxiety. This view is supported by much recent research, as will be seen in the next chapter.

Treatment techniques

Part two of this book aims to present a range of techniques commonly used in the treatment of anxiety. For ease of reference, the techniques have been divided according to the systems and, or, skills, which they primarily target, i.e. physical, mental, integrated and active relaxation techniques. This separation does not imply that a physical technique does not also induce mental relaxation or vice versa. An outline for a group-based anxiety management course is also included.

7

The relaxation phenomenon

Diana Keable

THE DUAL NATURE OF RELAXATION

Although there are many different routes to relaxation, the ultimate effect is similar. Some techniques, like the meditative, hypnotic and cognitive methods, rely primarily on the mental dimension to achieve relaxation. Others, based on muscle relaxation and conditioning processes rely more on physiological function to bring about the relaxed state. However, it will be seen that each relaxation technique depends in some degree on both bodily and mental parameters. This is consistent with the understanding that the anxiety state comprises both mental and biological symptoms. Thus, all relaxation techniques, whatever their procedural emphasis, must incorporate both aspects.

Relaxation is a difficult concept to describe. It is not merely an absence of anxiety or mental and physical arousal. Some of its possible effects are listed below.

Mental relaxation:

- passive attitude to worries or distracting thoughts
- enhanced ability to focus attention on one object, word or thought
- increased mental discipline
- enhanced awareness of mental and physical internal processes
- accelerated alpha brain waves (slow frequencies associated with the relaxed state)
- agreeable feelings of well-being and peacefulness.

Physical relaxation:

- reduced breathing and gaseous exchange rates
- reduced heart rate, blood pressure and volume
- reduced output of sweat and blood flow to skeletal muscles
- reduced blood cholesterol and lactate levels
- reduced electrical activity in the muscles and skin
- reduced muscle tension
- reduced beta brain waves (rapid frequencies associated with arousal)
- increased digestive efficiency
- increased immune system efficiency.

Wilson gave the following apt description of the elusive concept of relaxation: 'relaxation is not so much the opposite of activity as its complementary state'.[1] Relaxation, therefore, is not simply a negative condition, but a meaningful and recuperative experience. The continuum and harmony between the mind and body is nowhere demonstrated more strikingly than in the phenomenon of relaxation. The ability to induce the relaxed state at will is therefore a powerful tool in combating the deleterious effects of stress.[2]

As far as the theories proposed to explain the relaxation phenomenon are concerned, again, there is no clear consensus. Lichstein[3], in his extensive review of relaxation techniques, gave the following summation:

No single theory of relaxation reigns superior. Indeed an adequate theory of relaxation could not be constructed without summoning most of the views reported herein. Each captures a unique, indispensable facet of this multivariate phenomenon, and the entire relaxation enterprise threatened when any one element is wanting.

RELAXATION TECHNIQUES COVERED IN THIS BOOK

The purpose of the next three chapters is to introduce a range of different relaxation techniques, many of which may be adapted for use as components of an anxiety management programme. It is not intended to be an exhaustive list — such an undertaking would be of prohibitive length

and of doubtful value. Various styles of anxiety management will also be described. In each case an attempt will be made to show the theoretical bases upon which the techniques have been founded, and to comment on their clinical application. The techniques covered in this book are organised under the following headings:

1. *Physical and mental techniques* — discussed in Chapters 8 and 9.

a. The physiological approach:

- progressive relaxation
- biofeedback
- simple relaxation
- differential relaxation

b. The meditative approach:

- the relaxation response

c. The hypnotic approach:

- autogenic training
- visualisation.

2. *Integrated programmes* — discussed in Chapter 10.

a. Cue-controlled relaxation
b. Systematic desensitisation
c. Anxiety/stress management.

TREATMENT TECHNIQUE SELECTION AND EFFECTIVENESS

There is still no consensus regarding the relative effectiveness of one technique over another. However, combined programmes, such as those based on the cognitive behaviour therapy model are generally more effective than relaxation training alone.[3,4] Considerable evidence exists to support the 'specific effects' model[5] which places the responsibility onto the therapist to select the critical components to suit each individual's needs. For example, where the symptomatology is mainly of physiological origins, then the programme should emphasise physiological techniques such as biofeedback and muscle-relaxation training. Similarly, where cognitive features are foremost, the treatment programme should emphasise cognitive restructuring. Combined programmes are at their most effective when the components are harmonious. One exception that has been identified is combined hypnosis and biofeedback, which appears to have a weaker effect than either component used singly. The mechanism by which different combinations of techniques facilitate, or militate against, treatment effectiveness remains unclear.[3,4]

MODELS OF RELAXATION PROCESS AND OUTCOME

Finally, it should be pointed out that competing theories have been advanced in the attempt to explain how relaxation training works. The benefit of the 'specific effects' model[5] has been disputed in favour of the 'relaxation response' model.[6] However, it is argued that all the relaxation techniques involve certain critical components in common and these produce the same characteristic 'relaxation response'.

It has also been contended that the specific effects of different techniques are built upon a general relaxation response.[7] Building on this, a new 'hierarchical' model has been put forward by Smith.[8] This theory posits that the state of relaxation involves a continuum of skills of increasing difficulty and complexity. Thus, the skill of muscle relaxation appears at the bottom of the hierarchy, requiring the least challenge to acquire. The next steps involve acquiring cognitive skills, as well as skills in the use of more self-directed and unstructured procedures, and so on. The most difficult level is held to involve a state of complete passivity, without the use of a focal device such as a mantra.

REFERENCES

1 Wilson M 1983 Occupational therapy in long-term psychiatry. Churchill Livingstone, Edinburgh
2 McCormack G L 1992 The therapeutic benefits of the relaxation response. Occupational Therapy Practice 4(1):51–60
3 Lichstein K L 1988 Clinical relaxation strategies. John Wiley, New York
4 Lehrer P M, Woolfolk R L 1993 Specific effects of stress management techniques. In: Principles and practice of stress management, 2nd edn. The Guilford Press, New York
5 Davidson R J, Schwartz G E 1976 The psychobiology of relaxation and related states: a multiprocess theory. In:

Mostofsky D I (ed) Behaviour control and modification of physiological activity. Prentice-Hall, Englewood Cliffs, New Jersey
6 Benson H 1983 The relaxation response and norepinephrine: a new study illuminates mechanisms. Integrative Psychiatry I:15–18
7 Schwartz G E, Davidson R J, Goleman D T 1978 Patterning of cognitive and somatic processes in the self-regulation of anxiety: effects of meditation versus exercise. Psychosomatic Medicine 40:321–328
8 Smith J C 1988 Steps toward a cognitive–behavioral model of relaxation. Biofeedback and Self-regulation 13:307–329

8

Physiological relaxation techniques

Diana Keable

PROGRESSIVE RELAXATION TRAINING

Background and methodology

This approach, proposed by Jacobsen in the 1930s is probably the most well-known technique, and was the forerunner of many other modern relaxation training methods.[1] The technique hinges on the development of advanced muscular skills aimed at recognising and releasing minute amounts of tension. Through progressive relaxation an exceptionally deep level of muscle relaxation can be achieved. A long training period is required, and daily practice sessions lasting 1–2 hours are recommended. Different types of muscle work, e.g. movements involving flexion and extension, are practised over all muscle groups.

Jacobsen proposed that a powerful feedback loop exists linking the skeletal muscles and the brain. As a result of his early experiments, Jacobsen was able to show that when a subject's muscles were relaxed, they reported subjective feelings of calm. In anxious subjects, however, levels of muscle tension were invariably high and correlated with subjective feelings of tension. Thus, he argued that if a subject could be trained to relax their skeletal muscles, subjective tension and anxiety would diminish simultaneously. In other words, if the mind has the power to affect the state of muscles, then, equally, the muscles can affect the state of mind.

Jacobsen's progressive relaxation has, perhaps unfortunately, been widely confused with contrast relaxation'. This technique was evolved from Jacobsen's original method by Wolpe in 1958 for use as a component of his 'systematic desensitisation' procedure for the treatment of specific phobias.[2] Contrast relaxation involves exaggerated 'tense–release' exercises and is probably the most widely used relaxation technique in clinical and educational settings. Although this technique is quick and convenient for use in many situations, it is a comparatively crude approach. The tense–release exercises are held to provide a kind of platform from which to make the 'leap' into relaxation.[3] The author has so far failed to collect sufficiently convincing evidence to confirm the truth of this notion in practice. Instead, clinical observation has often indicated that the opposite case is true. This has shown that prior tensing may only serve to reinforce existing tension, and that rather than providing a platform for relaxation, the manufactured tension may be difficult to release in itself. In such cases, the original tension has only been increased by the treatment intervention! One recent study[4] also supports the view that tensing muscle groups prior to relaxation is physiologically detrimental to the relaxation process. Interestingly, this was also Jacobsen's position on the matter. Not surprisingly, several studies suggest that contrast relaxation is less effective than true progressive relaxation.[5]

Clinical usage

True progressive relaxation is almost certainly far too lengthy and complex a technique to be appropriate for use within most general clinical settings. While it is an admirably thorough training regime, more immediate and flexible methods are usually preferable in this context. Contrast relaxation has been adopted very widely for this reason, although, as has been stated, its effectiveness is in some doubt. However, contrast relaxation may be useful in the initial stages of an anxiety management programme to facilitate perception of muscle tension and the feelings associated with it. The importance of attaining this recognition cannot be overstated; contrast relaxation is uniquely structured to facili-

tate its achievement. For these reasons, a set of instructions for contrast relaxation is given in the client packs which can be found in the Appendix (see Client Pack 1 Supplement).

BIOFEEDBACK
Background and methodology

Many authors have contributed to the body of knowledge relating to the use of biofeedback in relaxation training over the last two decades. Miller, in 1969, was one of the first proponents of biofeedback.[6] This technique relies on the use of various kinds of equipment which provide the individual with continuous biological information about his internal processes. Such information may be communicated in a variety of immediate ways via bleeping sounds, flashing lights, oscilloscope or meter readings. The equipment may be used to monitor various modalities associated with arousal levels, e.g. heart rate, galvanic skin conductance/resistance, brain-wave activity, gut motility, blood pressure, skin temperature and voluntary muscle tension in selected sites.

Using biofeedback it has been demonstrated that individuals can learn to control autonomic responses as well as voluntary muscle activity. Biofeedback is thought to work by providing information about internal processes which does not otherwise reach consciousness. Using this information, the individual learns to develop control over these processes through operant conditioning. The exact mechanism by which biofeedback enables individuals to affect their own visceral or autonomic activity is still not yet clear. For instance, are the changes brought about by cognitive manipulation or by purposeful skeletal muscle changes which indirectly affect the autonomic modality under study? In other words, the simple act of thinking peaceful thoughts may be enough to reduce the heart rate. Credidio[7] and Goldberg[8], and others[9,10] have argued that while an individual can learn to reduce arousal in the specific site or system selected for biofeedback, this arousal reduction does not necessarily generalise over the body as a whole. Disappointing treatment outcomes have therefore led to some scepticism about the effectiveness of biofeedback.[9,10,11]

Clinical usage

Biofeedback has several disadvantages in the clinical situation. Firstly, accurate and reliable equipment is generally costly and large, rendering it inconvenient for use within the group situation. Although some cheap and portable equipment is available, e.g. GSR and skin temperature monitors, they are unlikely to be accurate enough for assessment or research purposes. Secondly, individuals differ according to which physiological systems react most to stress. For example, a skin temperature measure might be a good index of arousal level in one person, but in another heart rate is the best indicator. In group situations it is rarely possible to assess the psychophysiological reaction profile of each individual and then provide the appropriate piece of equipment for each client! Thirdly, it has been argued that, ultimately, ordinary relaxation training is more effective in reducing arousal than biofeedback.[11] In spite of these drawbacks, biofeedback can be a powerful teaching tool when used as part of an anxiety management programme. In the author's opinion its most effective application lies in its value as a demonstration and teaching aid. Hamilton[12] has described ways in which biofeedback has been used in occupational therapy to treat a variety of problems that involve elements of anxiety. However, the sophistication of biofeedback should not beguile the clinician into believing that it is necessarily superior to more simple methods of relaxation training. An alternative approach, which may be termed 'human biofeedback', is an excellent teaching procedure for learning how to recognise and relax muscle tension.[13] Instructions for 'human biofeedback' are given in Chapter 12.

SIMPLE (PHYSIOLOGICAL) RELAXATION

Background and methodology

Designed by Mitchell[14], a physiotherapist, this technique involves precise movements of the agonist muscle groups rather than the opposing antagonist muscle groups. It is the antagonist groups, usually the strong flexors, which are responsible for moving the body into the typical postures associated with anxiety. Some examples include: raised shoulders, frowning facial expression, crossed legs and arms, clenched fists. The Mitchell method is based on the principles of reciprocal inhibition relating to voluntary (skeletal) muscles. Accordingly, when the agonist muscle group moves the body part into the relaxed position, the antagonist group *must* relax or the movement cannot take place. When one muscle group moves, its opposer 'switches off' in order to accommodate the change of position.

The technique also comprises the following elements:

- natural breathing movements, slow and low in the chest
- mental registering of the new positions of 'ease' produced by the agonist muscle movements
- individual choice of cognitive activities, which may involve a sequence such as a poem or prayer; unpleasant thoughts or worries to be consciously ignored.

Unlike the commonly used contrast relaxation, Mitchell's technique does not involve tensing exercises since she does not accept that muscle tension can be consciously perceived. Instead, she stresses the role of the proprioceptors and skin pressure receptors which have pathways reaching beyond the subcortex to the higher brain, unlike muscle tension receptors. Thus, the activity of proprioceptive and skin pressure receptor organs are exploited in her technique to help train the individual to recognise the relaxed position. This is achieved by encouraging the individual to focus attention upon the changes of position.

Clinical usage

Mitchell's technique offers a refreshing alternative to the more well-established approaches to physiological relaxation. It is quick and simple to learn and teach in the clinical situation. The method also lends itself readily to differential application in daily living situations. This is enhanced by the learning of 'key' positions or movements which can be used to initiate generalised relaxation during activity.

As a physiological approach to relaxation, Mitchell's technique appears promising but does not appear to have been subjected to any controlled trials of its effectiveness. One study[15] confirmed its effectiveness in treating muscle tension in women with rheumatoid arthritis, but further studies are required to support these findings. However, a similar alternative — 'stretch-based' relaxation training[16] — has recently been described in the literature, and outcome studies have shown promising results. As with other physiological methods, the technique cannot be relied upon to deal adequately with the cognitive symptoms and emotional distress associated with anxiety disorders. However, this technique has a useful role in relaxation training and, as part of an AMT programme, in tackling the physiological aspects of anxiety. Among the physiological approaches, it is the author's technique of choice.

The technique does not require dimmed lighting or softly spoken instructions from the therapist, and the technique can be practised virtually anywhere that is sufficiently warm and comfortable. The instructions for simple relaxation are given in Client Pack 2 (Supplement) which can be found in the Appendix. Three positions are suggested for training, and these are described in the clinical guidelines section of Chapter 14.

DIFFERENTIAL RELAXATION
Background and methodology

Differential relaxation is the term employed to denote the application of relaxation skills to activities of daily living, particularly those which are stress-inducing. It is insufficient to learn how to relax when lying down in a quiet, secluded and dimly lit environment. The ultimate objective of relaxation training is to extend skill learning beyond the training situation, so that it can be used to help the individual control tension while carrying out daily activities. For example, many anxious clients experience high levels of tension while shopping, using public transport, in social situations, or at work.[13]

Mitchell[14] Jacobsen[17] and Alexander[18] have all described differential applications relating to their techniques. Jacobsen emphasised the need to distinguish between 'primary tension' levels — i.e. tension required to perform an act — and secondary tension — i.e. tension which is excessive and superfluous for the task in hand. Jacobsen's technique, which he called 'self operations control', involves training the individual to learn to relax non-essential muscles during activity, and to reduce the level of tension in working muscles to the degree actually required to perform the task. The renowned Alexander technique describes the 'use' and 'misuse' of the body while carrying out an action or posture. Misuse results from inappropriate learning of excess tension habits. Training is lengthy and concentrates largely on correcting posture and body alignment during simple actions like sitting and standing. Musicians, actors and athletes have been among those to use the Alexander technique to enhance their performance. Mitchell has also emphasised the need to apply her technique to daily living situations such as driving and using the telephone. She suggests the development of personal 'key' postures and movements to initiate relaxation discreetly in stressful situations.

Clinical usage

Differential relaxation training progresses from passive states, such as lying/sitting in non-stressful environments, to standing, walking and carrying out activities under busy, stressful conditions. Guidelines on the application of differential relaxation appear in Chapter 12.

REFERENCES

1 Jacobsen E 1938 Progressive relaxation, 2nd edn. University Press, Chicago

2 Wolpe J 1958 Psychotherapy by reciprocal inhibition. Stanford University Press, Stanford

3 Bernstein D A, Borkovec D 1973 Progressive relaxation — a manual for helping professionals. Research Press, Illinois

4 Lucic K S 1991 Progressive relaxation training: muscle contractions before relaxation? Behavior Therapy 22:249–256

5 Lehrer P M 1982 How to relax and how not to relax: a re-evaluation of the work of Edmund Jacobsen. Behaviour Research and Therapy 120:417–428

6 Miller N E 1969 Learning of visceral and glandular responses. Science 163:434–445

7 Credidio S G 1980 Stress management with a psychophysiological profile, biofeedback and relaxation training techniques. American Journal of Clinical Biofeedback 2:130–136

8 Goldberg R J 1982 Anxiety reduction by self-regulation: theory, practice and evaluation. Annals of Internal Medicine 96, pp 483–487

9 Lehrer P M, Woolfolk R L 1993 Specific effects of stress management techniques. In: Lehrer P M, Woolfolk R L (eds) Principles and practice of stress management, 2nd edn. The Guilford Press, New York

10 Hawton K, Salkovskis P M, Kirk J, Clark D M (eds) 1989 Cognitive behaviour therapy for psychiatric problems — a practical guide. Oxford University Press, Oxford

11 Silver B V, Blanchard E B 1978 Biofeedback and relaxation training in the treatment of psychophysiological disorders: or are the machines really necessary? Journal of Behavioral Medicine 1(2):217–239

12 Hamilton A M 1983 Electromyography: potential use in occupational therapy. British Journal of Occupational Therapy 146(11):316–318

13 Marquis J N, Ferguson J M, Barr Taylor C 1980 Generalization of relaxation skills. Journal of Behaviour Therapy and Experimental Psychiatry 11:95–99

14 Mitchell L 1977 Simple relaxation. John Murray, London

15 Jackson T 1991 An evaluation of the Mitchell method of simple physiological relaxation for women with rheumatoid arthritis. British Journal of Occupational Therapy 54(3):105–107

16 Carlson C R, Curran S L 1994 Stretch-based relaxation training (review). Patient Education and Counselling 23(1):5–12

17 Jacobsen E 1964 Anxiety and tension control. J.B. Lippincott, Philadelphia

18 Gelb M 1981 Body learning (manual on Alexander technique). Aurum Press, London

9

Mental relaxation techniques

THE RELAXATION RESPONSE
Background and methodology

Meditation is a widely recognised activity but our concern in this context is purely its relevance to relaxation. Some relaxation techniques, based on the meditative approach, have been specifically designed for use in the clinical setting. Benson's regime, the 'relaxation response', is probably the most well known and widely used example.[1] Benson evolved his technique from the study of a variety of ancient religious practices and modern research on stress physiology. He noted that certain factors common to such activities as prayer and meditation produced a phenomenon which he termed the 'relaxation response'. In his experiments with transcendental meditators, he consistently recorded reductions in physiological arousal e.g. oxygen metabolism, heart rate, blood pressure and muscle tension. Based on these studies, he developed a simple technique with which he achieved similar results in non-meditators.

The technique involves four main elements:

- sitting in a quiet, comfortable environment
- preliminary muscle relaxation with closed eyes, cultivating an easy, natural breathing rhythm
- a passive attitude to mental distractions or worries
- using a neutral focal device to engage the attention, usually the silent repetition of a word such as 'one'.

Practice sessions should be carried out twice daily for 10–20 minutes.

Clinical usage

Benson's technique is comparatively easy and convenient to learn and teach in the clinical situation. Once learned, the technique can be applied to a variety of everyday situations, e.g. travelling on public transport. However, there are two main disadvantages in using the technique with severely anxious clients. Firstly, clients with acute symptoms of anxiety are likely to find difficulty in adopting a passive attitude. Secondly, such clients may also be unable to concentrate on the focal device, finding themselves overwhelmed by distracting cognitive activity during relaxation practice. Clearly, the autonomous use of a focal device and the adoption of a passive attitude are essential components of the technique. Because of this, clients should be selected carefully for training in this method. Alternatively, the technique may be more useful in the later stages of an anxiety management course, once some basic relaxation skills have already been mastered. However, a great advantage of this method is that client dependence on the therapist is avoided from the start because practice is client-controlled throughout.

HYPNOSIS AND AUTOGENIC TRAINING

Background and methodology

Hypnosis is becoming an increasingly established practice within medical and psychiatric settings; perhaps one of the best-known users of hypnotic techniques was Sigmund Freud, himself. However, it has had a rather unfortunate history in the popular world of entertainment. This, coupled with a certain aura of mystique which has surrounded the practice of hypnosis, has engendered a general feeling of suspicion towards it. Nevertheless, it is reassuring to note that hypnosis cannot make people do anything they do not want to do — the cooperation of the subject is essential.

In the clinical setting, hypnotic techniques may be used in a number of ways, e.g. psychoanalysis, facilitation of behavioural/attitudinal change, relaxation induction and to treat psychosomatic conditions.[2] The method considered here, 'autogenic training', was evolved in the 1920s by Schultz and Luthe from hypnotic techniques used in the medical setting.[3] Although clinically standardised hypnotic induction methods are available, autogenic training provides a self-help alternative. After a period of training this can be used independently by the client. Only the first six basic exercises are described here; these are aimed at achieving generalised relaxation. More advanced stages involve visualisation, fantasy and problem-orientated suggestion, ultimately focusing upon deep psychic conflict and trauma. Consequently, specialised training should be sought in order to practise the technique; this is especially important in view of the fact that the advanced stages of the technique are essentially a psychoanalytical procedure. Contact addresses for further information about courses can be found at the end of Chapter 14. The use of autogenic training with clients suffering from psychosis is inadvisable.[4]

The process by which techniques based on hypnosis achieve their effects are not clearly understood. However, the element of suggestion is thought to be the key factor.

Clinical usage

Given the proper training of carefully selected clients, autogenic training may be one of the more powerful ways of inducing relaxation. There are, however, certain disadvantages. Firstly, it is not suitable for more disturbed clients, e.g. those suffering from any form of psychosis. Secondly, as specialised training is required, the technique is less accessible for many therapists. Thirdly, careful selection of clients is also important due to the high levels of cognitive discipline required. Clearly this technique is best presented in the later stages of treatment, when acute anxiety has abated and the client has already achieved some skill in the more basic relaxation techniques.

Autogenic training — first stage instructions

The basic autogenic training exercises utilise suggestive phrases in order to induce the relaxed state or trance:

- 'I am at peace'
- 'my right arm is heavy'
- 'my right arm is warm'
- 'my solar plexus is warm'
- 'my pulse is calm and strong'
- 'my breath is calm and even'
- 'my forehead is pleasantly cool'.

Note that the heaviness and warmth exercises move on from the right arm to the left, and from thence to the right and left legs in turn. A few minutes is spent contemplating each phrase. Two fairly short practice sessions daily are recommended. A passive or spectator-like attitude towards anxious thoughts or worries is cultivated during practice. The client is encouraged to regard such cognitive distractions as a beneficial process by which the mind discharges anxiety.[4]

VISUALISATION

Background and methodology

Alternative techniques utilising the mechanism of suggestion and imagery include visualisation and guided fantasy. The use of visualisation is becoming increasingly widespread in psychological and general medicine, orthodox and otherwise, e.g. holistic cancer regimes and pain management. It is an infinitely flexible and, reputedly, powerful technique which can be applied creatively to meet the needs of a particular individual or group. Payne[5] described imagery as: 'thinking in pictures as opposed to thinking with words'. She points out that many of our greatest thinkers — e.g., Aristotle, Einstein

and Jung — considered imagery a key component of creative thought processes and a vital link with the unconscious. Visualisation is held to be associated with activity in the right cerebral hemisphere, but exactly how the process works in treatment applications is unknown.[5]

Clinical usage

The careful application of visualisation is particularly useful in the context of an anxiety management training programme. Visualisation may be a valuable tool in helping clients to gain independent control over their symptoms. A wide variety of techniques exist, in which visualisation is used to assist in the achievement of specific goals[5,6,7] or to promote general relaxation and self-awareness.[5,8] For example, visualisation can be used to rehearse feared situations imaginally, thus bringing about a degree of desensitisation prior to exposure. It may also be used to assist in deepening relaxation in a variety of ways, e.g. to imagine the muscles softening and lengthening as they relax.

As with any technique which involves fantasy, visualisation should not be used with psychotic clients. In psychosis, the ability to distinguish reality from fantasy is impaired. Visualisation involves elements of suggestion and fantasy which may exacerbate psychotic symptoms.

Care should also be taken not to encourage dependence on the therapist through the use of such techniques. Therapist-led guided fantasy is usually more suitable for experiential and drama-related activities than for relaxation training. After all, the ultimate aim is to encourage clients to gain independent control of their anxiety symptoms.

Refer to the supplement sections of Client Packs 4 and 5 for examples of how visualisation can be used in anxiety management.

REFERENCES

1 Benson H 1976 The relaxation response. Collins, London
2 Barber X T 1993 Hypnosuggestive approaches to stress reduction: data, theory, and clinical applications. In: Lehrer P M, Woolfolk R L (eds) Principles and practice of

stress management, 2nd edn. The Guilford Press, New York
3 Schultz J M, Luthe W 1969 Autogenic therapy. Vol. 1 Autogenic methods. Grune & Stratton, New York

4 Rosa K R 1976 Autogenic training. Victor Gollancz, London

5 Payne R A 1995 Relaxation techniques — a practical handbook for the health care professional. Churchill Livingstone, Edinburgh

6 Fanning P 1988 Visualization for change. New Harbinger, Oakland, California

7 Shone R 1984 Creative visualization. Thorsons, Wellingborough, Northamptonshire

8 Achterberg J 1985 Imagery in healing: shamanism and modern medicine. New Science Library, Boston

10

Integrated programmes of anxiety management

Diana Keable

CUE-CONTROLLED RELAXATION
Background and methodology

Cue-controlled relaxation involves two main components:

- muscle relaxation (usually contrast relaxation)
- a cue word stimulus, such as 'calm' or 'control', to induce a relaxed response.

Cue-controlled relaxation is based on a behavioural conditioning rationale in which the cue word acts as a conditioned stimulus to relax.[1] The client is first trained in basic muscle-relaxation skills. Practice in the silent repetition of the cue word while breathing out then follows. This must be done while the client is in the relaxed state. Daily, self-directed practice sessions should be carried out over a period of 4–5 weeks. During each session the client repeats 20 pairings of the cue word with exhalation. Following training, the cue word is used as an anxiety-control device whenever anxiety symptoms are noted, until relaxation follows. The cue word is held to prevent arousal by invoking a relaxed response to the anxiety stimulus. Thus, the anxiety stimulus is divested of its power to produce an anxious response.

Several outcome studies of cue-controlled relaxation have produced some disappointing results regarding its comparative effectiveness.[2] However, before it is safe to dismiss the technique, the following factors must be borne in mind:

- prior training in muscle relaxation must be

thorough and there is evidence that in many studies this was not the case

- the muscle relaxation technique commonly used in conjunction with cue-controlled relaxation is the 'contrast' method, which may be comparatively ineffective.

Clinical usage

'Cue-controlled' relaxation has several advantages:

- it can be used as a method of self-help
- it is convenient and simple to teach and learn in both group settings and on an individual basis
- it is easily adapted for use as part of an anxiety management programme
- the addition of the cue word may help to increase the effectiveness of muscle relaxation for clients with marked cognitive anxiety
- the technique can be applied in a variety of daily living situations
- it may be used as an emergency anxiety control technique in highly stressful situations.

However, a fairly high level of skill in physical relaxation is required before the technique as a whole can be expected to be effective. The cue-controlled method usually involves the use of contrast relaxation — a relatively weak technique (see the discussion at the beginning of Chapter 8). Thus, it may be worthwhile to consider using the cue-word approach with an alternative physiological method of relaxation training, e.g. simple physiological relaxation.[3] One of the greatest advantages of cue-controlled relaxation is its utility for in vivo application. Two further alternatives, emergency relaxation and breathing control, are given in Client Pack 3 in the Appendix.

SYSTEMATIC DESENSITISATION
Background and methodology

Systematic desensitisation was designed by Wolpe[4] in 1958, and is based on behavioural conditioning principles, i.e. reciprocal inhibition or counter-conditioning. It involves two main elements:

- prior training in contrast relaxation, an abbreviated form of Jacobsen's[5] progressive relaxation
- progressive exposure to a hierarchy of fear stimuli while in the relaxed state.

The technique is designed for the treatment of specific phobias such as claustrophobia, fear of spiders or snakes. It is inappropriate for use in generalised anxiety.

The technique works by gradually accustoming the client to increasing intensities of exposure to the fear stimulus. Wolpe asserted that if the client could be trained to relax in the presence of the fear stimulus, then its power to induce anxiety would be weakened. According to the counter-conditioning rationale, relaxation is antagonistic to anxiety, so that one cannot be anxious and relaxed at the same time. Thus, if a client who fears lifts learns to relax when using them, lifts will cease to stimulate fear in that client. Exposure to the fear stimulus is regulated by the fear hierarchy, previously worked out by the client and therapist. Exposure is carried out imaginally in the early stages of treatment and then progresses to real-life contact with the fear object or situation. The client should learn to be completely relaxed at each stage on the fear hierarchy before progressing to the next level.

Clinical usage

More recently, graded programmes of simple exposure are the preferred method of treatment for phobic clients, the relaxation component often being discarded. However, phobic problems frequently present with panic anxiety, and this, in turn, is strongly linked to hyperventilation. Where this is the case, breathing retraining is an essential part of treatment. Finally, the desensitisation element can also be used imaginally, as part of an anxiety management programme. It is particularly useful in preparing clients for stressful situations through imaginal rehearsal of coping skills before exposure (see Client Pack 5, supplement section).

ANXIETY MANAGEMENT
Background and methodology

The general term 'anxiety management' has increasingly been used to denote the new comprehensive programmes designed to deal with generalised anxiety problems. These arose during the 1970s and some of the best known of these are: 'anxiety management training' by Suinn and Richardson,[6] and 'stress management/innoculation' or 'cognitive behaviour modification' by Meichenbaum.[7] The range of anxiety-management regimes appear to fall broadly into three categories.

1. Those emphasising physiological arousal control — e.g. self-control desensitisation,[8] applied relaxation[9] and anxiety management training.[6] This group relies heavily on training in relaxation as a coping skill, usually progressive relaxation or its abbreviated form, contrast relaxation. Methods based on arousal control include some elements of differential application in vivo.

2. Those emphasising cognitive control — e.g. systematic rational restructuring[10] and cognitive modification.[11] These regimes are based on the view that negative and irrational cognitions are the basic mediator in anxiety disorders, particularly the mislabelling of physiological arousal symptoms. For example, a tension headache might be taken to indicate the existence of serious brain disease by some severely anxious clients. Systematic rational restructuring has its roots in Ellis's rational emotive therapy[12] which is described in Chapter 3. Cognitive modification represents the cognitive portion of stress inoculation[7] described below. Cognitive modification is a systematic programme of education, rehearsal and application phases, designed to promote the identification and replacement of faulty cognitive responses. Cognitive control techniques involve the practice of coping skills within the training setting, and then differentially, in vivo.

3. Those combining cognitive and arousal control skills — e.g. stress inoculation or cognitive behaviour modification.[7] In combined programmes clients are trained to apply both physiological arousal and cognitive control skills

as appropriate to the situation in which anxiety arises. Such programmes are the most comprehensive of all self-control approaches to the treatment of anxiety. Combined anxiety management courses may comprise several types of relaxation, cognitive restructuring elements and behavioural skills training. The following components might be included in a typical comprehensive anxiety management course:

1. Education about the causes and effects of anxiety upon the mind, body and behaviour, with special emphasis on accurate identification of arousal symptoms.
2. A variety of relaxation methods, e.g. contrast relaxation, breathing exercises, emergency stress control, differential relaxation, meditative relaxation and visualisation.
3. Cognitive restructuring or rational emotive therapy approaches, with special emphasis on the identification of faulty cognitive patterns such as irrational or negative self-talk.
4. Realistic goal-setting.
5. Problem-solving techniques.
6. Social skills and assertiveness training.

The cognitive behaviour modification model acknowledges that anxiety is a multidimensional problem and attempts to deal with symptoms on all levels, i.e. physiological, cognitive, social, occupational and behavioural. The replacement of negative coping responses with an array of positive strategies or coping skills with which to deal with stress is emphasised. In this way clients are encouraged to achieve personal control or self-mastery over their own symptoms. Internal locus of control has been acknowledged as a powerful tool in overcoming anxiety and enhancing coping competence.[13,14,15]

Clinical usage

Anxiety management is not one single technique, but a structured programme of several different but complementary approaches. For this reason, a comprehensive anxiety management course is a comparatively complex regime, requiring effort and forethought to set up. Attention should be paid to the following considerations:

1. In order to achieve continuity, treatment should be presented in a closed-group setting in the form of an ongoing course of sessions. This necessitates more careful planning than for single-session relaxation, and usually involves the setting up of a waiting list of appropriate clients.

2. Since so much educational material is involved, the preparation of written handouts or tapes is required to reinforce information given within sessions and guide practice of the coping skills.

3. Regular homework assignments must be given and monitoring sheets can be used to record progress and check that home practice is actually being done.

4. Feedback sessions in which clients can discuss their individual progress are an essential part of each session.

Anxiety management programmes can be readily adapted to suit a wide range of needs and abilities. For example, the pace of the programme may be adjusted to suit the needs of each client group. It is most important that clients are allowed sufficient time to master basic relaxation skills before moving on to more advanced skills. The actual course components themselves can also be used selectively to produce various course combinations to suit different client groups. An eight-module anxiety management programme is described in the following chapter, along with advice on ways of adapting it to suit different needs.

ACKNOWLEDGEMENTS

Some of the material contained in this and the preceding three chapters has been based upon three previous publications by the author: Keable D 1985 Relaxation training techniques — a review. British Journal of Occupational Therapy.

Part one: What is relaxation? 48(4):99–100

Part two: How effective is relaxation training? 48(7):201–204

Keable D 1988 Relaxation training in occupational therapy. In: Scott D W, Katz N (eds) Occupational therapy in mental health — principles in practice. Taylor & Francis, London, ch 10, pp 133–143

REFERENCES

1 Cautela J 1966 A behaviour therapy approach to pervasive anxiety. Behavior Research and Therapy 4:99–111

2 Lehrer P M, Woolfolk R L 1993 Specific effects of stress management techniques. In: Lehrer P M, Woolfolk R L (eds) Principles and practice of stress management, 2nd edn. The Guilford Press, New York

3 Mitchell L 1977 Simple relaxation. John Murray, London

4 Wolpe J 1958 Psychotherapy by reciprocal inhibition. Stanford University Press, Stanford

5 Jacobsen E 1938 Progressive relaxation, 2nd edn. University Press, Chicago

6 Suinn R M, Richardson F 1971 Anxiety management training: a nonspecific behaviour therapy program for anxiety control. Behavior Therapy 2:498–510

7 Meichenbaum D 1977 Cognitive behavioural modification. Plenum Press, New York

8 Goldfried M R 1971 Systematic desensitisation as training in self-control. Journal of Consulting and Clinical Psychology 37:228–234

9 Zeisset R M 1968 Desensitisation and relaxation in the modification of psychiatric patient's interview behaviour. Journal of Abnormal Psychology 73:18–24

10 Goldfried M R, Decenteceo E T, Weinberg L 1974 Systematic rational restructuring as a self-control technique. Behavior Therapy 5:247–254

11 Meichenbaum D H 1972 Cognitive model of test anxious college students. Journal of Consulting and Clinical Psychology 39:370–380

12 Ellis A 1962 Reason and emotion in psychotherapy. Lyle Stewart, New York

13 Hiroto D S 1974 Locus of control and learned helplessness. Journal of Experimental Psychology 102:187–193

14 Johnson J H, Sarason I G 1978 Life stress, depression and anxiety: internal–external control as a moderator variable. Journal of Psychosomatic Research 22:205–208

15 Anderson C R 1977 Locus of control, coping behaviours and performance in a stress setting: a longitudinal study. Journal of Applied Psychology 62:446–451

FURTHER READING

Blowers C, Cobb J, Mathews A 1987 Generalised anxiety: a controlled treatment study. Behavior Research and Therapy 25(6):493–502

Childs-Clarke A, Whitfield W, Cadbury S 1989 Anxiety management groups in clinical practice. Nursing Times 85(30):49–52

Deffenbacher J L 1988 Some recommendations and directions. The Counseling Psychologist 16(1):91–95

Meichenbaum D H, Deffenbacher J L 1988 Stress inoculation training. The Counseling Psychologist 16(1):69–90

Ost L 1987 Applied relaxation: description of a coping technique and review of controlled studies. Behavior Research and Therapy 25(5):397–409

Suinn R M, Deffenbacher J L 1988 Anxiety management training. The Counseling Psychologist 16(1):31–49

11

A group anxiety management course outline

Diana Keable

This chapter presents a plan for an eight-module anxiety management course (AMC). It is hoped that therapists wishing to run courses of their own will find this plan a useful guide. However, as the needs of different groups of patients vary so widely, it must be emphasised that the course should be adapted to suit each client group. Guidance notes on the clinical application of the course, together with advice on how it can be adapted to different needs, will be covered later in this chapter.

The AMC described here has been designed along cognitive behavioural modification (CBM) lines.[1] It incorporates behavioural techniques and specific skills such as relaxation training with cognitive approaches, e.g. cognitive modification[1] and rational emotive therapy.[2] The overall accent is on education about the realities of physical and psychological anxiety symptoms and on training the patient in 'coping skills' to deal with them.

CBM regimes generally emphasise three main components: education, skills rehearsal and action. This AMC has been organised in relation to these headings.

WHAT THE COURSE INVOLVES — AN OVERALL OUTLINE

Education

The educational element of the course covers the following topics:

- causes and effects of anxiety and stress
- how relaxation works

- recognition of physiological cues of arousal e.g. hyperventilation
- the benefits of regular exercise
- negative and irrational thinking and their effects on anxiety levels (including 'catastrophising', unhelpful assumptions, unrealistic expectations of self/others)
- avoidance and its reinforcing properties in relation to anxiety
- realistic goal-setting
- problem-solving techniques
- social skills and assertiveness as ways of improving confidence in dealing with relationships and social situations.

Skills rehearsal

The rehearsal element of the course covers the following arousal-control skills.

1. Physical relaxation methods:

- contrast relaxation
- Mitchell method — simple relaxation
- correct breathing
- emergency relaxation
- differential relaxation.

2. Mental relaxation methods:

- meditative relaxation (Benson's relaxation response)
- visualisation.

3. Cognitive control activities:

- imaginal desensitisation exercises
- role-play of stressful situations
- recognition of faulty thinking; challenging and coping with anxiety symptoms; cognitive control exercises.

Action

The action element of the course refers to the application of techniques outside sessions and includes:

- relaxation methods as appropriate to the situation and individual client's needs

- self-help task assignments relevant to the stage of the course to consolidate the material covered
- completion of daily diaries and rating scales, e.g. recording stressful situations, personal reactions and ways of coping, progress in developing relaxation skills
- setting and tackling behavioural goals set during the course.

A basic outline of the content of each module follows and is intended as a guide for therapists. Detailed educational material as well as instructions for the techniques are given in the client packs in the Appendix and in the next chapter on active relaxation. The client packs also contain the self-rating scales and diary sheets referred to in the homework sections.

COURSE PLANNING NOTES FOR THERAPISTS

An overview of the eight-module AMC is shown below:

Module 1 Introduction: what is anxiety?
Module 2 Physical tension control
Module 3 Relaxation in action
Module 4 Mental tension control
Module 5 Coping with life stresses
Module 6 Goal-setting and problem-solving techniques
Module 7 Improving your social life
Module 8 Keeping up the good work.

Module 1: Introduction: what is anxiety?

Aim To introduce the general concepts relating to anxiety and to teach a relaxation method to facilitate recognition of muscular tension.

Education Round of introductions. Briefly obtain examples from group members concerning how stress/anxiety has affected their lives using brainstorming techniques. The use of a flip chart/blackboard is suggested. This aims to encourage identification and promote group cohesion as well as serving as an ice-breaking exercise.

Talk Educational content of the module, given by the therapist, including brief overview of the following main points:

1. How the course aims to help you. What is anxiety management training?
2. What is anxiety? What do we mean when we talk about 'nerves' and 'stress'.
3. What causes anxiety — past events, inaccurate/insufficient learning, inadequate or inappropriate coping methods? Do the reasons for anxiety really matter? Pragmatic approach to dealing with anxiety in the here and now is more fruitful.
4. What happens to our bodies when anxious? Fight/flight reaction, stress hormones, etc. Emphasise that some anxiety is normal and positive.
5. Faulty thinking — loss of confidence and self-esteem due to negative and irrational thoughts. Catastrophising, unreasonable assumptions, expectations, etc.
6. Lifestyles and relationships — effects of stress in daily living include avoidance, unhappiness, poor communication, poor work-related performance, lack of assertiveness, overdependence on others or lack of trust. How unrealistic goals lead to failure cycle. Role stresses.

Skills rehearsal Demonstrate contrast relaxation method and briefly explain its rationale. End session with feedback from clients and give instructions for self-help assignments.

Action: self-help assignments

1. Practise contrast relaxation and make a list of personal physical 'tension spots' for the next session.
2. Complete daily diaries and rating sheets to record stress levels and relaxation training progress.

Client Pack 1 Includes general information on anxiety and its effects, as well as reiterating the rationale and aims of the AMC, including what is expected of the patient. The Supplement gives contrast relaxation instructions.

Module 2: Physical tension control

Aim To impart the concepts relating to the physical signs and symptoms of anxiety and teach the main physical relaxation method to be used in the AMC.

Education Feedback: discuss clients' experience of the self-help assignments from the previous session and note personal tension spots. Check progress of relaxation practice. Therapist to advise and comment on feedback as appropriate.

Talk To cover the following:

- how relaxation works in relation to 'fight/flight' responses
- characteristic stress positions — increase personal awareness of these
- the benefits of exercise in anxiety reduction.

Skills rehearsal

1. Testing for tension in pairs — 'human biofeedback' exercise (see active relaxation techniques, Chapter 12).
2. Loosening-up exercises to disperse tension and restlessness (pre-relaxation).
3. Demonstrate Mitchell's 'simple relaxation' method.

End with feedback and instructions for next self-help assignments.

Action: self-help assignments

1. Practise simple relaxation method.
2. Complete ratings and diaries as before.
3. Make a list of early-warning signs noted prior to an increase in arousal — physical cues to use relaxation.

Client Pack 2 Includes a general introduction to physical techniques of tension control and guidelines on usage. Basic relaxation theory. The Supplement gives instructions for Mitchell's method of relaxation.

Module 3: Relaxation in action

Aim To teach differential relaxation methods and advise on the application of physical relaxation skills to everyday activities.

Education Feedback — discuss self-help assignments from previous session including early-warning signs of tension. Check progress of relaxation practice.

Talk To cover the following:

1. Different stressful situations — obtain suggestions from group, e.g. supermarkets, buses, etc. Discuss ways of dealing with them and adapt relaxation skills in various settings.
2. Basic principles of muscle work, tension and relaxation, reciprocal inhibition.

Skills rehearsal

1. Teach differential relaxation — sitting, standing, walking, doing a simple task. Modelling of relaxed versus tense styles of activity by therapist. Clients practise during session.
2. Teach controlled, deep, slow breathing and emergency relaxation technique.

Note: To enhance learning, a small portable biofeedback indicator of arousal may be used if available, or, alternatively, patients can be taught how to measure their own respiration and pulse rates. Muscle tension can be detected in pairs using human biofeedback as previous session.

End with feedback and instructions for next self-help assignments.

Action: self-help assignments

1. Practise differential and emergency relaxation and report on progress using the specially structured form in Client Pack 3.
2. Note mental stress triggers, thoughts and feelings for next session, particularly negative automatic thoughts e.g. 'I can't cope'.
3. Continue diaries and ratings as before.

Client Pack 3 Includes more information on physical tension control — putting relaxation into practice. The Supplement provides instructions for differential and emergency relaxation methods.

Module 4: Mental tension control

Aim To describe the concepts of faulty thinking and teach mental relaxation methods.

Education Feedback: sharing of examples of personal negative thoughts from the self-help assignments by the group members. Check relaxation practice progress. Give short irrational

beliefs test;[2] score and discuss as introduction to talk.

Talk To cover the following:

1. Causes and effects of faulty thinking. The various forms it takes — negative and irrational thoughts, catastrophising, unrealistic/inappropriate assumptions and expectations. Relate to examples from group members' self-help assignments.
2. How to control faulty thinking — use of positive thinking and challenging irrational thoughts.

Skills rehearsal

1. Choose one example of faulty thinking from the group and work it through on flip chart/blackboard encouraging group members to re-evaluate realistically and suggest alternatives and challenges.
2. Demonstrate mental relaxation techniques e.g. Benson's relaxation response and visualisation.

End session with feedback and instructions for next self-help assignment.

Action: self-help assignments

1. Note faulty thinking occurring when anxious and challenge on specially structured form.
2. Practise mental relaxation techniques.
3. Continue ratings and diaries.

Client Pack 4 Includes information on faulty thinking and how to challenge it. Instructions for mental relaxation techniques are given in the Supplement.

Module 5: Coping with life stresses

Aim To reinforce the recognition of, and ability to challenge, faulty thinking in stressful situations. Teach imaginal desensitisation techniques.

Education Feedback: discuss examples of faulty thinking and challenging responses from the self-help assignments. Check relaxation progress as before.

Talk To cover the following:

- brainstorm stressful situations and life events in group

- the life events inventory (see p. 61) could be used to demonstrate points; e.g. that ordinary events, even relatively pleasant ones involving change, can be highly stressful
- discuss avoidance of particular situations — how it reinforces fear
- improving positive coping skills is the most effective way of dealing with stress and adverse life events.

Skills rehearsal Imaginal desensitisation (imaginary rehearsal) practice using physical and mental relaxation techniques combined. Intensive practice in session — each client to choose three situations which arouse anxiety and work through these from the least to the most fear-provoking using coping techniques imaginally to control anxiety.

End group with feedback and instructions for next self-help assignment.

Action: self-help assignments

1. Continue imaginal desensitisation practice as in session. Write out 'hierarchy' of situations to work through by next session. Start using physical and mental techniques together to aid coping.
2. Compile a list of personal goals in order of difficulty for next session.
3. Continue diaries and ratings.

Client Pack 5 Includes information on the life stresses of modern times and ways of coping with them. The Supplement contains guidance notes on imaginal rehearsal exercises.

Module 6: Goal-setting and problem-solving techniques

Aim To teach practical goal-setting and problem-solving methods and their application to personal problems.

Education Feedback: discuss self-help assignments related to personal goals and check relaxation practice as before.

Talk To cover the following:

1. Goal-setting — setting realistic targets and breaking main goals down into smaller, more achievable stages. Discuss group members' goals in relation to these guidelines.
2. Select one problem from the group and work through the problem-solving technique using the group to brainstorm and select options.

Skills rehearsal In small groups or pairs, write down one common problem and practise setting realistic goals and using the problem-solving approach.

End session with feedback and instructions for next homework assignment.

Action: self-help assignments

1. Make a list of problems and work through problem-solving method on form provided for at least one.
2. Practise goal-setting on form provided for problem chosen, as above.
3. Commence action decided upon to solve at least one problem and report back next session on progress.
4. Continue ratings and diaries.

Client Pack 6 Includes information on realistic goal-setting and problem-solving. How to put into practice.

Module 7: Improving your social life — coping confidently and effectively in social situations

Aim To teach basic social skills' principles and rehearse their appropriate use through the role-play of difficult situations common to group members.

Education Feedback — group members to report on self-help assignments — difficulties encountered carrying out problem-solving technique. Check on relaxation practice progress.

Talk To cover the following:

1. Why we need to socialise, seek and maintain relationships and hobbies.
2. Social skills — getting to know people, shyness, etc. Non-verbal and verbal behaviour relating to social skills.
3. Assertiveness — versus aggressive/submissive behaviour.

4. Brainstorm a list of difficult social situations from group members' experiences.

Skills rehearsal

1. Each group member to choose one example of a stressful social scenario to role-play (5 minutes each). This should be of easy to moderate difficulty — not too intense or emotional, especially at first.
2. Each person to describe a scenario roughly to the group, stating how they have actually coped with that situation in the past, what didn't work, how they would like to improve it. Protagonist to choose auxiliary egos from group. Group members can be asked to use coping techniques to manage anxiety about the role-play. The therapist might suggest: 'if you can do a role-play, most ordinary situations will be easier. In any case the anxiety tends to subside the more you get involved in the role you are tackling.'

End session with feedback and instructions for next self-help assignment.

Action: self-help assignments

1. Decide on another problem for final role-play next session: 'don't forget this will be your last chance!'
2. Complete feedback questionnaire sheet on the course — aspects most/least helpful, etc.
3. Complete test sheet to assess how accurately concepts taught have been learned. (These are considered as part of the final session of revision so that any misunderstandings can be cleared up before the course finishes).
4. Note down any aspects individuals feel they require revision on for final session.
5. Continue ratings and diaries.

Client Pack 7 Includes information on social skills and assertiveness — coping with people. Role demands.

Module 8: Keeping up the good work

Aim To revise and reinforce the main points covered throughout course and to complete individual role-plays.

Education Feedback: sharing of views from group members about the course using feedback questionnaires.

Talk To cover the following:

- going through revision tests as a group and dealing with any questions arising from this as well as queries from individual group members
- summing up main concepts
- instructions on maintaining use of coping techniques effectively until follow-up.

Skills rehearsal

- final role-plays as previous session
- round of appreciations/resentments before group finishes.

Client Pack 8 Includes revision notes summarising points to remember, plus the consolidation and continuation of the techniques learnt. After session: complete post-course tests and arrange follow-up appointments for 6 to 12 weeks' later.

NOTES ON THE CLINICAL APPLICATION OF THE AMC

Many of the issues mentioned in the brief outline given below are discussed more fully in Chapter 14: Teaching resources and Chapter 15: Troubleshooting — some common problems. The author assumes that therapists attempting to run the AMC will already be conversant with the principles of group facilitation and have had prior experience in running groups. Further reading on group work is also given at the end of Chapter 14.

Session length

As a rough guide, it is envisaged that the material in each module will normally take approximately one and a half hours to cover. However, the overall length of each module and its components can be allotted time as appropriate to each group's needs. As regards how much emphasis to place on each component, the education section should normally take about one third of the total time available, leaving the bulk of session time for rehearsal and feedback. More in-depth coverage of the educative portions are provided in the client packs. (Also see the section below: Adapting the course format for different needs.)

Setting

The setting used for anxiety management sessions will vary according to the facilities available to therapists and most situations can readily be adapted. However, it is advisable to choose a venue relatively free from interruptions and affording sufficient privacy for the relaxation content of the sessions. This can usually be assured by attaching a 'relaxation in progress' notice outside the room. The therapist should not worry unduly about the existence of moderate amounts of extraneous noise. This presents a realistic situation since clients must ultimately learn to relax in noisy environments.

It is not necessary to darken the room, although this may be helpful in the initial stages. Strip lighting can sometimes be extraordinarily irritating, however, and can simply be turned off during relaxation practice. It is important that the room used should be sufficiently warm since the body temperature tends to drop during relaxation and a cold environment interferes with relaxation. Adequate ventilation is also required.

It is important to have reasonably comfortable chairs available for relaxation practice, preferably with head- and arm-rests. Alternatively, ordinary chairs can be pushed up against a wall to support the head. Additionally, it is helpful for mats and pillows to be made available so that relaxation can be practised lying down. Mats can be expensive, so if they are unavailable a carpeted floor or blankets will serve the purpose adequately. For differential relaxation practice a larger space such as a gymnasium, large room or outdoor area is useful to accommodate standing and walking practice.

Presentation

Since anxiety management is basically an educative technique, a didactic but empathic teaching style of delivery is appropriate.

Once the group has developed some cohesion, there may be a tendency on the part of its more vocal members to draw out the feedback and discussion times, leaving insufficient time for the teaching material to be covered fully. This should be tactfully avoided so that the course structure is adhered to as closely as possible (see 'discussion times' below).

Simple visual aids such as flip charts can usually be cheaply and easily made to enhance the delivery of educative material. Simple cartoon drawings to accompany key phrases can be eye-catching and memorable.

Selection criteria

The inclusion criteria for the AMC is broad. For the majority of clients with psychiatric problems, anxiety is an important contributing factor. However, it is expected that most clients will experience some degree of difficulty in learning anxiety reduction skills. For example, those clients with poor hearing or those with extra-pyramidal side-effects associated with phenothiazine medication, may find the techniques hard to master. In such cases, the therapist's skill and imagination in adapting his or her approach to individual needs is invaluable. Lundervold's study[3] provides an example of how a behavioural relaxation training course was used with a mentally handicapped adult.

However, there are certain contraindications. Relaxation training and related techniques should not be used with those suffering from florid psychosis or acute mania. Other clients who would be unlikely to benefit include those exhibiting the following:

- disruptive/disturbed behaviour
- substantial cognitive impairment e.g. advanced dementia
- poor verbal skills
- monosymptomatic/simple phobias
- excessive 'state' anxiety.

Adapting the course format for different needs

Although the course has been designed as a

cohesive whole, usually given over a period of eight consecutive weeks, this format may not suit all client groups. The following are some examples of how it can be adapted.

1. The course could be split into two sections. The first half (Client Packs 1–4), could be used as a basic course and the second half (Client Packs 5–8) could be used as an advanced course. The same group of clients could attend both courses with a gap of several weeks in between courses for consolidation. Clients who had not found the first course useful need not join the advanced course. Alternatively, for clients who are thought unlikely to benefit from the advanced course, the therapist might choose to use the basic course only.

2. For a group who are likely to take longer to master the concepts and procedures involved, the number of sessions could be doubled. At the rate of one shorter session per week, the whole course would last 16 weeks. Alternate sessions of teaching and consolidation could be employed in an extended course format. The consolidation sessions could be used to reinforce material taught at the previous session, thus allowing more time for discussion, feedback and practice of the techniques within the sessions. This structure also gives more time for clients to adapt the techniques and concepts to their daily lives, and effect realistic change.

3. Conversely, for a more advanced group, a faster pace may add momentum. For such clients, up to two sessions per week could be given so that the complete course lasts four weeks. This structure allows less time for consolidation and the carrying out of personal assignments. However, the shorter time may give rise to a reduced drop-out rate.

Follow-up

It is important that long-term follow-up assessment is carried out at some point after the course terminates. This enables the therapist to gauge the effectiveness of treatment over time. It is not realistic to assume that treatment effects have persisted unless this is done. From similar courses, there is also evidence that treatment effects continue to improve for some time after the course has finished.[4] A period of three months after treatment is suggested as a suitable interval for follow-up, at which time assessment can be repeated and compared with pre-course and post-course results.

Course structure

The AMC presented here is intended to be delivered as a series or course of sessions spanning a pre-determined period of weeks with the same client group. This demands considerable planning. In order to arrange an AMC course, sufficient numbers of suitable clients have to be gathered and interviewed well in advance. This necessitates a waiting list and liaison with referring agencies. A certain amount of administrative work is also involved. Conversely, conventional relaxation training may be delivered on a single-session basis so that clients can be introduced to treatment immediately and receive as many sessions as the therapist thinks fit. This kind of relaxation training is often a component part of a weekly treatment programme into which clients are allocated as they are referred e.g. in a day hospital setting.

Another alternative is to set up a rolling programme of anxiety management sessions. Accordingly, clients may start at any stage and remain on the course until all modules have been covered. Thus, a client presenting at Module 5, will stay on the course through all eight modules, terminating after Module 4. Although this arrangement appears to lack progression, it works surprisingly well for many clients and is often a better option than waiting weeks or months to start treatment. This necessitates an 'open' style of group which may reduce cohesiveness. However, the greater flexibility means that clients who take longer to master the techniques can stay longer and repeat sessions if necessary.

In the writer's opinion, however, the extra work involved in setting up an AMC is well worth the effort and improves the ultimate standard of treatment considerably. In the closed group, course format, clients are able to take part in a more cohesive group, thus increasing their motivation and also following a more logical, graded progression in the learning process. Conventional relaxation training may also be considerably enhanced if delivered in a similar course format.

Client numbers

In order to ensure a viable group size it is recommended that the course begins with around 15 members. In the writer's experience the drop-out rate is often around 50%. This is particularly the case with hospital out-patient groups. Sufficient numbers need to be maintained to ensure that a workable core group remains, usually around 6–10 members. Where numbers fall below this, the group process may be adversely affected, detracting from the potential richness of material which the clients themselves may bring to the group. However, groups of more than 10 members may be less effective. This was confirmed by one study[5] which compared large and small group AMT formats.

Written material

Clients may have initial problems completing the self-help assignment forms. This must be expected for the first few sessions and they should be explained clearly on repeated occasions. It is suggested that therapists ask for assignments to be handed in regularly each week so that they can be checked. Individual clients who have filled in the forms incorrectly can then be tactfully advised.

Self-help assignments

Some clients may not do their homework for a variety of reasons, usually associated with lack of motivation. This should be sympathetically but firmly followed up. Most groups will usually need repeated reminders about the importance of the self-help assignments. It is suggested that the therapist emphasise clearly that homework is the client's own responsibility and that it is the most crucial part of the treatment. Many clients report difficulties with relaxation when practising on their own. This is partly due to a tendency to depend on the therapist and can often be avoided by placing the emphasis on autonomous practice from the outset. Such clients should be encouraged to persevere and reminded not to expect instant success — relaxation is a skill like any other and requires considerable practice before mastery can be achieved. It may be useful to add that some people unfortunately give up too soon and thus fail to reap any benefits. Throughout the course it may be necessary often to restate the fact that relaxation is not a soft option and requires persistent hard work on the client's part. (Also see the section entitled 'Homework: adherence to practice' in Chapter 15.)

Discussion times

Free discussion and sharing in a cohesive and supportive group is of great benefit. However, there may be a tendency to bring a preponderance of emotional material to AMT sessions, which may be difficult to deal with appropriately within that context. This may also leave little time for the main business of the sessions — anxiety management training. It may be necessary for therapists to assist such clients in identifying and accessing more legitimate outlets such as support groups or counselling in order to meet their needs more appropriately. Attempts must be made to achieve a sympathetic but sensible balance in this matter. Unstructured / aimless discussion may also be destructive if it reinforces negative / irrational beliefs about anxiety symptoms rather than the possibility of change.

Occasionally the therapist may encounter some 'resistance', often at the half-way stage when some clients may feel confronted and challenged by the course to take responsibility for tackling their own symptoms. Some hostility may be expressed at this point and clients affected may drop out of the course or attend only sporadically. This can be linked to psychological investment in the maintenance of symptoms which are crucial to personal dynamic equilibrium. An alternative approach, usually within an individual setting may be more appropriate in such cases. Chapters 14 and 15 consider this issue more fully.

Setting-up schedule

This check-list may be useful as a guide for a therapist setting up the course.

1. Decide on the client group to be treated and carefully define it, noting inclusion and exclusion criteria.
2. Set out specific aims of treatment for the client group.
3. Prepare appropriate assessment battery; e.g. standardised instrument, structured interview schedule.
4. Decide on the following:
   a. day, time, frequency and length of sessions
   b. format of course
   c. find suitable venue
   d. allocate course therapists (at least two are recommended with one for back-up support in case of staff absence)
5. Start collecting clients. Notify referral sources — describe aims of course and type of clients suitable.
6. Start interviewing / assessing clients as they are referred.
7. Check equipment availability / suitability e.g. mats, pillows, chairs, client's training material.
8. Prepare visual aids, e.g. flip charts or transparencies for overhead projector.
9. Check that the number of suitable clients is sufficient. This is crucial as the drop-out rate is often around 50%, so that, for a minimum core group of eight clients, 16 clients are required initially.
10. Set commencement date for course, then notify clients and relevant staff.
11. Evaluate pre-course data in order to arrive at a profile of the group, e.g. levels of anxiety, previous relaxation experience, clinical diagnoses and medication.
12. Carry out course.
13. Administer post-course assessments. Check correct names and addresses of clients are recorded for follow-up.
14. Compare results before and after treatment.
15. Arrange follow-up interviews. Repeat assessment batteries and compare with previous results.

REFERENCES

1 Meichenbaum D H 1972 Cognitive model of test anxious college students. Journal of Consulting and Clinical Psychology 39:370–380
2 Ellis A 1962 Reason and emotion in psychotherapy. Lyle Stewart, New York
3 Lundervold D 1986 The effects of behavioral relaxation and self-instruction training: a case study. Rehabilitation Counseling Bulletin 30(2):124–128
4 Deffenbacher J, Suinn R 1982 The self-control of anxiety. In: Karoly P, Kanger F (eds) Self-management and behavioural change. Pergamon Press, New York
5 Daley P C, Bloom L J, Deffenbacher J L, Stewart R 1983 Treatment effectiveness of anxiety management training in small and large group formats. Journal of Counseling Psychology 30(1):104–107

12

Active relaxation techniques

Diana Keable

This chapter describes the procedures for further activities which may be used to promote relaxation through action. These are intended for use either as part of the anxiety management course described in the previous chapter, or in general relaxation training. These approaches differ from conventional relaxation techniques in that the accent is on the application and/or release of tension through activity. The first two techniques are designed to reinforce the skill of muscle relaxation and demonstrate how it can be applied to daily living. The remaining methods use vigorous physical activity to release accumulated tension and/or to heal its adverse effects. Active techniques are often especially useful for those clients who find the more passive forms of relaxation difficult to utilise. This may be due to one or more of the following reasons:

- high levels of state/acute anxiety
- residual psychotic symptoms
- side-effects of medication causing symptoms such as muscle rigidity/tremor
- restlessness
- tight, painful musculature
- limited concentration span
- preoccupation with distressing thoughts.

The activities included here are:

- 'human biofeedback' (residual tension check)
- differential relaxation exercises (sitting, standing, walking, task performance)
- pre-relaxation exercises
- aerobic exercise.

HUMAN BIOFEEDBACK

This exercise is based on an excellent and powerful means of teaching patients an awareness of tension which was described by Marquis, Ferguson and Barr Taylor.[1] The exercise assists in identifying the difference between tension and relaxation using verbal feedback.

It may be carried out by the therapist treating individual clients or in group settings. In the latter case, the group divides into pairs, one client in each pair taking the role of 'therapist'. The other client takes the role of 'patient' and the pair work through the procedure. At the end, they swap roles and repeat.

The 'therapist' starts by asking the 'patient' to be seated and to relax as much as possible. The 'therapist' then goes through the procedure described below.

Procedure for 'therapists'

General signs of tension

Look at your patient: notice any visible signs of tension such as a clenched jaw, furrowed brow, tense posture, etc.

Talk to your patient: notice any signs of tension in the voice.

The pulse and respiration may also be checked if appropriate and this should be slow and regular.

Shoulder girdle and upper limbs

Firmly but gently supporting the weight of the limb, place one hand under the elbow and one just above the wrist. Then lift the arm and perform the movements described below, palpating for muscle tension and noting any resistance. This may be felt as tightness and pressure against the grip.

1. Gently hinge the elbow back and forth.
2. Using circular movements, rotate the shoulder.
3. Grasp the arm just above the wrist, with both hands, and carefully shake the hand in all directions.

If the patient is completely relaxed, the limb or part should feel very heavy, limp, soft and move freely. To check whether the patient is artificially assisting the movements, make an unexpected change of direction.

Abdomen

Firmly press the abdominal wall with a finger. This should feel soft and yield to pressure.

Hip and lower limbs

Place one hand under the knee and one behind the ankle. As for shoulder girdle, hinge the knee, rotate the hip and shake the foot.

Head and neck

Place both hands under the head, just above the back of the neck. Invite the patient to allow the weight of their head to fall back onto your supporting hands. Gently roll the head from hand to hand.

This exercise may be more comfortably and easily performed if you kneel on the floor and rest the patient's head on your lap. This helps to achieve a more secure position for the patient's head and makes it easier for you to support the weight of the head — which is deceptively heavy.

Tension spots

Individual muscles can be palpated to check for tension if necessary.

While you are checking the limb or body part for tension you should be continually informing the patient of the current state of tension in the muscles and encouraging and reinforcing the patient to achieve deeper relaxation. Naturally any signs of overt anxiety such as sweating and trembling should only be remarked upon cautiously and tactfully in a group situation.

Points to consider

As this technique involves touch, issues concerning trust and intimacy should be carefully considered before its introduction in group or individual situations. For example, it is unlikely to be suitable for acutely ill clients or those with a seriously disturbed body image. The exercise is also more likely to succeed when some rapport and familiarity has developed between the therapist and the client / clients. However, the exercise can serve as a good way of increasing trust and cohesiveness in group settings, often producing some constructive but infectious amusement as well. It is best to use the technique when some relaxation skills have already been taught — perhaps at a mid-way point in a relaxation / anxiety management course. Finally, the technique also serves as an invaluable tool for the therapist to assess client progress in muscle relaxation skills.

DIFFERENTIAL RELAXATION

The aim of this series of graded exercises is to encourage application of skills to everyday living situations. It is helpful to have clients rehearse differential skills within the clinical setting initially. Once the basic concepts and techniques have been understood, clients will be better able to apply relaxation in their daily lives. The links between basic relaxation and its practical usage usually require considerable reinforcement.

Differential relaxation is generally taught when some mastery has been achieved in the supine position. It usually starts with sitting relaxation, although, some trainees will have started learning relaxation from a sitting position in any case. After sitting, relaxed ways of standing, walking and doing simple to complex tasks are taught. Environmental and stress elements can gradually be added such as light, noise, people and activity as the patient progresses. The therapist should also discuss with the group ways of adapting differential relaxation to individual problem situations, such as telephoning, driving, shopping and standing at bus stops.[1,2] (Also see Client Pack 3.)

Presentation suggestions

Here are some suggestions for leading clients through a series of differential relaxation exercises.

Sitting relaxation

'Choose a comfortable, supportive chair to begin with. Wriggle the small of your back right into the chair — feel it supporting your weight so that you can relax your back muscles. Find a comfortable place to support your arms and wrists, either arm-rests or lap. Make sure that your arms are not tightly pressed to your sides or crossed over your chest — slide them a little away from you. Let your head rest on the back of the chair or, if it is not high enough, push the chair against a wall to rest your head. Unclench your hands. Pull your shoulders down. Centre your head on your shoulders and raise your chin slightly. Keep both feet directly below your knees and flat on the floor. Watch your breathing — check that it is *low* in the chest and *slow*.'

The client can later progress to relaxed sitting while performing tasks such as writing or telephoning, and in more stressful situations such as bus journeys.

Standing relaxation

'Choose a space for yourself to stand, anywhere in the room, preferably without shoes. Feel your feet firmly placed on the floor, a little apart and parallel. Close your eyes and stand comfortably. Notice how your whole body feels when you're standing, note any feelings of strain or discomfort. Now imagine that there is a straight line running right through you from the top of your head down to the floor, finishing between your feet. In the standing position, try to centre yourself around the line. First adjust your head, neck and chin. Then your shoulders, arms and trunk — pull your shoulders down and let your arms hang loosely at your sides. Then centre your bottom, spine and legs. Especially notice your knees — allow yourself to sway very slightly as you centre yourself but keep your feet firmly planted on the floor. Feel the weight of your body from the top of your head, downwards, through your feet to the floor.

Now I am going to walk around the room slowly and help you all check that you are really standing in a relaxed way. I shall gently push each person from the side. You should feel flexible but not rigid. Allow yourself to give slightly in response to my push, but try to keep steady so that you do not stagger. If you find this difficult, steady yourself, let go of unnecessary tension, be aware of your weight and allow it to be supported by the floor.'

Walking relaxation

Use as large a room as possible for this activity, such as a gym, or even better, use rough grass out in the open.

'First use your standing relaxation, pull your shoulders down and free your arms, let them hang beside you. *Very slowly* move off, firmly but gently placing each foot on the floor. Imagine that you are moving like a cat. Imagine that you are flowing along. Feel your legs swinging forward slowly from the hip, by their own momentum. Only use enough effort to keep up the slow walking pace and no more. Check that every part of you is relaxed except the working parts. If you find that you tend to stagger a little when you move slowly, concentrate harder on placing each foot down deliberately and feel the floor under your foot with each step. Feel your weight being supported by the floor with each step. Do not be tempted to speed up. Appreciate every step that you take, noticing the myriad sensations that you are receiving from the soles of your feet.'

Relaxing while carrying out a simple task

Any fairly straightforward task such as peeling a potato or making a paper clip chain can be used.

'Use your sitting relaxation, pull your shoulders down, wriggle your back into the chair and allow it to take your weight. Place your pile of paper clips in front of you or on your lap, within arm's reach. Slowly start to link the clips together one at a time, using forearms and fingers, but only with as much effort as absolutely necessary. At the same time notice what the rest of your body is doing — are your shoulders raised, your thighs clamped together, your arms stuck to your sides? What about your head, neck, face, jaw, mouth, eye-lids, forehead and scalp? For

example, ensure that you are not frowning, thrusting your head forward or clenching your teeth. Survey your whole body and check that you are expending no more energy than the amount that you need to do the job. Enjoy carrying out your task — notice the skill of your fingers and eyes as they coordinate your movements.'

PRE-RELAXATION EXERCISES

These are simple exercises designed to rid the body of residual tension before the relaxation session. For particularly restless clients, it is useful to recommend that these exercises are carried out prior to each relaxation practice session.

Loosening-up movements

Instruct clients to feel themselves shaking out their tension as they perform the exercises.

Vigorously shake your right hand as if shaking off drops of water, allowing your hand to become completely floppy. Continue the shaking movements up the arm until the whole arm and shoulder is involved.

Repeat for the left hand, arm and shoulder.

Repeat for the right, then left leg as for the arm.

Instruct clients not to worry too much if they wobble about a bit, but, if there is any difficulty or fear, to steady themselves with one hand on a wall.

Some vocalisation can be added here for further tension release or simply ask clients to take a deep, slow breath to finish and feel themselves breathing away the tension as they exhale.[3]

Gentle stretching

A series of basic stretching exercises can also be a very useful way of releasing accumulated tension prior to relaxation. Such exercises should aim to rebalance muscle tension, working through all the major muscle groups, involving upper and lower limbs, trunk, back, hips, shoulder and neck. The stretching exercises described by Payne[4] are a highly recommended example.

The use of yoga postures or T'ai Chi movements are also recommended for this purpose, provided that access to properly trained instructors can be arranged.

AEROBIC EXERCISE

A growing body of evidence indicates that regular aerobic exercise improves psychological as well as physical health. Several studies have reported the following benefits:

- reduced anxiety, feelings of stress/tension, depression, fatigue and depression
- improved alertness, concentration, mood, energy levels and resistance to infection
- improved appearance (including weight loss and physical fitness), confidence, self-esteem, as well as increasing social contact and enjoyment.[4,5,6]

What causes the mood-enhancing effects of aerobic exercise is still unclear. However, two possible chemical mechanisms have been identified. The first is the action of the endorphins, naturally occurring opiates, which help to moderate pain perception and elevate mood. The second factor may be that exercise simply has the effect of 'burning off' stress hormones, such as the corticoids, which have accumulated in the blood. The primitive fight/flight syndrome has the effect of preparing the individual to take vigorous physical action. This rarely occurs in response to modern day stresses, leaving a residue of excess stress hormones which take longer to disperse in passive states. Finally, the old adage: 'a healthy body means a healthy mind', may turn out to contain a great deal of truth. The strong link between physical and mental health is now incontrovertible, and may best be described as a two-way feedback loop. In the opinion of the writer, much more emphasis should be placed on physical fitness interventions for those with mental-health-related problems.

Access to properly qualified instruction is, of course, essential. It is only necessary, therefore, to give a few further guidelines here.

1. Those unaccustomed to vigorous exercise should have a medical examination prior to embarking on any fitness programme.
2. The golden rule is to *build up slowly*. No-one should suddenly start exercising significantly beyond their accustomed limits. Intensity and duration of exercise sessions should be gradually increased over a period of time.
3. All exercise sessions should include a comprehensive warming-up section to prepare the body for exercise, and also a gradual winding-down section at the end. This enables the body to adjust its demands on heart and respiration rates, blood pressure and volume more gradually and safely.
4. Ideal exercise programmes should include a mixture of aerobic and anaerobic exercise. Aerobic exercise is held to increase general stamina, promote weight loss, enhance mood and reduce anxiety/tension. Anaerobic exercise is more efficient for muscle toning, strengthening and joint suppleness.
5. Starting an exercise programme is the most difficult phase. Strong incentives are needed to persist until the habit is established and the benefits begin to appear.
6. Exercise should be strictly avoided during an infection/fever, including the common cold.
7. Exercise should never exceed the individual's tolerance level; it is essential to develop an awareness of what is a comfortable limit and remain within it. Exercise tolerance will necessarily vary according to age and physical capacity; older people need to exercise more cautiously.
8. It is best to exercise frequently and regularly, rather than for lengthy, intensive bouts. At least three times weekly for 20–30 minutes is recommended.[4,5]

REFERENCES

1 Marquis J N, Ferguson J M, Barr Taylor C 1980 Generalization of relaxation skills. Journal of Behaviour Therapy and Experimental Psychiatry 11:95–99

2 Mitchell L 1977 Simple relaxation. John Murray, London

3 Bond M, Kilty J 1982 Practical methods of dealing with

stress. Human potential research project, University of Surrey, Surrey

4 Payne R 1995 Relaxation techniques — a practical handbook for the health care professional. Churchill Livingstone, Edinburgh

5 Sadgrove J 1994 Exercise: why bother? The Observer supplement 11.12.94 (14:Body Mechanics). Observer, London

6 Byrne A, Byrne D G 1993 The effect of exercise on depression, anxiety and other mood states: a review. Journal of Psychosomatic Research, 37(6):565–574

Clinical applications

Part three of this book aims to address some of the major challenges faced by therapists using anxiety management techniques in a variety of different clinical settings. Information, practical resources and advice is offered along with several chapters providing a more in-depth focus on different clinical groups. The final chapter, on occupational stress and burnout, is devoted to the needs of the therapists themselves.

13

From assessment to evaluation: procedures and practicalities

Sue Hutchings

ASSURING EFFECTIVENESS

No anxiety management programme would be complete unless methods to evaluate effectiveness were incorporated into the implementation process. Effectiveness is not simply completing the originally agreed number of sessions, but whether real changes have occurred in the behaviours of the participants. The process of evaluation also entails a critical appraisal of programme structure, methods, delivery and use of resources, both in terms of therapists' time and teaching materials.

This can be an uncomfortable time for even the most diligent and conscientious therapist who has always endeavoured to provide a quality service to programme participants and referral agencies. As the previous chapters in this book demonstrate, anxiety management programmes can be an organised and theoretically sound way of providing practical, client-centred solutions to the everyday problems that clinical anxiety can create in people's lives. However, this is no excuse to become complacent and the discerning therapist should continually be striving to answer the following questions about their clinical practice:

- does this anxiety management programme work?
- how do I know it works?
- who does it work for — the therapist? the participant? the family? the referral agency?
- if this anxiety management programme works, does all of its component parts work equally well?

- if only certain parts of the programme seem to work, could the next programme be modified in order to further enhance effectiveness?
- can I demonstrate the programme's effectiveness to others?

The questions posed above serve as the basis for this chapter and it is evident that comprehensive evaluation cannot rest with the therapist's best hunch or immediate impression. Thorough and impartial evaluation involves the systematic scrutiny of the structure, methods, delivery and resourcing of an anxiety management programme and that it has retained its client-centred focus (Fig. 13.1). Once well established, anxiety

management programmes can become familiar and certain territory for the experienced therapist who could begrudge the notion of programme modification unless it was supported by objective evidence.

To many therapists, evaluation is a logical part of the problem-solving process and is a natural constituent of good professional practice. However, good evaluative procedures require clear assessment to act as a baseline for change. It is a fallacy to assume that any intervention or programme can be successfully evaluated as an afterthought. Evaluation that is merely tagged on to the end of an anxiety management programme lacks sufficient rigour to be taken as serious clinical evidence of effectiveness. Without thinking through how a programme will be evaluated in the initial planning stages, the end result could bear little relation to the programme's original objectives.

Including the opinions and perspective of the participants is an important but time-consuming part of this evaluation process and one that requires a clear focus. Empowering and enabling the participants to evaluate a programme entails a careful consideration of methods and delivery, as well as ensuring an atmosphere of mutual trust and genuine collaboration. It could be tempting for the busy, over-stretched and under-resourced therapist to conclude that effective evaluation takes up too much time and energy, and that it is easier to comply with the impetus of a regular routine of established and well attended anxiety management programmes. However, effective evaluation could equally save valuable time by identifying possible modifications and clearly justifying therapeutic value to the client, to other professional colleagues and to referral agencies.

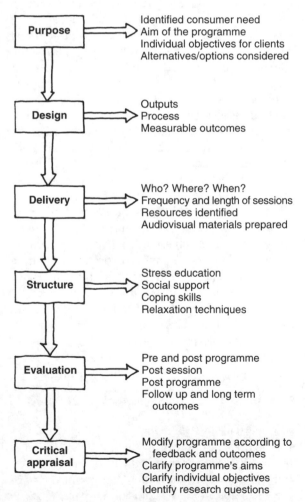

Figure 13.1 The assessment and evaluation cycle.

ESTABLISHING A BASELINE

The relationship between assessment and evaluation

As already indicated, the constructive evaluation of an anxiety management programme starts at the initial planning stages. In order to demonstrate clearly changes in the behaviour of participants, effective assessment procedures help to identify a baseline which can illustrate the 'before and after' differences. If assessment procedures are ad hoc, informal and largely descriptive, these methods alone do not generate enough rigorous objective data to act as an indicator of behavioural change.

The necessity for assessments to provide a baseline for change requires the therapist to select data collection tools prudently. Although different assessment methods for clinical anxiety are now widely available, the therapist needs to select those which will generate qualitative and quantitative data, and provide a coherent baseline profile of the individual client. It can be easy to be somewhat seduced into relying mostly on interviews that allow plenty of scope for recording the subjective view of the client, and one which allows the client to articulate their views, concerns and aspirations. Although this biographical information is important in order to retain a client-centred focus and to add a 'human face' to clinical interventions, it cannot stand alone as sufficient baseline data.

When deciding on appropriate assessments, the therapist needs to select tools which provide a balance of descriptive information (qualitative data) and numerical measures (quantitative data). Although the concept of numerical measures may be an anathema to the humanistic philosophic principles of some therapists and one that seems to negate the individuality of the client, numerical data can act as a useful complement to more qualitative data. Besides acting as an effective illustration of pre- and post-group change, data can be accumulated on an individual client basis, as well as providing useful information on the cohorts of anxiety management groups, thereby helping to guide future planning and resourcing.

The types of measures used by assessment tools vary and produce different levels of numerical data. Straightforward 'tick the box' questions which may only require a 'yes' or 'no' answer yield data in terms of categories (nominal data). More sophisticated measures require the client and/or the assessor to rank responses according to points on a scale or continuum (ordinal data). More refined numerical measures involve the use of a scale which uses intervals of equal value (interval data), and scales which make use of an absolute zero as well as equal intervals (ratio data). Although this is a very simplistic summary of the types of numerical measures used, and may necessitate further reading, a basic understanding of these differences is fundamental to formulating focused research studies. Even if identifying and investigating a research question is not on the therapist's agenda, being informed and clear about the type of numerical data presently collected could save time in designing a protocol at a later date.

When endeavouring to select appropriate assessment tools for particular clients in a particular setting, high-quality objective assessments should:

- be clear and easily understood by the client and assessor
- have a definite structure that allows for the systematic collection of quantitative or qualitative information, or a combination of both (semi-structured interviews may include opportunities for biographical information as well as requiring a ranking of responses)
- be valid and reliable and not subject to the bias of the individual assessor (for example, standardised tests have been scrutinised to ensure that they are rigorous and allow for the interpretation of results)
- have a comprehensive way of recording results and with clear documentation
- use an appropriate index of measurement which allows for the meaning of results to be apparent
- be specific and sensitive to the particular client group (in terms of age/gender/clinical setting)
- help the therapist formulate focused objectives for the individual client
- assist the therapist in identifying overall aims for an anxiety management programme.

It is evident from this list that the therapist may well select a number of assessment tools, as one assessment method alone is unlikely to meet all of the above criteria. The danger of this is that a large assessment 'battery' of tests, interviews and questionnaires can overwhelm the client and be time-consuming to implement. Therefore, judicious selection of two or three of the most appropriate assessment tools needs to be paramount. Although it is tempting to establish a highly detailed baseline profile of each client, focused assessment will enable the evaluation process to produce results that are evident, explainable and accessible.

Setting objectives

Following the completion of a baseline assessment profile of an individual client, the next crucial step is the setting of clearly defined objectives. This is the process of articulating in measurable terms what it is you are hoping to achieve with an individual client. The art of focused objective-setting may already be a highly practised skill of the experienced therapist, but in today's health and social care climate of accountability, it is the absolute bedrock of determining the value of therapeutic interventions.

The language of this stage of the problem-solving process varies across the health care professions, but essentially what is fundamental is to distinguish between the general purpose of the anxiety management programme (goal or aim) and the specific outcomes for the individual (objectives). Carefully formulated objectives go beyond well-meaning good intentions, rather they enable the therapist to plan effectively by considering such important variables as the measurable achievement, the timescale and the input of the client and/or therapist. These elements can be succinctly described as the 'what, when and who' factors involved in effective objective-setting.[1] Naturally, objectives should be established in conjunction with the client and therefore need to be relevant to the individual and realistically attainable.

It is important at the objective-setting stage to clarify that outcomes do not simply mean attendance at a series of anxiety management sessions. Although comparatively straightforward to measure, diligent attendance does not auto-matically imply that real behavioural change has occurred. Motivation to attend and participate in anxiety management sessions is essential in the process of change, but achieving measurable outcomes requires the individual client to go beyond the 'classroom'; it means making changes in their everyday lives and actively demonstrating that they can apply new knowledge, skills and attitudes to novel situations. The way anxiety management is delivered, described as the 'outputs' of therapy, is important to monitor, but needs to be accountable to the end-results of intervention. A well-organised and efficiently implemented anxiety management programme consisting of eight sessions may account for resources, time and money, but unless achievable results can be clearly demonstrated, its ultimate effectiveness is unproven.

When setting objectives for individual clients, it may be helpful to be clear about the following distinctions:

- what are the outputs of the anxiety management programme? (in terms of number of sessions/hours of therapy)
- what processes are involved in the implementation of the programme? (from referral to the discharge of a client)
- what are the outcome measures of the programme that indicate its effectiveness and what is the most appropriate timescale? (the end of a session/end of a series of sessions/at a later follow-up period of a specified number of weeks or months)
- what is the overall purpose or aim of the programme?
- what are the specific objectives for each individual client and do these contain tangible parameters such as behavioural measures, a timescale, location and people involved.

Being this thorough at the initial stages of running an anxiety management programme may seem a little over-indulgent and perhaps frustrating to the enthusiastic therapist who is keen to implement new ideas. However, laying firm foundations for such a therapeutic programme makes good sense in the long term, ensuring that the programme's purpose and value are less vulnerable to cost-cutting exercises or the scrutiny of clinical audits.

Methods of evaluation

As anxiety is a multifactorial phenomenon with a variety of cognitive, physiological and social consequences, there are a range of assessment methods which may be appropriate. Each method has its relative strengths and drawbacks, and as previously discussed, generates data of differing types and levels. What follows is an overview of the different assessment methods with comments on their possible clinical usefulness.

Interview schedules

These may be either structured or unstructured, in relation to the explicit format of the interview and the specificity of the questions. Most commonly in use are semi-structured interviews, which offer the interviewing therapist a definite framework to follow but allow for relevant subjective details, making the process pertinent to the individual client. Although the interview is typically used to gather initial descriptive data, some schedules also require the therapist and/or client to rank or rate their degree of dysfunction, thus generating additional quantitative data.

Naturally, the interview offers the therapist all the obvious opportunities to initiate a therapeutic relationship with an individual client. Its particular strength is that it is an assessment process which allows the client to 'tell their story' and put across a personal perspective of the presenting problems. The particular pitfalls with interviews is that unless monitored, they can be time-consuming and unfocused, resulting in the client unloading every conceivable difficulty and not giving an adequate answer to the questions. The interviewing therapist may indeed collude in this process by allowing this to happen and not directing the client back to the task in hand at an appropriate juncture.

Although therapists may wish to design and utilise their own interview pro forma, this is a complex and time-consuming enterprise. It is more practical to use a well-established interview schedule and if it is not strictly relevant, adapt it according to the requirements of the client group and clinical setting. The drawback to adapting an existing assessment tool is that it may weaken its validity and reliability, so a fine balance is required between pragmatism and scientific rigour.

Given these considerations, using an unstructured approach in an interview may seem an attractive and less fraught option. The experienced therapist who has worked a lot with people who have clinical anxiety may have developed a highly intuitive instinct for what questions to ask a newly referred client, in order to establish the nature and degree of the presenting problems. However, the drawbacks here are that this process does not easily translate to baseline data that may inform the team management of the individual case. It is also a highly 'customised' approach to assessment and specific to the individual therapist who cannot always guarantee absolutely to be able to implement an anxiety management programme from beginning to end for every newly referred client. A more structured approach to interviewing not only ensures objectivity of results, but assists continuity of programme delivery.

Self-rating questionnaires

The advantage with questionnaires are that they are designed to be completed by the client, therefore enabling active participation in the assessment process. The type of data ultimately collected may vary from different levels of quantitative data (more closed questions) to eliciting subjective information (open questions), or may consist of a combination of these methods. Questionnaires are straightforward to administer and therefore can be an effective use of time, as well as yielding useful data from an individual or group.

Despite these attractive advantages, a questionnaire is only as good as its design: unclear instructions, a confusing and long-winded format and ambiguous questions do not assist the data-gathering process, no matter how well intentioned. In that respect, before using a questionnaire as a major part of an assessment repertoire, it is wise for the therapist to have personally 'road-tested' its suitability, or to have piloted it with a small group first.

Both interview schedules and questionnaires are widely used in the assessment of anxiety-related problems. In both procedures, self-ratings can be obtained concerning how anxiety in all its forms affects the individual's life. The use of a simple visual analog scale, e.g. a line calibrated from 0–10, can be quite effectively used to self-rate even complex aspects of anxiety. The frequency or degree of the cognitive, behavioural, physiological or social manifestation of anxiety can be recorded and monitored by the client and therapist in this way. For example, an analog scale may be used to record changes before and after relaxation training or to note homework progress.[2] Although this self-rating method is subjective and specific to the individual, in many cases it is a useful tool as it allows the client to reflect and 'own' their experience of anxiety and to be in charge of monitoring changes.

Observation techniques

Informal observation is a constant, ongoing process and part of the therapist's clinical toolkit of skills. The observant therapist is continually noting how an individual is behaving and responding to interventions, both on a one-to-one basis and in a group setting. The therapist's interpretation of a client's behaviour may develop into a hunch or impression which may provide a useful counterpoint to the more formalised assessment methods, and add to the richness of baseline data by reflecting the uniqueness of an individual client. Such intuitions, built on the therapist's observations, do need to be grounded and to be related to the broader assessment strategy in order to avoid unhelpful bias and misinterpretation.

More formal, structured observational methods of assessment can also provide useful data on the effects of therapeutic interventions. This entails a more systematic approach to observing and recording behaviours by requiring specific target behaviours to be identified. The process of identification involves a precise description of the behaviour to be monitored so that it can be effectively distinguished from other behaviours and reliably recorded by more than one therapist. The method of recording behaviours may vary in terms of timescale (in viva setting, one session or part of a session) and whether information on the frequency or duration of the behaviour is being elicited. To do justice to structured observational methods, the video-taping of a session or role-play may enable a more detailed analysis, though use of a two-way mirror and a non-participating observer can also be an effective way of gathering data.

Again, in order to benefit from the richness of observational data, the therapist needs to be clear which behaviours to target and why the information may be clinically useful. This can be greatly facilitated by selecting a comprehensive method of recording observations and being able to interpret the results in a meaningful way.[3] Although these more formalised observational methods can be initiated and started from 'scratch', it can entail a lot of groundwork and preliminary pilot studies in order to arrive at a system which operates smoothly. It is always an astute move to investigate fully what structured and standardised behavioural assessments tools are already in existence before embarking on the creative but time-consuming process of 're-inventing the wheel'.

Testing

This approach is often used to measure the physiological changes which occur in relation to the relaxation response. A variety of physiological 'markers' may be measured, such as pulse and respiration rates, blood pressure, muscle tension and skin temperature or electrodermal activity. One or several of these variables are measured pre and post relaxation (per session or per series of sessions) and record the individual's arousal levels. If relaxation training has been effective, then the measures should record a decline in arousal levels and present a graphic illustration of physiological changes as a result of intervention. The greater number of modalities measured, the more accurate and sensitive the results are likely to be, appropriately reflecting each client's individualised and often idiosyncratic response to stress and relaxation.

The measuring of such tangible physiological variables can often be a very useful part of an assessment repertoire. Some clients who may feel overwhelmed by anxiety and powerless to effect any change can respond positively to this kind of monitoring and feedback. Making a small but significant start in coping with clinical anxiety may be symbolised by the client learning and practising a relaxation technique which has a demonstrable effect on their physiological arousal levels. The drawbacks for the therapist are that the measuring of such physiological variables may require specialist equipment which can be expensive and time-consuming to set up and operate efficiently.

Although the measurement of physiological variables can provide what appears to be clear and objective data, in reality the therapist has to be circumspect regarding both the reliability and validity of any results. For example, the individual's arousal level in a relaxation session could be influenced by external factors such as the time of day, an upsetting confrontation earlier in the week or what they had for lunch. Although under test conditions the objective assessor would endeavour to account for and exclude the effects of such external factors and to provide a uniform relaxation environment, it is clearly impossible to screen out every idiosyncratic variable which may influence results.

The size and meaning of the results may also be relative and need to be seen in a context and not as a pure indicator of a 'success' or 'failure'. This relates to the 'law of initial values' which has already been discussed in Chapter 2. For example, if a client is extremely anxious prior to starting relaxation training, a drop in arousal levels may be apparent but may not be numerically significant enough to indicate the effects of relaxation. On the other hand, if a client is already reasonably relaxed, only a small reduction in arousal may be demonstrated. However, this small change may represent a more meaningful

and significant level of relaxation than the larger reduction shown by the more anxious client. Finally, we cannot assume that arousal reductions are due to the relaxation training; they could be attributable to the effects of time and habituation.[2]

As with the other assessment methods we have discussed, it is evident that no one method has any sort of superiority in terms of ease of use or clinical usefulness. Each method, if it is to be used effectively, needs to be clearly appraised for its relative strengths and limitations, and ultimately selected on an informed basis by the therapist and/or the team. Despite the pitfalls of physiological testing, it is worth remembering that it may be the physical symptoms of anxiety which can often be the most salient and distressing features for the client. It may be hyperventilation or tension headaches which initially caused the client to seek help, therefore the very real physiological consequences of anxiety need to be acknowledged and addressed in the data-collection process.

LEVELS OF CHANGE

Another factor to consider when selecting relevant assessment methods is the level of change being targeted by the therapeutic intervention. The notion of 'change' pervades the ethos and delivery of all psychological interventions and resides in the fundamental difference between a 'cure' (cessation of the disease process) and a therapeutic effect (a shift in a person's self-awareness and altered lifestyle). Consequently, the concept of change is difficult to define precisely, as it depends on the individual and the amount, durability and type of change being anticipated.

Targeting levels of change in anxiety management may be dictated to some extent by the prevailing model or theories of stress used to underpin the programme's philosophy and subsequent delivery. Some models represent stress as a cause and effect response, whereas other models see stress as an all-encompassing phenomenon. These differing views of stress ultimately influence the way the person with clinical anxiety is perceived and assessed. The prevailing model of stress will also provide an explanation of what particular stress management techniques are effective therapy and why they may work. The crux here is that the therapist needs to be well aware of the preferred model of stress used to guide and inform the anxiety management programme being proposed. This process of clarifying the theoretical foundations could be affected by the dominant theories used by other team members or the particular frame of reference used by the unit or department. In both cases, the therapist needs to determine that the levels of change being targeted for therapeutic intervention are compatible with personal and professional goals.

Micro-levels of change

Micro-levels of change really focus on the symptoms of clinical anxiety. In order to ascertain whether change has occurred at this level, measurement and recording of presenting symptoms is required so that symptom reduction can be effectively demonstrated. Change at this level is usually construed as the reduction or lessening of particular physiological manifestations, such as fewer tension headaches, less frequent panic attacks or less muscular discomfort. Gaining ground over these small constituents of the larger clinical picture of anxiety may indeed be the very goal a client wishes to achieve; it can therefore help them feel a sense of mastery over their problems.

Macro-levels of change

These are the more global aspects of change, and may incorporate the view that environmental factors need to be modified if clinical anxiety is to be fully addressed. This could entail considering a person's work environment and encompass the health-promotion strategies that a company or workplace follows for its employees. A more feasible focus might be improving the individual's quality of life and facilitating a better understanding of the role anxiety has played in family and personal relationships. At this level of change, symptom reduction may not be the primary focus, or indeed the result of therapeutic intervention, but the client's ability to recognise and anticipate the causes and effects of stress may lead to a more positive reframing of the clinical problem. Although the symptoms of clinical anxiety may still persist, the client may feel more able to cope and make full use of support networks and self-help strategies.

Timescale of change

This is acknowledging that the point at which the therapist decides change has occurred can be significant and vary according to the aims and goals of the particular anxiety management programme. For example, one interpretation of change is to monitor session-by-session change.[4] The value of evaluating the session impact of an anxiety management programme is that it can give the therapist useful immediate feedback and can be more precisely monitored than post-intervention follow ups after several months.

Stiles, in 1980,[5] devised criteria for evaluating session impact which consisted of session depth (value to client), session smoothness (degree of psychological comfort for the client) and positivity (post-session mood of client). If carried out consistently and comprehensively with clients on a session-by-session basis, this sort of approach would generate a considerable amount of useful data on the relative effectiveness of a programme's design and delivery.

An alternative strategy is to evaluate change after the completion of the programme and during the last session in the series. This enables clients to reflect what they have achieved over the weeks and to acknowledge that mastery of certain techniques, such as relaxation, have taken place. Although this appears to be an obvious point at which to evaluate change, it can also be deceptive. Evaluating change in the context of a supportive and familiar group environment may indicate immediate gains, but may not be a realistic indication of the client's ability to utilise coping skills on a regular daily basis.

Post-intervention change is a strategy for

recording change weeks or months after the anxiety management programme has ended. This gives a clearer picture of what stress management techniques the client is habitually using and what level of improvement has been maintained over time. This particular time perspective certainly gives the client, programme organisers and purchasing agencies hard proof of clinical effectiveness, but again has some inherent difficulties. Firstly, the logistics of organising individual follow-up appointments can be time-consuming and may not always guarantee attendance and client cooperation. Secondly, it cannot always be demonstrated that any evident changes in behaviour are exclusively attributable to the anxiety management programme, but could be due to a combination of factors which may be hard to unravel.

Non-specific factors influencing change

As indicated above, there may be other non-specific factors that contribute to a client's change of behaviour which can cloud the clarity of the evaluation process. The most apparent non-specific factors that influence changes in behaviour are the availability of group support and the opportunity for clients to meet others with similar problems. The therapeutic value of sharing experiences with others and feeling understood is not to be underestimated, as a client with anxiety may have become increasingly socially isolated and withdrawn.

Though difficult to arrange or to evaluate deliberately, the therapist can certainly enhance the interpersonal opportunities within a programme. Clients could be encouraged to 'pair up', for example, and to keep in touch between sessions. Any genuine friendships that develop could help clients to continue practising stress management techniques in their own time as useful homework. These informal social networks grow according to how the group is facilitated. If the therapist facilitates group cooperation and mutual trust at the beginning of a programme, it is more likely there will be a safer and more cohesive group climate.

FROM EVALUATION TO APPLIED RESEARCH

Diligent and systematic evaluation procedures can pave the way for the therapist to embark on more applied research. Unless the anxiety management programme has well-established assessment and evaluation strategies, then applied research may seem more like a quantum leap into the unknown rather than a natural progression of clinical reasoning. Applied research is essentially about critical enquiry within a clinical or work setting, not a laboratory, and seeks to address issues which help to develop good practice.

In addition, good research in the field of anxiety management and within the health care professions is all too scarce. Sound applied research is needed to improve and validate methods and techniques to demonstrate their effectiveness clearly. Although anecdotal and descriptive case study material has its uses and is a starting point, the hallmark of quality applied research is that it generates results that makes us scrutinise current practice with an objective eye.

Identifying a research question

The first step in the process is to identify the research question. This requires the therapist to be extremely precise and specific about the focus of the study, and to keep the proposed research within realistic parameters. Small-scale research projects may seem less glamorous and exciting than their more ambitious counterparts, but the scale of a study can be so overwhelming and unruly that any meaningful results may not be apparent or may simply get lost in the organisational complexities.

The research question may stem from an issue highlighted by the evaluation process and may be a way of systematically investigating the phenomenon further. It can be helpful at this stage to brainstorm around the subject in order to leave no intellectual stone unturned. This could be a collective exercise involving colleagues and co-therapists, and requires basic assumptions to be checked out thoroughly. You may ask yourself:

- what is the problem?
- when does it occur?
- where does it occur?
- who is affected?
- how does it occur?
- why does it occur?

The more time that is devoted to this stage, the better. This 'problem-setting' stage is crucial to focused applied research. There can be a tendency to select data-collection methods and to proceed with the practicalities so rapidly that any subsequent results fail adequately to address the initial research question.

If embarking on applied research in the clinical context, the therapist also needs honestly to appraise the practical considerations. This is where well-designed, small-scale projects triumph, as they make more realistic demands on time and resources. Ask yourself the following questions:

- can I work collaboratively with another colleague?
- what support will I get from my manager / department / service?
- what time do I have available?
- are there any deadlines to meet?
- what additional resources will I need?
- will I have any funding to help towards costs such as buying needed equipment / materials?
- do I need to get formal approval from my department / hospital? (e.g. ethics committees)
- where and how will I present my results?

All of the above questions are more easily answered if you have clarified your research question, so that you have a well-informed idea of how your project will take shape. In order to avoid the danger of 're-inventing the wheel', a thorough and comprehensive literature search is essential. This provides the researcher with a detailed background on what aspects of anxiety management have been researched before and what methods have been used. Careful reading of the discussion sections in particular may give useful insights into how to design your particular project and the pitfalls to avoid. In some cases, you may feel it is appropriate to replicate a study in your own clinical setting or to build on a previous study by acting on the stated indications for future research.

Designing a research project

Once sufficient time and energies have been devoted to exploring the feasibility of a research project, the next stage is to clarify the various components of the intended research. Even a clearly articulated research question does not automatically ensure a robust set of results unless the whole design is fully considered. This entails selecting the most appropriate data-collection method and devising a systematic way of conducting the research that is consistently impartial and objective. The following aspects require particular consideration:

- formulating the research question — this needs to be precise and unambiguous
- identifying the aims of the project — a few well-focused goals that are realistic and achievable
- acknowledging the limitations of the project — recognising that practical constraints exist and allowing for these in the research design
- identifying the target population and selecting a research sample — this will need to include precise inclusion and exclusion criteria, viable numbers and the method of selection
- devising an appropriate research methodology — this may need to include the piloting of a questionnaire or test in order to ensure valid and reliable results
- deciding on the most appropriate way of analysing results — this is to make sure that your findings can be interpreted into meaningful conclusions
- completing the research cycle — returning to your original research question to see if it is now possible to generate answers or whether further investigations are needed.

Following through the research cycle does enable the research project to retain some sort of momentum without getting too drawn out or side-tracked. This also helps to keep the researcher's own motivation and enthusiasm for the project at maximum levels, as it is easy to get frustrated by set-backs and disillusioned by the amount of time it takes to complete the various stages satisfactorily.

Another important consideration is whether the proposed study requires a control group in order to produce valid and reliable results. In the pure terms of empirical science, this means that any results can be compared with a cohort of subjects who were not exposed to whatever intervention was implemented with the identified experimental group. The opportunity to compare the effects more clearly differentiates the intervention as the change-producing agent and that any therapeutic effect is not merely a random occurrence.

This sort of scientific rigour is to be commended and can work in settings where variables can be strictly monitored and controlled. Devising a project that requires a control group works less well in a clinical setting and with interventions involving people, not laboratory rats! As suggested previously, working with human subjects requires the researcher to be mindful of the many subjective, idiosyncratic variables that may influence outcomes. A good number of these variables would be impossible to screen out of the research process if based in a clinical setting. Even the most diligent of researchers would be hard pressed to ensure a completely water-tight and empirically valid experimental and control group outside a laboratory setting.

The answer to these research dilemmas can rest in choosing a more 'quasi' form of experimental research or using a more subjective, qualitative approach. In busy clinical settings, one option for a control group is to utilise the people on the waiting list as research subjects. This can be a successful and more ethically acceptable way of validating results and effectively demonstrating that therapeutic change has not been an ad hoc, incidental event.

Types of evaluative research

Although it is not the intention of this chapter to discuss in detail the different types of research, a starting point may be that most therapists have a vested interest in evaluative research in particular. Robson[6] defined evaluation as 'an attempt to assess the worth or value of some innovation or intervention, some service or approach'. Most therapists delivering anxiety management programmes would probably recognise their own aspirations in that definition, though the impetus may vary from the demands of professional accountability, the requirements of clinical audit or the genuine desire to give an improved service to clients.

Robson also described evaluative research as being either formative or summative.[6] Formative evaluations are an effective way of helping the development of a programme and to identify possible modifications. Summative evaluations assess the overall impact of an intervention by appraising its effectiveness. Although summative evaluations may seem the more natural choice, formative evaluations can play a part in matching the most appropriate anxiety management strategy for an individual client or group. It can be disheartening for the conscientious therapist to complete a summative evaluation of an anxiety management group that has not been particularly effective when a formative evaluation may have highlighted options that could have minimised later difficulties.

Future research directions

At present, research into anxiety management is just beginning to gather momentum. The questions that still need to be addressed include the extent of change brought about by therapeutic interventions and how these changes occur. Particularly, how change can be maintained over time and successfully generalised to a client's everyday life once the support and learning opportunities provided by regular attendance at an anxiety management group have stopped. Current research practices are becoming increasingly mindful of producing hard empirical evidence of change as well as striving for meaningful clinical outcomes for clients.

The following ideas for further research on anxiety management are offered as a way of indicating the scope of future research:

- comparative studies of different methods of relaxation training
- the therapeutic value of the different component parts of an anxiety management programme
- the correlation between attendance at anxiety management groups and outcomes
- the effect homework assignments have on outcomes
- the development of an assessment tool to evaluate the impact anxiety has in the performance of daily living tasks
- the correlation between the number of sessions and the learning curve of the individual client or group
- the generalisation of stress management techniques and the optimum time for a follow-up or 'top-up' session.

CONCLUSION

There is little doubt that working to help clients overcome often very disabling anxiety is a richly rewarding field of clinical practice. The ability to empower individuals to conquer their psychological fears and physical symptoms lies at the heart of good practice. Perhaps somewhat overlooked in the devising and delivery of anxiety management programmes are the needs and strengths of the therapist — as a group leader, as a role model and as a human being. The phenomenon of stress can pervade everyone's life, although how we choose to perceive and cope with it makes a palpable difference. Supportive measures such as co-leadership or regular supervision are essential ingredients in providing an effective service, and the need for them is a professional reality not a personal frailty.

REFERENCES

1 Whalley-Hammell K R 1994 Establishing objectives in occupational therapy practice. British Journal of Occupational Therapy 57, 1 & 2: 9–13, 45–48
2 Keable D 1989 The management of anxiety. Churchill Livingstone, Edinburgh
3 Martin P, Bateson P 1993 Measuring behaviour, 2nd edn. Cambridge University Press, Cambridge
4 Reynolds S, Taylor E, Shapiro D A 1993 Session impact in stress management training. Journal of Occupational and Organisational Psychology 66(2):99–113
5 Stiles W B 1980 Measurement of the impact of psychotherapy sessions. Journal of Consulting and Clinical Psychology 48:176–185
6 Robson C 1993 Real world research. Blackwell, Oxford, p 171

FURTHER READING

Bailey D M 1991 Research for the health professional. F.A. Davis, Philadelphia
Clegg F 1982 Simple statistics: a course book for the social sciences. Cambridge University Press, Cambridge
Ottenbacher K J 1986 Evaluating clinical change: strategies for occupational and physical therapists. Williams and Wilkins, Baltimore
Payton O D 1994 Research: the validation of clinical practice, 3rd edn. F.A. Davis, Philadelphia
Robson C 1993 Real world research. Blackwell, Oxford

Examples of Assessments
Hassles and Uplifts Scale
Kanner, Coyne, Schaefer, Lazarus 1981
Self-report questionnaire using a 4 point scale. Hassles and uplifts scale. NFER-Nelson
Timescale: within the last month
Data: frequency and severity
117 hassle items
135 uplift items

May be time-consuming to complete but can yield useful information. Hassles scale provides information on the frequency and severity of daily stressful events (not major life events) which may be underestimated, yet can accumulate and prove anxiety-provoking. The Uplifts scale could be used in health promotion and 'stress proofing' strategies.

Clinical Anxiety Scale (CAS)
Smith, Bough, Gayden, Hussain, Sipple 1982 Clinical anxiety scale (CAS). NFER-Nelson,
Rating scale using 5 point scale
Timescale: within past 2 days
Data: intensity and severity
6 items plus a panic attack rating scale
Comprehensive and relatively concise assessment, though a little wordy. Can be used to collect baseline data and provide outcome measures.

Fear Questionnaire
Marks, Matthews 1979 Fear Questionnaire. NFER-Nelson,

Self-report questionnaire using a 9 point scale
Timescale: non-specific
Data: intensity and severity
20 items plus 2 items allowing client to identify most feared/other situation not included in questionnaire.
Short one-sided A4 questionnaire that is quick to complete. Generates a global phobic score and is chiefly targeted at those with agoraphobia, social phobia and blood-injury phobia. Useful for baseline assessment and outcome measurement.

Mobility Inventory for Agoraphobia
Chambless, Capito, Jasin, Gracely, Williams 1985 Mobility inventory for agoraphohia. NFER-Nelson,
Self report questionnaire using a 5 point scale

Timescale: non-specific
Data: frequency and severity
One question asks for total number of panic attacks in last 7 days to be recorded
29 items organised into 5 categories
Asks client to assess severity of avoidance behaviour and to differentiate between when accompanied and when alone. Client required to select the 5 most anxiety-provoking situations out of those identified in questionnaire. Estimated 20 minutes to complete. Useful for baseline assessment and outcome measurement.

14

Teaching resources

Diana Keable

CLINICAL GUIDELINES

CHOOSING THE RIGHT TECHNIQUE

The main considerations that the therapist will usually need to take into account are:

- how effective is the technique?
- how appropriate is the technique for the client/client group in question?
- what are the contraindications?

Technique effectiveness

Unfortunately, regarding the first question, there is no easy answer. Insufficient evidence exists to suggest that any one technique is clearly superior to another.[1,2] This is despite the fact that a number of comparative research studies have been carried out in an attempt to resolve this issue. The lack of conclusive evidence may be partly due to the complex difficulties which beset clinical research in this field. What we do know is that relaxation training in general is an effective and safe treatment for anxiety disorders, especially in view of the attendant difficulties with anxiolytic drugs.[3,4,5] It is now widely accepted that minor tranquillisers are not only of limited effectiveness in the long term, but may also cause serious psychological and chemical-dependency problems. However, traditional relaxation training has shown disappointing long-term effects, possibly because clients do not persist in practising the technique, or because the technique fails to tackle the cognitive and behavioural elements of anxiety.[5] By comparison, the few available studies of the new comprehensive anxiety management regimes have shown more consistently promising results.[2,6,7,8] These findings are not surprising since AMT programmes adopt a more thorough-going approach, tackling application as well as skills training. They also deal with the symptomatology of anxiety more comprehensively by targeting physical, mental and behavioural aspects. However, a full anxiety management programme may not always be indicated or possible in every clinical situation. Issues concerning the comparative effectiveness of techniques are discussed further in Chapters 7–10.

Technique suitability

As far as individual techniques are concerned, there is now some evidence that techniques should be selected according to specific problems.[2,9] Thus, the therapist must decide which technique has the most appropriate 'fit' for each individual. For example, phobic clients, or those with highly specific fears, may be helped more by a systematic programme of exposure to the phobic object than by anxiety management. The reverse case is equally true — systematic desensitisation has little relevance for those with generalised anxiety. Some clients emphasise their distressing physical symptoms, others are more concerned with worries and unpleasant anxious thoughts. Identifying the key systems which support the total anxiety reaction will help to indicate which technique/s to use. Also, both physical and mental anxiety may affect behaviour adversely, and are commonly associated with avoidance. The technique selected should also tackle the anxiety-related behaviour pattern involved. Chapters 7–10 consider further the issues concerning technique suitability.

As mentioned previously, not all clients are able to cope with ambitious anxiety-reduction programmes. In many cases, if a client is subjected to a regime that is too high powered, this will do more harm than good and reinforce a sense of failure. In choosing which technique is appropriate for each client one simple guideline is helpful:

the technique should fit the client's needs, and not the other way around. Clients inevitably demonstrate idiosyncrasies that may force the therapist to teach a technique which, for theoretical reasons, he or she may consider inferior. Personal preferences should also be taken into account when choosing the right technique for a client. If the therapist is conversant with a selection of methods, and able to teach them effectively, his or her clients will be able to make an informed choice about the method which best suits their individual needs.

Contraindications

Concerning contraindications, it should be noted that relaxation training may not always be an innocuous treatment, despite the fact that neither drugs, nor psychoanalytical elements are usually involved.[10] One of the major problems concerns the use of relaxation techniques with psychotic clients.[11,12] Although relaxation training can be used with psychotic clients, it is not advisable to include those demonstrating florid symptoms, or while in an acute phase of the illness. Clients who are in the grip of an acutely disturbed state are unlikely to be able to benefit from formal relaxation training and some may be adversely affected by it. This is because many relaxation methods, particularly those which demand some degree of visualisation, may serve to aggravate symptoms in clients who are unable to distinguish reality from fantasy. Further, the intimate nature of the relaxation session may, for psychodynamic reasons, prove distressing to some extremely withdrawn clients.

Once acute psychotic symptoms have settled down, the use of a structured approach focusing on behavioural activities is to be recommended, e.g. active or differential relaxation and physical exercise. It is certainly wise to avoid techniques involving imagery, such as guided fantasy journeys. Nonetheless, residual anxiety can become the major feature in an otherwise well-controlled clinical picture for many schizophrenic clients.[13] The existence of persistent low-grade anxiety may render affected clients vulnerable to breakdown when subjected to very small amounts of stress. It is, therefore, essential that an attempt is made to provide appropriate anxiety-reduction treatment for this group, and appropriately adapted AMT can be used very successfully with psychotic clients.[14]

A recent trend has developed towards working more directly on challenging psychotic delusional belief systems using cognitive therapy.[15] This is highly skilled work, usually requiring specialist training. Such an approach would rarely be attempted in the general context of an AMT course.

DECIDING ON SESSION LENGTH AND FREQUENCY

Individual sessions may comprise several components:

- a short introductory section
- an educational section
- practice of relaxation, or other technique
- a concluding feedback section.

The relaxation practice portion should usually only take up about 20–30 minutes of the session, which is also a realistic length of time for client's home practice sessions. Following this structure, the complete session need only last for around one hour. More extended sessions may be required for anxiety management courses to give sufficient time to cover the educational material and practise the techniques.

Expecting clients to practise relaxation solidly for a whole hour at a time is unlikely to be therapeutic. Concentration is bound to wander, and clients may lose sight of the aims of the session. Some clients may fall asleep and others may experience an increased level of anxiety during overlong sessions. It should be borne in mind that the major aim is to train the client to reach the relaxed state within progressively shorter periods of time. When clients are facing stressful situations outside the session, e.g. coping in a crowded supermarket, they will usually be unable to stop and spend an hour relaxing!

Regarding frequency, although it is often only feasible to hold teaching sessions once weekly, clients should practise on their own at least once

daily. This structure allows for consolidation of learning between one session and the next and helps to avoid the creation of dependence on the therapist. For client's home practice, several short sessions each day may be a better arrangement than one long one. Wilson[16] has also recommended short and frequent relaxation practice sessions for use in the long-term psychiatric setting.

CORRECT POSITIONING FOR RELAXATION PRACTICE

The three positions for relaxation described by Mitchell[17] are highly recommended. These are:

1. Lying supine with a small cushion or pad under the head. This position can be made blissfully comfortable by placing additional pillows under the knees and elbows. This arrangement is exceptionally supportive and helps to promote relaxation before the exercises have even started! However, it is preferable to use the floor rather than a soft bed or mattress, to discourage falling asleep.

2. Sitting upright on a supportive chair. The chair should have a head-rest if possible, but if not, the chair can be pushed up against a wall. Arm-rests are also useful to support the wrists; otherwise the wrists may be rested on the lap. The knee joints should be at right angles with the feet flat on the floor.

3. Sitting at a desk or table with a pillow on top of the desk. The client then relaxes head and arms forward onto the pillow. Again, the knee joints should be at right angles and the feet flat on the floor.

These positions are illustrated in Figure 14.1.

During teaching sessions clients can be encouraged to experiment with each position until they find the one that works best for their individual needs. Positions used should also be varied according to the situation in which practice is carried out, and according to individual requirements. For a client experiencing sleep difficulties, the supine position may be the most advantageous. For clients who are experiencing stress at work or study, the desk-top position may be

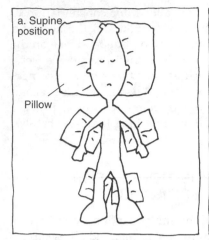
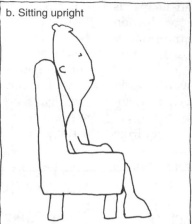
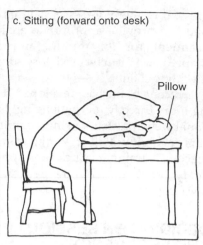

Figure 14.1 Positioning for relaxation practice.

indicated. This is always assuming, of course, that sufficient privacy can be ensured.

However, clients must eventually learn to relax in many different positions during daily life, as well as in stressful situations. Differential relaxation addresses this need, and encourages clients to keep tension down to the minimum necessary for carrying out everyday tasks. For this reason, clients should be discouraged from practising relaxation in only one position. Differential relaxation is described in Chapter 12.

PREPARING CLIENTS FOR RELAXATION

Clients who are new to relaxation techniques benefit greatly from a careful introduction before the treatment begins. The introductory facts may be presented either as part of an initial interview or in the form of a simple handout — preferably in both forms. The more accurate the clients' expectations of treatment are, the more likely they will be to accept the therapy and benefit from it.

Introductory remarks to the actual session itself should be designed to set the scene for the educative information to follow as well as rehearsal of the techniques themselves. If the session is the first of a series, it is helpful to introduce the group members and encourage sharing of common problems in a fairly neutral way, e.g. a group brainstorming exercise. Subsequent sessions can begin with feedback on their independent practice, discussing problems and reinforcing successes.

Before the relaxation practice portion of the session, the following points should be communicated:

1. The correct positioning for the exercise (which was described in the previous section).

2. Preparation of clothing if appropriate, e.g. loosening of restrictive waistbands or collars, discarding of shoes and spectacles.

3. Explanation that as this is a teaching session, it is important for clients to stay awake. It is best to warn clients before relaxation starts that should they inadvertently fall asleep, the therapist will lightly tap them on the arm or foot.

4. Requesting clients to be silent during the exercises. Should anyone wish to attract the therapist's attention for some important reason they should quietly raise their arm.

5. Encouraging clients to adopt a passive attitude towards extraneous noise or interruptions. The author usually does this by asking clients to: 'allow any noises simply to be there, and don't try to fight them; but do tell yourself that you are not going to let any noises disturb your relaxation'.

6. Allow clients a few moments to settle down before the relaxation exercises begin. It is helpful to encourage clients to clear their minds of current pre-occupations — perhaps by imagining leaving these in a pile outside the room while they are relaxing. During this initial period clients should focus their attention upon bodily sensations, like the rhythms of breathing.

However, when appropriate, it can be beneficial to lead the group in some gentle loosening-up exercises prior to relaxation, such as those described in Chapter 12. Exercises are particularly useful for excessively restless clients in order to help drain off excess tension.

PRESENTATION OF RELAXATION INSTRUCTIONS

Firstly, many people assume that the successful relaxation therapist is one who has the ability to soothe clients to sleep using soft and gentle monotones! It is true that some methods do still recommend this style of presentation and specific styles of vocalisation are certainly important in hypnosis. However, in the author's opinion this is quite unnecessary in the anxiety management or relaxation training context. After all, we do not want to risk encouraging clients to become dependent on the therapist's soft soothing voice in order to relax — and many clients do so only too readily! Laura Mitchell has mentioned this issue in connection with her simple relaxation method.[17] She recommends a fairly brisk delivery of the instructions or 'orders'. In any event, for most relaxation techniques, normal tone and volume should be quite acceptable for the delivery of relaxation instructions.

Secondly, how long should the therapist pause between each separate instruction? There are two possible pitfalls. If pauses are too short this will not allow sufficient time for clients to focus upon each movement and to absorb the sensory feedback which results. This, of course, is an essential part of learning the skill of relaxation. A tendency to rush the pauses may occur if the therapist is tense or has allowed insufficient time for this part of the session. On the other hand, overly protracted pauses may result in clients falling asleep or losing their concentration on the activity. Thus, it is important to achieve an optimum timing for pauses between instructions and the use of a watch can help to monitor the pace of delivery.

Thirdly, for the sake of standardisation, and particularly for research applications, it is important to stick fairly rigidly to the given procedure and phraseology for each technique. These have usually been carefully worked out to be consistent with the rationale of the technique. For instance, many techniques suggest phrases to facilitate the recognition of relaxation which are an integral part of the technique. However, while some techniques suggest giving each instruction twice, as treatment progresses it may only be necessary to give each instruction once.

Finally, the therapist need not remain in one spot during the session. It is entirely in order to move around observing and quietly correcting client's positions and movements throughout the session. After all, the main aim of the session is to *teach* relaxation, and this is of necessity an active process.

FEEDBACK AND DISCUSSION TIMES

It has already been suggested that each relaxation or anxiety management session should contain a section devoted to discussion and, in particular, client feedback on personal progress in skill learning. The feedback part of the session allows for the exchange of vital information between clients and the therapist. Through feedback the therapist may monitor progress and pick up individual difficulties. These can be used as teaching points in the group, and misconceptions can be clarified immediately. Additionally, if the importance of feedback is emphasised and clients are made aware that they will be asked to report back on their progress, this is likely to have a motivating effect.

However, it is important that feedback or discussion times are handled as constructively as possible and this is not always an easy task.

The following problems commonly arise:

- some clients may tend to dominate the discussion while others may be unforthcoming
- some groups may be largely unresponsive and depend too much on the therapist to prompt discussion
- some groups may tend to use the time to bring up irrelevant material or discuss personal symptoms at length.

It is assumed that most therapists in the psychiatric setting will be conversant with issues relating to group dynamics, and will have experience in applying the necessary skills. Consequently, only a few general points will be made here which relate to this particular kind of group work.

Relaxation training and anxiety management are based on teaching models, so these may require a more directive approach from the therapist than is usual in group therapy settings. If a group is experiencing difficulty in participating in the discussion, its members may require initial prompting from the therapist. The therapist may use his or her own observations of individual client's progress during the session, noting obvious signs of tension or relaxation and feeding these back. It may be helpful to ask open questions like: 'How did everyone find the session this time?' Or questions inviting individual difficulties: 'Did anyone find they didn't relax at all this time?' The therapist may have to work quite hard in the early stages of the group's life to build up trust, rapport and cohesion. However, the therapist should avoid dominating the group so that its members are prevented from discovering, and building on, their own potential to help themselves and each other. It may take great skill on the therapist's part to avoid being forced into taking too much responsibility to lead discussion. One useful way of facilitating more group participation is to encourage members to comment on, and share in, each other's problems by making suggestions and providing support.

On the other hand, while discussion must be encouraged it should be limited, tactfully but firmly, to pre-set time boundaries. This is especially important for groups containing members who attempt to dominate the discussion. In these cases, much of the material brought up is likely to be neither constructive nor relevant. It is helpful to keep in mind not only the aims of the treatment programme as a whole, but also those of each session in order to ensure that they are achieved within the time allotted. The therapist may need to remind the group of these objectives from time to time.

While therapists should obviously endeavour to be well-informed in their 'teaching' role, clients may ask legitimate questions, or raise problems, for which the therapist has no immediate or adequate answer or solution. It is perfectly acceptable to acknowledge this honestly and this is certainly a better policy than attempting to 'fob clients off' with vague, confusing, inaccurate or inadequate answers. Such a response would only serve to detract from treatment credibility and, consequently, treatment efficacy. Often, the required information can be followed up and supplied at the next session. Alternatively, group members may themselves be able to make useful suggestions and should be encouraged to do so.

HELPING CLIENTS TO RECOGNISE AND CHALLENGE PATTERNS OF THOUGHT WHICH INCREASE OR MAINTAIN ANXIETY

Background

Briefly, the cognitive model of anxiety describes two major types of disturbed thinking which characterise and maintain anxiety disorders. These are:

- negative automatic thoughts (NATs)
- dysfunctional assumptions (DAs)

NATs involve stereotypical and undermining thoughts such as 'I can't cope'/'everyone thinks I'm stupid'. DAs are similar to irrational beliefs as described by Ellis.[18] They refer to general rules or beliefs which predispose the individual to perceive and respond to situations maladaptively. Ellis argued that it is the way we respond to events, rather than the events themselves, that is responsible for the distress, anxiety or depressive responses experienced. Beck[19] pointed out that anxiety disorders are fuelled by a preponderance of danger-related ideation, where the level of threat inherent in a situation is consistently over-estimated. Thus, the cognitive behaviour therapy approach to anxiety has three main phases.

Phase one: Assisting clients to recognise their own faulty thinking patterns and understand how these contribute to the maintenance of anxiety symptoms.

Phase two: Teaching ways of modifying and challenging anxious thinking patterns/beliefs.

Phase three: Reducing maladaptive behaviour which reinforces anxiety, e.g. avoidance, and reinstating adaptive, positive goal-orientated behaviour.

Presentation

Some simple ways of presenting ideas concerning negative and irrational thinking can be found in Client Pack 4 in the Appendix. Checklists of typical anxious thoughts and beliefs together with ways of challenging them are given in pages 138–139 of this chapter. However, it should be acknowledged that these concepts are frequently the most difficult for clients to digest both emotionally and intellectually. Giving clear information about anxiety and how it is supported by negative/irrational thinking styles is indispensable. In order for this approach to be successful, clients must not merely recognise the relationship between cognition and anxiety in general, but identify specific examples that apply in their own case. The treatment process also involves teaching the client to question and challenge their faulty cognitions, and then to develop more positive and realistic styles and strategies to manage associated anxiety such as distraction.[20]

The final stage involves putting this into practice through the use of goal-setting procedures, so that the client tackles progressively stressful situations using the new cognitive strategies. Some additional techniques, suitable for group and individual settings, which may be used to facilitate this process include:

- self-rating scales
- thought diaries
- brainstorming sessions
- group discussion
- imagery/visualisation of anxiety-provoking scenarios
- role-play
- check-lists of typical anxious thought patterns/irrational beliefs
- recounting recent stressful experience and associated ideation.[20]

DECIDING WHEN TO DISCONTINUE TREATMENT

This is frequently a difficult decision. It is rarely realistic to expect 'total cures', and indeed such dramatic changes scarcely ever happen in the clinical setting. Clients with severe anxiety disorders are often left with some residual problems at the end of any course of treatment. It may, or may not, be reasonable to continue treating these, according to the circumstances in question.

One of the ways in which this apparently messy situation can be clarified is through the setting up of realistic aims prior to treatment. These aims should be based as closely as possible on the anxiety-related problems of which the client is complaining. Often clients present their problems in a vague and woolly manner and need help to define the difficulties clearly. For example, perhaps the client is saying that he 'feels bad when he is in social situations'. It should be ascertained exactly what 'feeling bad' means, in physical, cognitive or subjective terms, and in precisely which social situations. Having done this, clear objectives which specify the nature of the change required, whether behavioural, cognitive or physical, can be drawn up.

Once treatment begins, objective means of monitoring the progress of treatment and measuring its ultimate outcome are required. Various self-rating scales, evaluation tools and assessment procedures may be needed for this task (see Chapter 13). One advantage of objective measurement of change is that the decision to terminate treatment can be based upon sound evidence rather than subjective opinion. Having set up clear, realistic goals and assessed treatment outcome objectively, the decision to discontinue treatment is made easier. The client may fit into one of the following categories:

- none, or unacceptably few, of the aims set before treatment have been achieved
- all, or most, of the aims set before treatment have been achieved
- there has been a consistent failure to attend treatment sessions or complete the homework assignments set at an acceptable rate/level.

Of course, what is acceptable and what is not can also be defined with the client beforehand. Effort spent in the initial stages to engage the client as a partner in the treatment process will pay particular dividends in this respect. However, in each of the cases outlined above, the indication is that treatment should no longer continue, at least, not in its present form. There are many situations when terminating treatment is a positive thing to do, although some therapists may sometimes be reluctant to do so because it seems punitive. However, allowing clients to continue receiving treatment they no longer need may be positively damaging and militate against the development of independence. Allowing clients to continue in a treatment they are not benefiting from is also counter-productive and a waste of time. Similarly, if clients either fail to attend or otherwise fulfil their obligations towards treatment, this also indicates that it should stop.

Some clients may contend that they are still benefiting from relaxation, whilst from the therapist's observations this is not the case. However, it is not helpful to allow clients to 'coast' through treatment. Obviously, clients will differ in their speeds of learning and the length of training should be carefully matched to meet varying needs. Some clients may simply need more time to reach the goals of treatment.

Finally, there is ample evidence that learning continues long after treatment has ceased.[21] This highlights the need for long-term follow-up assessment procedures.

MAINTENANCE AND RELAPSE PREVENTION

Towards the conclusion of treatment the control and focus of treatment should gradually transfer from the therapist to the client. Follow-up sessions are an ideal setting for this process and function as a point of contact for clients to report back on their progress. The therapist's frequency of contact gradually fades while the client works independently on problem-solving and the consolidation of coping skills. Sessions should stress contingency planning and may be used to work on the following objectives:

- to identify highly challenging situations, including those which have precipitated relapse/aggravation of symptoms in the past
- to plan coping strategies for dealing with potential problems and preventing relapse
- to plan recovery from relapse, should it occur
- to practise the skills required in different settings and incorporate then into daily lifestyle.

It may be helpful to enlist the support of a significant other in maintaining treatment gains.

USING TEACHING ACCESSORIES
Books and handouts

There are various advantages in the use of written handouts and books to supplement information given in an anxiety management or relaxation training programme:

- they help to reinforce and expand upon material taught within the session
- they provide an aide-memoire for clients to refer to in between sessions
- some sessions may be missed in structured courses and written summaries of the material given in each session will help to fill in these gaps.

It is worth noting that some studies have used bibliotherapy successfully to present related techniques such as 'rational emotive therapy'.[22,23] However, the combination of live treatment followed up with reading material is the most efficient way to enhance learning.

Tapes

Various research studies have found that the taped presentation of relaxation training is an inferior mode of presentation when compared to live instruction.[2,24,25] The use of tapes does have some value, however, but must be used with the greatest caution if the creation of dependence upon them is to be avoided.

The main advantage of taped relaxation lies in the initial learning stages to reinforce live instruction. At this stage, clients often experience difficulty in memorising relaxation instructions. However, it is recommended that clients only use tapes for the first week or so, preferably using their own recorded voice rather than the therapist's. Clients often report that they find it difficult to relax autonomously, preferring an external voice to lead them. It should be pointed out that being able to relax independently is the aim of training. Additionally, relaxation skills must eventually be generalised for use in everyday living. Clearly tapes do not facilitate this well since they cannot be used in situations which demand personal interaction with the environment, e.g. during active socialisation, which is often experienced as highly stressful.

Visual aids

The use of visual aids to enhance the therapist's presentation of training material is highly recommended. A good diagram is worth a thousand words, especially when some of the material involved in anxiety management includes quite difficult concepts. Although visual aids may seem time-consuming to prepare, if they are done well, they can be used again and again in subsequent treatment courses. Suitable visual aids may include transparencies for use with an overhead projector, slides, flip charts and large felt-tipped pens, and even the humble blackboard and chalks. It is useful to have a combination available to augment the standard visual aids prepared beforehand, so that points can be

clarified visually as they arise. Finally, not all therapists feel confident enough to regard themselves as accomplished lecturers. If visual aids are used, not only do they enhance the therapist's presentation, but they also provide a ready prompt, so helping to ensure full coverage of the main points.

HEALTH PROMOTION TOPICS IN ANXIETY MANAGEMENT

The material presented here is intended as a brief guide to assist therapists in planning presentations on subjects relevant for inclusion in anxiety management or relaxation training sessions. Under each main topic heading a list of relevant issues to cover is suggested. Some of these topics are already included in the AMC, but where general relaxation training sessions are held, these can be improved by including a short talk on one of the topics as part of each session. Fuller information on many of these subjects is contained in the client packs and/or further reading suggestions are given at the end of the chapter.

All topics suggested are intended either to give specific information concerning anxiety, stress and relaxation, or to improve body awareness and provide general health education related to stress reduction.

Application

- daily living activities in which tension occurs: clients' examples
- principles of differential relaxation: energy-economic posture during activity
- relaxation strategies for daily living activities: sitting, standing, walking and performing tasks
- using personal relaxation triggers to cue relaxed response
- developing the habit of relaxation
- using 'emergency' relaxation in times of acute anxiety.

(See Client Pack 3, Chapter 12 and References 26, 27 and 28.)

Life events and stress

- what is 'stress'?
- examples from clients' experiences
- how ordinary events cause stress, even 'pleasant' ones like birth or marriage, because they initiate change
- change and life events: the Holmes and Rahe 'social readjustment rating scale'
- improving coping skills so that change can be adjusted to with less stress.

(See Client Pack 5, Chapter 6 and Reference 29.)

Avoidance

- what is avoidance?
- examples of common situations avoided from clients' experiences
- the effects of avoidance on quality of life and relationships
- how avoidance of, or escape from, a feared situation maintains and increases anxiety
- how staying in the situation and facing the fear gradually extinguishes anxiety
- overcoming avoidance in small, manageable stages.

(See Client Packs 1, 5 and 6 and pp. 125–133 of this chapter.)

Faulty thinking

- what is faulty thinking?
- negative thoughts and irrational beliefs
- examples from clients' experiences
- how faulty thinking increases anxiety
- how to recognise, re-evaluate and challenge faulty thinking.

(See Client Packs 1 and 4; pp. 125–133 of this chapter; Reference 30.)

Social skills and assertiveness

- what are social skills?
- non-verbal skills, e.g. eye-contact, posture, appearance
- verbal skills and encouraging other people to talk
- listening skills

- assertiveness is not the same as aggression
- using coping skills to reduce anxiety in social situations
- the benefits of rewarding relationships — why it's worth the effort.

(See Client Pack 7, Chapter 6 and Reference 31.)

Stress positioning

- the body language of stress
- demonstrate examples of tense sitting and standing postures
- invite clients to identify their own typical positions of tension
- how tense postures reinforce anxiety level
- how relaxed postures reduce anxiety, aid confidence and increase control
- typical activities in which group members adopt tense postures, e.g. telephoning, waiting in queues
- suggest and practise alternative positions.

(See Client Packs 2 and 3 and Reference 28.)

How relaxation works

- what is muscle tension?
- simple explanation and diagram showing how muscle fibres contract
- how muscle tension is communicated to the brain, and from the brain to the muscles, setting up a vicious circle of tension
- basic principles of muscle work: reciprocal inhibition, agonists and antagonists
- using the agonist muscle groups to 'switch off' the antagonist groups
- importance of recognising and releasing muscle tension
- difficulties experienced in relaxation, guidelines on practice routine.

(See Client Packs 2 and 3, Chapter 7 and Reference 28.)

Bodily effects of anxiety

- physical symptoms of anxiety, examples from clients' experiences

- fight/flight syndrome and its effects
- the bodily systems responsible and how they work together
- the two branches of the autonomic nervous system
- stress hormones e.g. adrenaline, thyroxine
- skeletal muscle tension
- physical stress reactions: patterns of responding unique to each individual
- importance of identifying personal stress symptoms in order to avoid mislabelling these as signs of illness
- relaxation techniques as methods of reducing bodily effects of anxiety.

(Client Packs 1 and 2, Chapter 2 and References 32 and 33.)

What are nerves?

- what are 'nerves'?
- elicit clients' ideas and perceptions
- simple explanation and diagram of a neurone
- where the nerves are situated, basic brain and spinal cord anatomy
- the function of the nervous system as a communication network between bodily systems and brain, relaying messages and initiating physical responses and movement
- how voluntary and involuntary (autonomic) control systems react during stress
- how relaxation works on the nervous system to reduce anxiety symptoms.

(See Chapter 2 and References 32, 33 and 34.)

Sleeping problems

- facts about sleep
- sleep cycles; Rapid Eye Movement 'REM' sleep and dreaming
- sleeplessness: not a catastrophe! we tend to underestimate the amount we sleep and overestimate the amount we need
- natural ways to invite sleep
- regulating sleep habits
- relaxation for getting off to sleep
- helpful and unhelpful beverages before sleep.

(See Chapter 16 and References 35 and 36.)

Breathing

- why we breathe
- role of oxygen and carbon dioxide
- simple explanation and diagram of upper respiratory tract, lungs and diaphragm
- how oxygen and carbon dioxide are exchanged in the lungs
- correct breathing method at rest: slowly and low in the chest, not rapidly or from the throat
- invite clients to check their own breathing movements
- exercises to improve breathing and enhance relaxation
- 'Emergency' anxiety-control breathing.

(See Client Pack 3 and References 34, 37, 38 and 39.)

Heart and lung function

- basic cardiovascular and pulmonary systems, how they work together to oxygenate the blood and body cells
- myths about the heart e.g. palpitations, 'missing a beat'
- invite worries and questions from clients about heart/lung function
- how heart/lung function is affected by anxiety
- benefits to the heart/lung system of correct breathing and regular, sensible exercise
- common-sense approach to diet and lifestyle to maintain health, e.g. reducing intake of saturated fats, sensible regular exercise.

(See Client Pack 2 and References 34, 37 and 40.)

Hyperventilation

- what is hyperventilation?
- recognised by rapid breathing movements in upper chest
- often occurs during panic attacks
- habitual hyperventilation associated with chronic anxiety
- basic chemical effects of hyperventilation: disturbs blood gas balance giving rise to excess oxygen and deficit of carbon dioxide
- resulting state of hypocarbia causes wide

array of symptoms, e.g. dizziness, palpitations, weakness and muscle pain
- may affect all main bodily systems causing 'undiagnosed/untreatable' illnesses
- how to correct: breathing regularly, slowly and low in the chest.

(See Chapter 5 and References 37, 38, 39 and 41.)

Driving and anxiety

- what factors do group clients find anxiety-provoking about driving, e.g. test-taking, fear of accidents, fear of getting lost?
- relaxation before journey
- route planning before journey
- correct positioning while driving
- attitude to driving to combat stress
- handling confrontations with other drivers.

(See References 28 and 42.)

Digestion

- basic digestive tract and how it works
- common problems related to anxiety e.g. stomach and abdominal pain, bowel sounds, constipation, frequent bowel movements and nausea
- how relaxation aids digestion
- importance of taking regular diet, dietary fibre and basic nutritional needs
- avoiding irritants, e.g. caffeine, fatty or fried foods.

(See References 40, 43 and 44.)

The skeleton

- muscles, bones and joints: basic anatomy
- importance of good posture to avoid pain and muscle fatigue
- how muscle tension increases pain
- relaxation to relieve pain e.g. back pain
- correct lifting techniques
- the importance of sensible exercise to strengthen muscles and protect joints.

(See Reference 45.)

Bladder and bowel function

- range of normal function: individual variations
- how these functions can be disturbed by anxiety, e.g. frequency, constipation
- suggestions for coping, e.g. relaxation and sensible diet.

(See References 34, 35 and 44.)

Physical exercise

- what exercise do group members regularly take?
- the benefits of exercise in reducing tension, related to fight/flight symptoms
- correct, healthy exercise habits
- 'Dos and Don'ts': start gradually if unused to vigorous exercise; do warm-up exercises before each session and wind-down gradually afterwards
- other benefits of exercise related to social and emotional well-being
- range of exercise and sporting activities and facilities available for different needs.

(See Client Pack 2, Chapter 12 and References 33, 46, 47 and 48.)

Goal-setting

- defining overall aims: 'what do you want to change?'
- invite clients' suggestions
- breaking down main goal into smaller, more achievable targets
- use one client example and break down into realistic, graded targets
- decide on plan of action needed and carry out
- importance of being specific about actual behaviour required to achieve goals
- pitfalls, what stops people from changing e.g. not being specific about problems, avoiding action
- using simple goal setting form to aid process.

(See Client Pack 6.)

Problem-solving

- defining problems
- examples from clients
- brainstorming techniques
- evaluation of solutions
- setting goals and plan of action
- using simple problem-solving form to aid process.

(See Client Pack 6.)

Panic attacks

- what are panic attacks?
- common symptoms: discuss examples from clients' experiences
- common fears during panic attacks, e.g. fainting, heart attack, other people noticing anxiety
- how to manage panic attacks using coping skills: relaxation and positive thinking
- hyperventilation
- avoidance/escape reinforces panic.

(See Client Packs 2, 3, 4 and 7; Chapters 1 and 5; References 37, 49 and 50.)

Lifestyle management

- stress in everyday living: examples from group members
- stress at work
- time management
- social and relationship problems, role conflict
- ways to reduce stress: re-organisation of work routines, planning and decision-making, finding hobbies and constructive outlets for tension
- inactivity/overactivity are equally stressful conditions
- planning regular periods for relaxation practice.

(See Client Pack 5 and References 27, 35 and 51.)

Medication

- correct use of medication i.e. as prescribed

- misconceptions about medication; drugs are only one part of therapy and should not be expected to remove all problems automatically, e.g. relationship problems
- the drawbacks of overdependence on minor tranquillisers
- coping with withdrawal from tranquillisers and sleeping tablets
- how relaxation can aid withdrawal and coping without tranquillisers.

(See Chapters 1 and 2; References 52, 53 and 54.)

Attitudes, beliefs and behaviour

- how our temperament, beliefs and ideas affect anxiety levels
- unrealistic expectations and assumptions about selves and others
- dynamic personal factors related to maintainance of anxiety: uncertainty and decision-making, suppression of feelings, resentment and acceptance, guilt and blame, relationship difficulties.

(See Client Pack 4; pp. 125–133 of this chapter; Reference 35.)

Stress triggers

- examples from group: 'what situations do you find stressful?'
- role conflicts
- relationship problems
- decision-making
- common situational causes of anxiety, e.g. shopping, queueing, confrontation
- individual symptoms/reactions when aroused: examples from group
- individual coping styles: constructive and destructive
- suggestions for coping with different stress triggers
- difference between stress and distress: seeking an optimal balance.

(See Client Packs 1 and 4; Chapter 6; Reference 27.)

Body/mind relationship

- body and mind not separate entities
- how the body and mind work together to produce an integrated stress response
- how physical symptoms can be caused by emotional distress, e.g. when we feel anxious our muscles automatically become tense and vice versa
- how emotional distress can make existing physical illnesses worse
- how to reduce emotional stress levels using physical relaxation and vice versa.

(See Client Packs 1 and 2; Chapter 5; Reference 32.)

FURTHER RESOURCES

CHECKLISTS

Typical anxious thinking patterns

- making small problems into big ones
- jumping to conclusions without taking all the facts/evidence/options into account
- making global judgements based on one example, e.g. that person must be totally nasty/wicked because they did 'X'
- exaggerating unimportant/irrelevant factors and underestimating the important/relevant ones
- thinking in extremes and ignoring the middle ground/compromise view, e.g. if you don't get top marks in a test, then you're a total failure
- looking at things from only one point of view, e.g. the negative one
- confusing facts with feelings
- forgetting that the way you think affects how you feel and behave
- assuming that you cannot change the way you think/behave
- predicting the future, e.g. assuming that the 'worst' will automatically happen
- underestimating how well you could cope if the 'worst' did happen
- forgetting to ask yourself whether the 'worst' would actually be as bad as you fear.

Negative/irrational attitudes to self/life

- believing that in comparison to everyone else you are weak/incapable/stupid, etc
- believing that you need someone/something strong to help you cope
- believing that, at all costs, you must never make mistakes
- believing that everybody else expects you to be perfect too
- when things do go wrong, assuming its all your fault
- putting yourself under unnecessary pressure, e.g. I should/must/ought to be/do better at this
- setting yourself standards that are either too high or too low: this allows you to continue believing that you really are a failure
- putting yourself down on the basis of flimsy, meagre or one-sided evidence
- believing that your past experiences have an automatic/inescapable influence on your future
- expecting everyone to approve of/like you all the time
- expecting events to go perfectly all the time and becoming very upset when they inevitably don't
- not recognising that it is the way we react to unfortunate events that usually causes the greatest distress, not the events themselves
- assuming that your needs are less/more important than everyone else's
- not looking at your strengths, only your weaknesses
- making allowances for everyone except yourself/vice versa
- taking things that others say/do too personally
- assuming that unfamiliar situations are always potentially harmful and therefore to be avoided at all costs
- wasting time asking yourself 'why'?
- believing that nothing can be done to change things for the better
- assuming that what is happening now will still seem as important in one/two years' time.

Some useful challenges

- am I taking all the facts into account?
- is there a more positive/useful way of looking at things?
- have I overlooked the important aspects?
- am I paying too much attention to unimportant aspects?
- am I underestimating myself and my abilities?
- am I judging myself too harshly/putting myself down?
- am I basing my reactions on feelings rather than facts?
- am I 'catastrophising'?
- am I thinking in extremes/jumping to conclusions?
- am I putting myself under pressure unnecessarily?
- am I expecting things to be perfect unrealistically?
- am I setting myself unrealistic goals e.g. too high/low?
- is there a more balanced/objective view?
- how would someone else see things?
- am I taking on too much responsibility for the outcome of situations over which I do not have full control?
- am I exaggerating the likelihood of the 'worst' happening?
- if the 'worst' did happen, would it really be as terrible as I think?
- will this really matter in one/two years' time?

Stress survival strategies

- increase your sense of control over stressful situations, for example, by applying stress management techniques
- accept aspects of stressful situations that you cannot change/control and try instead to change the way you perceive and react to them
- talk problems over with people that you trust, get another perspective
- learn to think rationally and positively
- look after your physical health during stressful periods: keep fit, eat wisely, get enough sleep and don't resort to drugs/alcohol

- develop satisfying recreational/creative and social outlets
- make relationships your priority
- seek out opportunities for fun and laughter
- do something nice for someone else
- make time to plan ahead, decide on your priorities and set your goals accordingly
- improve your time-management skills
- learn to say 'no'
- don't try to do everything yourself: delegate more
- stop trying/expecting yourself to be perfect
- develop relaxation skills and make relaxation a regular routine
- give yourself a break when you're tired/ill
- at times of conflict, avoid taking things personally/blaming others; try to distance yourself
- allow yourself to make mistakes without condemnation
- be kind to yourself: stop putting yourself down, and remember to treat yourself when you've achieved something
- live for the moment: don't waste time worrying about the future/regretting the past.

USEFUL CONTACTS

1. Booklet by Bond M, Kilty J 1982 Practical methods of dealing with stress. Write to: Human Potential Research Project, Department of Educational Studies, University of Surrey, Guildford, Surrey, GU2 5XH.

2. The British Holistic Medical Association, Rowland Thomas House, Royal Shrewsbury Hospital South, Shrewsbury SY3 8XF. Tel: 01743 261 155. Provides information and runs courses on a variety of health topics, including the use of relaxation techniques, e.g. biofeedback and autogenic training.

3. Centre for Autogenic Training, 100 Harley St, London W1N 1AT. Tel: 0171 935 1811. Provides courses for therapists wishing to practise autogenic training.

4. Relaxation for Living, Registered charity no: 264906. 12 New St, Chipping Norton, Oxon OX7 5LJ. Tel: 01608 646100. Provides regular newsletter, training courses and study days for

relaxation therapists, information leaflets and tapes for clients.

5. Health Education Authority (HEA), Health Promotion Information Centre, Hamilton House, Mabledon Place, London WC1H 9TX. Tel: 0171 413 1995. Provides information and courses on self-help methods of promoting health and fitness. Includes stress management methods.

6. MIND National Association for Mental Health, Granta House, 15–19 Broadway, Stratford, London E15 4BQ. Tel: 0181 519 2122. Apart from its general activities as a charity for the promotion of mental health, MIND produces a range of

relevant information leaflets and other publications, e.g. *Anxiety* – factsheet 9.

7. National Association for Staff Support, 9 Caradon Close, Woking, Surrey GU21 3DU. Produces a range of publications for health care staff and telephone advice line for members. Also organises database of local contacts, newsletter, workshops and conferences.

8. The Back Pain Association, 16, Elm Tree Road, Teddington, Middlesex, TW11 8FP. Tel: 0181 977 5474. Provides information, publications and support for those affected by back pain problems.

REFERENCES

1 Keable D 1985 Relaxation training techniques — a review. Part two: How effective is relaxation training? British Journal of Occupational Therapy July:201–204

2 Lehrer P M, Woolfolk R L (eds) 1993 Principles and practice of stress management, 2nd edn. The Guilford Press, New York

3 Goldfried M R, Trier C S 1974 Effectiveness of relaxation as an active coping skill. Journal of Abnormal Psychology 83(4):348–355

4 Peveler R C, Johnston D W 1986 Subjective and cognitive effects of relaxation. Behaviour Research and Therapy 24(4):413–419

5 Mclean J 1986 The use of relaxation techniques in general practice. The Practitioner 230:1079–1084

6 Butler G, Cullington A, Hibbert G, Klimes I, Gelder M 1987 Anxiety management for persistent generalised anxiety. British Journal of Psychiatry 151:535–542

7 Moores A 1987 Facing the fear. Nursing Times 83(27):44–46

8 Zurawski R M, Smith T M, Houston B K 1987 Stress management for essential hypertension: comparison with a minimally effective treatment, predictors of response to treatment, and effects on reactivity. Journal of Psychosomatic Medicine 31(4):453–462

9 Lichstein K L 1988 Clinical relaxation strategies. John Wiley, New York

10 Jacobsen R, Edinger J D 1982 Side-effects of relaxation treatment. American Journal of Psychiatry 139:952–953

11 Rosa K R 1976 Autogenic training. Victor Gollancz, London

12 Payne R A 1995 Relaxation techniques — a practical handbook for the health care professional. Churchill Livingstone, Edinburgh

13 Fairburn C G, Fairbairn S M 1979 Relaxation training in psychiatric admission units. British Journal of Occupational Therapy 42(11):280–282

14 Bloom L J, Gonzales A M 1981 Anxiety management with schizophrenic outpatients. Journal of Clinical Psychology 38(2):280–285

15 Kingdon D G, Turkington D 1991 The use of cognitive behavior therapy with a normalizing rationale in schizophrenia. Journal of Nervous and Mental Disease 179(4):207–211

16 Wilson M 1983 Occupational therapy in long-term psychiatry. Churchill Livingstone, Edinburgh

17 Mitchell L 1977 Simple relaxation. John Murray, London

18 Ellis A 1962 Reason and emotion in psychotherapy. Lyle Stewart, New York

19 Beck A T, Emery G, Greenberg R L 1985 Anxiety disorders and phobias. Basic Books, New York

20 Hawton K, Salkovskis P M, Kirk J, Clark D M 1989 Cognitive behaviour therapy for psychiatric problems — a practical guide. Oxford Medical Publications, Oxford

21 Deffenbacher J, Suinn R 1982 The self-control of anxiety. In: Karoly P, Kanfer F (eds) Self-management and behavioural change. Pergamon, New York

22 Kassinove J, Miller N, Kalin M 1980 Effects of pre-treatment with rational emotive bibliotherapy and rational emotive audiotherapy on clients waiting at a community health center. Psychological Reports 46:851–857

23 Horton A M N, Johnson C H 1980 Rational–emotive therapy and depression: a clinical case study. Perceptual and Motor Skills 51:853–854

24 Paul G L, Trimble R W 1970 Recorded vs 'live' relaxation training and hypnotic suggestion. Comparative effectiveness for reducing physiological arousal and inhibiting stress responses. Behavior Therapy 1:285–302

25 Borkovec T D, Sides J K 1979 Critical procedural variables related to the physiological effects of progressive relaxation: a review. Behaviour Research and Therapy 17:119–126

26 Marquis J N, Ferguson J M, Barr Taylor C 1980 Generalization of relaxation skills. Journal of Behavior Therapy and Experimental Psychiatry 11:95–99

27 Bond M, Kilty J 1982 Practical methods of dealing with stress. Human Potential Research Project: University of Surrey, Surrey

28 Mitchell L 1977 Simple relaxation. John Murray, London

29 Holmes T H, Rahe R H 1967 The social readjustment rating scale. Journal of Psychosomatic Research 11:213–218

30 Ellis A 1961 Reason and emotion in psychotherapy. Lyle Stewart, New York

31 Ellis R, Whittington D 1981 A guide to social skill training. Croom Helm, London
32 Pelletier K R 1977 Mind as healer — mind as slayer. George Allen & Unwin, UK
33 Morse D R, Lawrence-Furst M 1979 Stress for success. Van Nostrand Reinhold, USA
34 McNaught A, Callender R 1983 Illustrated physiology. Churchill Livingstone, Edinburgh
35 Chaitow L 1983 Relaxation and meditation techniques. Thorsons UK
36 Lloyd A 1981 Sound sleep sense booklet. Relaxation for living, Walton-on-Thames
37 Henryk Hrehorow Z 1984 Better breathing for health and fitness, revised edn. The Winslow Press, Buckingham
38 Cluff R A 1985 Chronic hyperventilation and its treatment by physiotherapy. Physiotherapy 71(7):301–305
39 Lloyd A 1980 Better breathing booklet. Relaxation for living, Walton-on-Thames
40 Briggs G M, Calloway D H 1979 Nutrition and physical fitness. Holt, Rinehart and Winston, USA
41 Lum L C 1981 Hyperventilation and anxiety state. Journal of the Royal Society of Medicine 74:1–4
42 Lloyd A 1981 Drive and survive booklet, revised edn. Relaxation for living, Walton-on-Thames
43 Mayer J 1977 A diet for living. Pocket Books, New York
44 Bingham S 1987 The everyman companion to food and nutrition. J M Dent, Melbourne
45 Anthony C P, Thibodeau G A 1983 Textbook of anatomy and physiology. The C.V. Mosby Company, St Louis, USA
46 Kraus H, Raab W 1961 Hypokinetic disease: diseases produced by lack of exercise. Charles C Thomas, Illinois
47 Cooper K 1970 The new aerobics. Bantam, New York
48 Mobily K 1982 Using physical activity and recreation to cope with stress and anxiety: a review. American Corrective Therapy Journal 36(3):77–81
49 Stampler F M 1982 Panic disorder: description, conceptualization, and implications for treatment. Clinical Psychology Review 2:469–486
50 Gelder M G 1986 Panic attacks: new approaches to an old problem. British Journal of Psychiatry 149:346–352
51 Beech H R, Burns L E, Sheffield B F 1982 A behavioural approach to the management of stress. John Wiley, Chichester
52 Haddon C 1984 Women and tranquilizers. Sheldon Press, London
53 Melville J 1984 The tranquilizer trap — and how to get out of it. Fontana, London
54 Stopforth B 1986 Outpatient benzodiazepine withdrawal and the occupational therapist. British Journal of Occupational Therapy 49(10):318–322

FURTHER READING

General: stress and anxiety

Dobson C B 1982 Stress: the hidden adversary. MTP Press, UK
Fisher S, Reason J 1988 Handbook of life stress, cognition and health. John Wiley, Chichester
Forgays D G, Sosnowki T, Wizesniewski K (eds) 1992 Anxiety — recent developments in cognitive, psycho-physiological and health research. Hemisphere publishing corporation, Washington
Klein D F, Rabkin J G 1981 Anxiety: new research and changing concepts. American psycho-pathological association series. Raven Press, New York
Levitt E E 1980 The psychology of anxiety, 2nd edn. Lawrence Erlbaum, USA
Sanders G S, Suls J (eds) 1982 Social psychology of health and illness. L. Erlbaum Associates, New Jersey
Sims A, Snaith P 1988 Anxiety in clinical practice. John Wiley, Chichester

Practical anxiety management and related methods

Butcher P, De Clive-Lowe S 1985 Strategies for living: teaching psychological self-help as adult education. British Journal of Medical Psychology 58:275–283
Cluff R A 1985 Chronic hyperventilation and its treatment by physiotherapy. Physiotherapy 71(7):301–305
Cullen B 1984 The management of anxiety. In: Wilson M (ed) Occupational therapy in short-term psychiatry, 2nd edn. Churchill Livingstone, Edinburgh
Hawton K, Salkovskis P M, Kirk J, Clark D M 1989 Cognitive behaviour therapy for psychiatric problems — a practical guide. Oxford Medical Publications, Oxford
Kennerley H 1995 Managing anxiety — a training manual, 2nd edn. Oxford Medical Publications, Oxford
Lehrer P M, Woolfolk R L (eds) 1993 Principles and practice of stress management, 2nd edn. The Guilford Press, New York
Lichstein K L 1988 Clinical relaxation strategies. John Wiley, New York
Marquis J N, Ferguson J M, Barr Taylor C 1980 Generalisation of relaxation skills. Journal of Behavior Therapy and Experimental Psychiatry 11:95–99
Michelson L, Ascher L M (eds) 1987 Anxiety and stress disorders — cognitive–behavioural assessment and treatment. Guilford Press, New York
Miller R J, Cullen B, O'Brien R 1981 'Are you sitting comfortably?' — Psychological approaches to the management of stress and anxiety. British Journal of Occupational Therapy 44(1):5–9
Moores A 1987 Facing the fear. Nursing Times 83(27):44–46
Payne R A 1995 Relaxation techniques — a practical handbook for the health care professional. Churchill Livingstone, Edinburgh
Roberts C M 1982 Rational emotive therapy — a cognitive–behaviour treatment system. Perspectives in Psychiatric Care 20(3):134–138

Psychotherapy/group skills

Bloch S, Crouch E (eds) 1985 Therapeutic factors in group psychotherapy. Oxford University Press, UK

Burnard P 1989 Counselling skills for health professionals, 2nd edn. Chapman & Hall, London

Rogers C R 1951 Client-centred therapy. Constable, London

Wright H 1989 Group work perspectives and practice. Scutari Press, Harrow

Yalom I D 1985 The theory and practice of group psychotherapy, 3rd edn. Basic Books, New York

Other recommended reading

Byrne A, Byrne D G 1993 The effect of exercise on depression, anxiety and other mood states: a review. Journal of Psychosomatic Research 37(6):565–574

Creed F, Mayou R, Hopkin A 1992 Medical symptoms not explained by organic disease. The Royal College of Psychiatrists and The Royal College of Physicians of London, London

Ellis A 1962 Reason and emotion in psychotherapy. Lyle Stewart, New York

Fransella F 1982 Psychology for occupational therapists. The British Psychological Society: The Macmillan Press UK

Grings W W, Dawson M E 1978 Emotions and bodily responses: a psycho-physiological approach. Academic Press, USA

Roberts G W 1995 Trauma following major disasters: the role of the occupational therapist. British Journal of Occupational Therapy 58(5):204–208

Seligman M E P 1975 Helplessness. W H Freeman, USA

Therapy Weekly 1995 Managing stress booklet. Special interest booklet no.1. Macmillan Magazines, London

Thompson R 1967 Foundations of physiological psychology. Harper and Row, UK

Van der Kolk B A 1987 Psychological trauma. American Psychiatric Press, Washington

Wilson M 1983 Occupational therapy in long-term psychiatry. Churchill Livingstone, Edinburgh

Yates A J 1983 Behaviour therapy and psychodynamic psychotherapy: basic conflict or reconciliation and integration? British Journal of Clinical Psychology 22:107–125

15

Troubleshooting — some common problems

Diana Keable

DEALING WITH DIFFICULTIES ARISING DURING RELAXATION SESSIONS

Clients who fall asleep/snore during relaxation

This may occur for a variety of reasons including:

1. Repetitive, aimless relaxation sessions which do not actively involve the clients in working progressively towards relevant goals.

2. Relaxation sessions in which clients are soothed to sleep in a dimly lit environment by the soft voice of the therapist!

3. Misunderstanding of the teaching aims of the session, usually evidenced by such comments as: 'that was wonderful — I fell right off to sleep — what on earth did you wake me up for?'

4. Inappropriate referral of clients for whom anxiety is not a significant problem.

5. Over-sedation causing excessive drowsiness.

6. Disrupted sleep cycle/insomnia causing drowsiness during the daytime.

States of demotivation and institutionalisation can be the unfortunate result of the repetitive, routine presentation of the same relaxation technique — especially if it merely involves putting on a relaxation tape. In such cases, where clients are seen to respond by falling asleep, this should be deemed as the least harmful outcome. The creation of client dependence is another likely complication and this is discussed in the next section. Techniques used should be selected with reference to specific and relevant therapeutic goals. Effort should also be made to ensure that clients are not referred to relaxation simply as a matter of course, but on the basis of clinical need.

Before training commences, the therapist should explain that, as this is a teaching session, the full attention of all clients will be required in order for them to learn the skills independently. It should be emphasised that relaxation skills are intended for use in stressful situations outside the session which clients will be unable to sleep through. Even where clients are using relaxation to combat sleeping problems, they will still need to stay awake during teaching sessions. Some clients may be troubled by excessive drowsiness due to over-sedation. In such cases it may become necessary to delay training until the medication has been adjusted. However, using the upright sitting position for relaxation and increasing the amount of light/voice volume in the practice environment may ease the problem. Finally, before the session begins, clients should be told that if they do inadvertently fall asleep the therapist will waken them with a light tap on the arm or leg. This will help to prevent clients being startled if they do have to be woken.

Following instructions incorrectly or not at all

Occasionally the therapist may observe that some clients are not carrying out the exercises or movements required during the session. There are several possible reasons for this including hostility towards treatment or the therapist, lack of motivation, inability to hear the therapist, and even embarrassment. The precise reason can be established tactfully during feedback after the session. Often, however, the problem can be identified and quietly dealt with during the session itself. It is usually quite acceptable for the therapist to move around during the session and encourage or correct clients' positioning. In the case of those with hearing problems, the therapist should first establish that the client has an appropriate hearing aid, in working order. The therapist can also try moving closer to any clients affected and giving instructions as clearly as pos-

sible. For those clients who are hostile towards relaxation, or who are poorly motivated, it may be necessary to set up an informal discussion outside the session, where the value of their continued attendance can be jointly reviewed. There may be other reasons for the apparent disinclination which the client needs assistance to express openly. As far as embarrassment is concerned, this usually fades after a few sessions provided the therapist does not draw too much attention to it.

Disruptive/disturbed/distressed behaviour during relaxation

Behaviour of this kind may strongly indicate that the type of relaxation being conducted is not suitable for that particular client. Disruptive clients should normally be excluded from the session if their behaviour disturbs other clients. The therapist may then need to consider an alternative approach to the treatment of clients who are excluded in this way. Occasionally some clients experience the soothing, intimate atmosphere of relaxation sessions as psychologically threatening, and may use disruptive behaviour as a defence. Others may experience marked emotional distress during relaxation and be unable to express the reason for this. This may occur just at the moment when they actually begin to relax. These phenomena may relate to early psychological trauma. In each case, relaxation may be contraindicated for those clients affected.

Dealing with acute anxiety states

Clients suffering from intense agitation or panic may be unsuitable for group relaxation training until the condition settles down. In the early stages of acute anxiety, or during a panic attack, the client may require individual attention from the therapist. Mitchell[1] has suggested how the therapist can approach intensely anxious clients and help them to relax in the immediate situation. Hyperventilation is often involved in acute anxiety and panic, and the therapist may be instrumental in training the client to overcome this. Finally, it is also worth noting that in exposure programmes for phobic problems, the client is usually encouraged to 'stay with the fear' until it subsides. Part of the therapist's role is to support the client through this process, and reinforce learning that anxiety decreases through progressive exposure to the feared situation.

WHY DOES TRAINING SOMETIMES FAIL?

It is inevitable that some clients will fail to benefit from relaxation training or anxiety management. Some of the most common reasons why training is impeded include the following:

- poor motivation
- cognitive problems, e.g. poor concentration span, learning problems
- inability to generalise learning outside sessions
- inadequate home practice rates
- staff-related problems, e.g. lack of continuity, expertise
- excessive acute/state anxiety
- client dependence on a particular therapist/voice/method/position
- florid psychosis/acute behavioural disturbance
- side-effects of phenothiazine medication e.g. muscle rigidity, dyskinesia
- the side-effects of sedative medication causing excessive drowsiness/tendency to fall asleep during sessions
- hostility towards therapist
- lack of credibility in the effectiveness of non-drug treatment
- use of muscle tension as a psychological defence mechanism, e.g. fear of 'letting go', lack of trust, fear of experiencing bodily pleasure
- psychological need to maintain symptoms for various dynamic reasons e.g. to ensure dependency needs are met, fear of change
- external locus of control which militates against a client's readiness to believe in the effectiveness of self-help treatment regimes.

Of course, many of the problems which prevent relaxation and related treatment regimes from succeeding also apply to other psychological treatment regimes. When clients are failing to benefit from treatment, it is essential that the therapist attempts to ascertain why. Having done this, the next questions to ask are:

- does the problem indicate that the type of treatment was unsuitable for the client in the first place?

and if so

- can I adapt the treatment, or offer an alternative approach, to meet the client's needs?

Clearly, some of the problems listed here as possible reasons of treatment failure — such as acute state anxiety or psychosis — are not problems which the therapist can or should tackle in a group-based relaxation training or anxiety management context.

Appropriate selection criteria are discussed in Chapter 11. However, the therapist should ensure that treatment is:

- of a high standard
- appropriate for the client group
- extended to lifestyle and problem areas outside the clinical situation.

Attention to these factors may provide at least part of the solution to many of the difficulties, e.g. staff-related problems, lack of credibility in non-drug interventions, lack of generalisation and other learning problems.

However, some of the most difficult, and common, stumbling blocks are associated with motivation, and complex psychological forces frequently operate in this arena. Clearly, motivational problems affect compliance levels, and in relaxation/anxiety management training, some degree of independent practice is crucial to success. These issues are discussed further in the next section.

Therapists will be aware that some compliance problems are unconscious on the part of the client and are not deliberate attempts to foil the therapist's efforts. Careful handling is required, particularly where the client is deemed to be psychological fragile and/or has been unable to engage in open and constructive dialogue about the personal dynamics maintaining symptoms. In such cases, a paradoxical approach may be instrumental in facilitating change. For example, instead of strenuously continuing to try and persuade the resistant client to put more effort into treatment, the therapist could suggest that a change of approach is now indicated. As the treatment seems to be doing no good / the symptoms are too severe, the client might feel better if he discontinued / did it more in his own way. This strategy may be helpful in shifting the focus of the client's motivation by removing the need to work against the treatment. Henceforward, it may be possible to engage the client in a more productive therapeutic partnership, in which the client controls and chooses what he wants to work on, and how.

Of course, almost everyone can benefit from learning to relax and control anxiety, including the therapist. After all, just as anxiety is a natural, and to a large extent normal, human reaction, so is the relaxation response. Accordingly, the referral criteria are wide.

For this reason, when problems are encountered it is essential that an attempt is made to establish possible reasons and solutions for the problem. However, once the therapist has ensured that the problem does not lie with herself or the treatment she is offering, the ultimate responsibility to benefit from treatment is the client's own. Although the therapist may be able to increase the client's motivation by various means, it is necessary to bear in mind where her responsibility finishes, and the client's choices must be respected. Finally, it is important to ensure that the aims and expectations of a particular client group are realistic. It is only against such a background that success or failure can be accurately measured. When teaching relaxation methods to a poorly motivated group of clients with added learning problems, goals should be set at a level that they can reasonably be expected to achieve.

HOMEWORK: ADHERENCE TO PRACTICE

Issues of compliance

Compliance rates with independent practice among adult populations have been shown to be approximately 50%.[2] Given this huge rate of attrition, it is vital to examine how this might be reduced. One relevant factor is the issue of fitting the technique to the client, taking individual preferences into account. Popularity of different techniques varies widely, and therapists would do well to study their client's reactions to techniques and recommend individually tailored treatment regimes accordingly. Other individual factors held to increase compliance include:

- expectation of success
- motivation to succeed
- internal locus of control
- ability to assimilate training material.[3]

Somewhat surprisingly, some studies have shown that intensive, frequent practice of relaxation techniques is not always necessary in order to achieve therapeutic benefits.[2,3] It is crucial, however, that some degree of practice is carried out, although the critical amount required varies according to the individual. In a study comparing 'frequent' and 'occasional practisers' of meditation, Carrington[2] found no differences in symptom improvement levels. When these groups were combined and compared to lapsed practisers and non-practising controls, the findings were highly significant. Subjects who did not practise at all showed no improvement, while those who did practise, even if only occasionally, showed significant improvement in stress-related symptoms.

Nevertheless, issues regarding effects of practice frequency have not yet been fully resolved and findings have been widely contradictory.[3] The simple assumption that the more practice you do, the more benefit you will gain, may now be considered suspect. A more complex picture in which various individualised factors play a role is beginning to emerge. For instance, some people may apply relaxation skills more strategically, increasing their use sporadically in times of stress. There is also some evidence that, once learned, relaxation may become a permanent coping skill to be summoned up as required.[3] This does not apply in all cases, however, and some individuals need to practise consistently in order to maintain the benefits. In summary, whilst therapists should continue to encourage frequent practice in every case, they may be reassured that the results will not necessarily be inferior where practice is infrequent.

Increasing compliance with homework

The therapist may increase the client's motivation to succeed simply by enumerating the positive benefits to be achieved. It is also vital that the therapist makes clear what is expected of participants from the start and agrees these expectations with clients before treatment. It should be strongly emphasised that the client is taking part in a self-help treatment, the results of which depend almost entirely on his own efforts.

It is frequently helpful to draw up jointly agreed homework contracts, based on a therapeutic alliance between the therapist and client. For example, clients might be asked to suggest a forfeit clause for themselves if they repeatedly default on attendance or fail to complete a sufficient number of homework assignments, this might be extra homework, or that treatment will be terminated pending review. However, this should not be carried out in a punitive spirit, rather, it should emphasise identification of the obstacles to adherence and a search for solutions. The nature of the strategies employed will, of course, depend on the needs of the client/client group in question. It is also crucial that treatment expectations are realistic at the outset so as not to set the client up for failure and further demotivation. Having laid this foundation, clients should be followed up assiduously if they fail to carry out agreed personal practice and homework assignments.

Peer group pressure may also assist in encouraging clients to do their homework. Feedback on assignments should be requested as part of each session along with the handing in of home practice record sheets and self-rating scales. If clients are aware that they will be expected to account for their progress within each session, this can act as a powerful spur. Having created a climate in which homework is seen as the most impor-

tant element of the total treatment package, the therapist should also ensure that:

- the client fully understands the assignment given
- the assignment is relevant and appropriate in relation to the client's individual problems and circumstances
- assignments are graded and progressive, moving at an appropriate pace from easy to more difficult tasks
- detailed written material has been given in relation to assignments, and to reinforce live training within the session
- clients are warned to expect some set-backs, and that these should be seen as a normal part of the process, not an indication to give up trying
- appropriate and positive reinforcement is given for all achievements
- monitoring of compliance is carried out using more than one method to ensure greatest accuracy, e.g. self-monitoring, direct observation, behavioural testing, monitoring by others
- where compliance rates are inadequate, genuine efforts are made to identify the nature of the problem and possible solutions
- as treatment progresses, more and more responsibility for the process is handed over to the client, e.g. in setting goals and assignments.[4,5]

AVOIDING CLIENT DEPENDENCE ON THE THERAPIST

This is a situation in which prevention is better than cure. Again, before training begins, clients should always be made aware that the treatment regime is a self-help method, the success of which depends almost entirely on their own efforts. The role of homework assignments is also crucial both to ensure treatment efficacy and to deter client dependence on the therapist.[2,3,4,5,6] It is advisable to inform clients of the great emphasis that will be placed on personal homework throughout the course, and their agreement to accept this responsibility should be obtained prior to training. Having done this, the motivation to continue carrying out homework may often be facilitated through the use of monitoring and self-rating techniques, e.g. relaxation practice diaries, log books and graphs of personal progress. These should be handed in and discussed at each session, during feedback. This process helps to discourage non-existent or vague attempts at independent practice. The giving of positive reinforcement for the client's efforts is also crucial. (Homework is discussed more fully in the previous section.)

Therapists can also avoid encouraging dependence by phasing out their own leadership role as swiftly as possible. If the aim of the treatment course is to teach clients to relax independently, once the basics have been mastered, the therapist should begin to withdraw. The focus of training should then shift from therapist-centred teaching to client-centred feedback about progress and practice outside the clinical setting.

The technique used, and its style of presentation, also requires consideration to evaluate whether it is facilitating independence or hindering it. With this in mind, the following points are worth noting:

1. Does the technique involve the therapist soothing clients into a relaxed state by speaking in a soft voice? They may grow to rely on her voice in order to become relaxed.
2. Is the technique always presented in a dimly lit and quiet room. Environmental interference — light and noise — should gradually be increased as relaxation training progresses.
3. Do clients always lie down to practise relaxation? They should be encouraged to vary the positions they adopt when practising, i.e. sitting in various postures and even standing for short periods.
4. Is the technique used always the same one? It is often valuable to teach a variety of techniques so that clients do not get 'stuck' on a particular method.
5. Is the technique composed of progressive stages, as in a course structure? This

encourages clients to move on and advance their level of skill.
6. Does the therapist always lead the relaxation portion of the session? Clients could also be encouraged to take a turn as leader of the relaxation sessions by giving the instructions to the group.

Finally, both therapist and client should seek to identify the nature of the obstacles which prevent the client from progressing independently, and address these directly. For instance, attitudes related to an external locus of control may undermine clients' ability to gain control of their own emotional reactions. Similarly, lifestyle or environmental problems may prevent effective practice/application of skills.

SUMMARY OF STRATEGIES TO FACILITATE SUCCESSFUL TREATMENT

1. Develop an adequate screening procedure to avoid inappropriate referrals.
2. Clients should not be accepted for treatment if they are unlikely to benefit, or do not see it as relevant to their problems.
3. Clarify what clients can expect from treatment before it commences. The more accurate clients' expectations of treatment are, the more likely they are to be satisfied with it and motivated to participate. It is vital to explain the self-help emphasis of the techniques and also to enumerate the benefits that can be gained, e.g. the ability to control distressing anxiety symptoms independently, increased confidence and self-esteem.
4. Clarify your expectations of clients before treatment. Gain clients' agreement, if appropriate, by jointly establishing individual treatment contracts. The therapist should aim to negotiate terms that clients themselves consider fair.
5. Present high-quality training sessions. Sessions should be well prepared, interesting and relevant to clients' needs. Training should aim to provide an empowering experience

which fully involves the clients it is attempting to reach. Therapists should acknowledge the value of the client's contribution to the therapeutic process.

6. Make client's homework assignments the most important part of the training process. Use every appropriate tool to achieve and monitor compliance with this, e.g. regular homework feedback sessions, daily practice self-rating scales, personal progress log books, intermittent graphs of personal progress, peer pressure, treatment contracts, positive reinforcement from therapist. Anticipate problems in homework adherence and plan accordingly.

7. Phase out therapist's leadership role as rapidly as possible. Relaxation techniques usually need to be demonstrated once or twice only (unless there are specific learning problems). The emphasis should then be placed on client-centred feedback about the practice of skills and progress outside the clinical setting.

8. Present relaxation techniques in a manner that does not reinforce dependence on the therapist. Some common pitfalls of this kind are described in the previous section on avoiding client dependence.

9. Enable clients to set specific, realistic goals related to the problems they are experiencing. Encourage clients to apply the skills they have learned in tackling real problems and improving their lifestyle outside the clinical setting. They should set concrete, achievable targets so that improvements can be readily identified.

10. Discharge clients at an appropriate stage in their treatment. It is better to discharge clients rather than create the additional problem of dependence. Clients with residual problems can be offered a course of follow-up sessions aimed at empowering them to deal with remaining problems independently.

11. Maintenance and relapse prevention. Anticipate set-backs and help clients to develop strategies for coping with them. Use a contingency planning approach in order to identify high-risk situations and positive responses for dealing with them. Encourage thorough consolidation of the coping skills required through rehearsal in a variety of different situations. Enlist the support of a significant other in maintaining treatment gains.

REFERENCES

1 Mitchell L 1977 Simple relaxation. John Murray, London
2 Carrington P 1993 Modern forms of meditation. In: Lehrer P M, Woolfolk R L (eds) Principles and practice of stress management, 2nd edn. The Guilford Press, New York
3 Lehrer P M, Woolfolk R L (eds) 1993 Principles and practice of stress management, 2nd edn. The Guilford Press, New York
4 Michelson L, Ascher L M (eds) 1987 Anxiety and stress disorders — cognitive–behavioural assessment and treatment. Guilford Press, New York
5 Hawton K, Salkovskis P M, Kirk J, Clark D M (eds) 1989 Cognitive behaviour therapy for psychiatric problems — a practical guide. Oxford University Press, Oxford
6 Hillenberg J B, Collins F L 1983 The importance of home practice for progressive relaxation training. Behaviour Research and Therapy 21(6):633–642

16

Working with physical disorders: the psychophysiological approach

Diana Keable

Kathryn Ashworth
Rosemary Johnson
(Pain management)

Kate Radford
(Cardiac rehabilitation)

THE TREATMENT APPROACH

Introduction

Psychophysiological models of anxiety are discussed in Chapter 5, including the development of psychosomatic medicine, its aetiology, and the role of personality in increasing vulnerability to disease. This chapter moves on to explore how anxiety management techniques can contribute to the treatment of somatic disorders in which anxiety plays a large part.

Dualism, in which the mind and body are seen as entirely separate entities, was first described by Descartes in the seventeenth century. Until relatively recently this notion was embraced within mainstream western medicine, and this has been blamed for its failure to treat the individual in holistic terms.[1] Much useful work has been done to bring about this state of enlightenment, particularly in the fields of psychosomatic medicine and liaison psychiatry. However, the term 'psychosomatic' disease has now begun to outlive its usefulness. More recently, the term 'psychophysiological' disease is being used in preference.[2] The psychophysiological approach allows a more fluid and individualised interpretation of the disease process than that originally propounded by the psychosomatic school. (See Ch. 5.)

It is now generally accepted that an indefinite number of somatic conditions may be precipitated and/or maintained by a mixture of somatic and psychosocial factors. For the purposes of this chapter, psychophysiological disorders are grouped as follows:

1. Somatic disorders, where a significant organic disturbance exists.

2. Somatic symptoms, where no significant organic disturbance exists e.g. illness behaviour, somatisation.

3. A mixed category in which an existing somatic disorder is aggravated disproportionately by psychosocial factors.

The first category might apply, for example, to an individual with a demonstrable physical disorder such as hypertension or gastric ulcer, which is compounded by the effects of a stressful lifestyle. The second category applies to those whose perception of the existence/severity of their symptoms is without basis in reality, e.g. hypochondriasis or hysterical conversion syndromes. The third category denotes an indeterminate mixture of the first two categories. An example of this might be a chronic back-pain sufferer with depression, anxiety and a contracted lifestyle. It must also be pointed out that the precise aetiology and extent of symptoms is frequently unclear, serving to complicate the picture still further, e.g. headache, pain, balance problems, respiratory problems and some forms of hysterical conversion.

Elements of good and bad practice

Before moving on to outline elements of good practice in dealing with each of the above categories, it may be helpful to ennumerate approaches which have been identified as antitherapeutic in this field:

- dismissive, hostile or judgemental attitudes on the part of the clinician, often characterised by expressions such as: 'just try and forget about it', 'pull yourself together', 'stop making such a fuss, you're wasting my time'
- denying that the client's symptoms exist at all: 'it's all in your mind', 'you're imagining it'

- attempting to reassure the client with irrelevant/confusing explanations
- discharging the client on the basis that there is nothing the clinician can do to help
- assiduously referring the client for a long series of investigations of doubtful value or relevance
- providing medication or other medical intervention for the sole purpose of placating the client
- failing to make basic enquiries about possible psychosocial factors involved
- failing to give clients a full and proper explanation about their condition, particularly the influence of psychosocial factors; this may sometimes be an attempt to avoid an angry or defensive response
- failing to refer the client for the appropriate psychological assessment at an early stage.

Many clinicians reading the above list will be in a position to recognise these approaches as unfortunately familiar occurrences. Clearly, while it is ideal for the whole treatment team to work in harmony towards the overall therapeutic goal, there is much that an individual clinician can do to set a good example in this area. This can make all the difference to ultimate clinical outcome and do much to restore the client's relationship with the service. The following suggestions are offered as elements of good practice in the treatment process when working with people with psychophysiological disorders.

1. Ensure that clients feel they have been properly listened to and understood.
2. Establish a positive working partnership between the client and clinician. At all costs, avoid the relationship becoming combative.
3. Convince clients that the clinician takes their pain/symptoms seriously. Even where there is no demonstrable physical origin for the symptoms, the client's experience is nonetheless real.
4. Provide accurate, clear information in order to fill the gaps in the client's understanding of the relevant disease process. Identify appropriate links between the physical and emotional state.

5. Find out what the client believes is causing/aggravating the pain/symptoms, and upon what evidence he has based his conclusions.
6. Where appropriate, help the client to review, question and test out this evidence. The use of questionnaires and self-monitoring tools are of great assistance in this process.
7. Assist clients to develop a new, more realistic understanding of their symptoms by reframing them in a holistic manner; include psychosocial factors which precipitate or maintain the illness.
8. At each stage, check that clients have thoroughly understood what has been discussed and how it relates to their own situation.
9. Assist clients to identify and tackle behaviours/lifestyle factors which aggravate the problem, e.g. diet, activity levels, occupation, medication abuse, avoidance.
10. Assist clients to develop positive behavioural and psychological coping strategies to aid self-management of the problem.

Where a significant organic disorder exists, treatment should emphasise education about how stress can affect the physical condition and the need to make vital lifestyle changes. This approach will be exemplified later in this chapter (p. 155). Where problems are primarily psychogenic, treatment should emphasise helping the client to conceptualise their symptoms more appropriately and to develop positive coping strategies.[3] In such cases, the psychological elements of treatment are paramount and no time should be lost in getting the relevant assessments and interventions under way. If the client's attitudes are allowed to become entrenched, a chronic condition may develop.[2,3]

Partridge[4] has suggested that the treatment process should take into account factors concerned with motivation. Accordingly, treatment should be organised with emphasis on achievement-related tasks, incorporating consideration of the following factors:

- affiliation needs
- levels of aspiration
- knowledge of results
- emotional reactions to illness
- perception of illness
- coping strategies.

In a recent review of the literature, Lehrer and Woolfolk[5] drew the following conclusions in relation to the treatment of psychophysiological disorders:

1. Stress management interventions are effective treatments or adjuncts for a wide variety of somatic disorders.
2. Anxiety-reduction techniques are more effective when applied specifically in relation to the relevant symptomatology, e.g. muscle relaxation for muscle tension pain and cognitive therapy for problems with a primarily cognitive presentation.
3. Non-pharmacological interventions, e.g. AMT programmes, are preferable since they avoid chemical dependence and are more likely to be effective in the long term.
4. Treatment should be geared to produce the change required, i.e. is it important to change what the client actually feels, or what they believe, in relation to their symptoms? In the first case, relaxation skills may successfully reduce perceived symptoms relating to muscle tension, for example. In the second case, a change in the client's interpretation of/attitude to his symptoms may be more important.
5. Combinations of techniques — as used in most comprehensive AMT courses — are more effective in treating psychophysiological disorders.
6. Although treatment should be individualised, some of this work can be done successfully within a group context.[6]

The remainder of this chapter will be devoted firstly to the subject of pain management, and secondly to the treatment of some common psychophysiological disorders, i.e. cardiac, musculoskeletal and general medical problems, using AMT.

CHRONIC MUSCULOSKELETAL/ RHEUMATOLOGICAL DISORDERS

The background

This group of disorders contains some of the most common and intractable problems that therapists are likely to encounter. Examples include:

- chronic back pain
- chronic neck/shoulder conditions
- rheumatoid arthritis
- chronic trauma-related conditions
- repetitive strain injury.

The effects of such conditions upon the patient's well-being can be devastating. Wide-ranging problems may result affecting all aspects of the individual's lifestyle, including physical, psychological, social, occupational and behavioural areas of function.[7] The following list gives some of the common effects:

- pain
- restricted mobility in and out of the home
- reduced independence in personal self-care activities
- reduced independence in home management tasks e.g. shopping and housework
- reduced independence in child-care activities
- restricted lifestyle, including fewer social and recreational outlets
- relationship problems, e.g. family, marital
- restricted sexual activity
- sleep disturbance
- financial hardship
- loss of job/reduced job options
- disrupted/reduced work output
- depression/anxiety
- suicidal ideation
- reduced self-esteem and confidence.

Clearly, the deleterious effects are not limited to the individual alone — the ripples spread to include partners, family members, work colleagues and those beyond. For example, the huge economic costs of musculoskeletal disorders are not only borne by those directly affected.[8,9] The annual cost of back injury to British industry has been estimated at £5.1 billion per year.[9] The Health and Safety Executive[10] has recently stated that musculoskeletal disorders are the largest form of work-related ill health in the UK. It estimated that 5.4 million working days were lost in England and Wales during 1990 due to musculoskeletal problems.

In many cases, however, these disorders are relatively transient and do not become chronic or substantially disabling. What factors contribute to the development of chronicity? Even where the condition is by its nature a chronic one, each individual varies in the extent to which their psychosocial function becomes disrupted. This depends upon a number of factors. One argument holds that there is a link between severity of pain and the development of depression.[11,12] Conversely, it has been proposed[13] that depression only results when maladaptive cognitive responses are used to cope with the pain. Weiser and Cedraschi[14] reviewed numerous studies of psychosocial factors associated with the development of chronic low back pain. Various factors including personality type, cognitive styles, social support, life events and compensation status were found to be significant influences in chronic disability states. However, many of the studies were adversely affected by inadequate methodology. Thus, it was not possible to draw firm conclusions about the relative importance of any one of these factors in predicting chronicity.

Finally, while some factors confirmed expectations, others were surprising. As expected, outstanding compensation claims may indeed hamper successful outcomes in rehabilitation, but so may the existence of supportive social circumstances. Supportive spouses were shown to play a significant role in reinforcing pain behaviour.[15,16,17] In such cases the illness may have a role in maintaining or stabilising family dynamics. The contribution of the family in the development of chronic illness has been highlighted as an important area for further study.[14]

Treatment formats

A wealth of studies has shown that cognitive behaviour modification (CBM) is an effective treatment strategy for musculoskeletal and rheumatological conditions.[8,14,18,19,20,21,22] The CBM model holds that cognitive factors such as coping style, attitudes, beliefs and expectations have a major impact on pain and disability levels. These factors are susceptible to modification through learning and CBM programmes aim to decrease maladaptive (pain) behaviours and increase those which are adaptive.[8] Examples of pain behaviours include repetitive descriptions/complaints of pain, reduced activity levels, avoidance of responsibility, reliance on pain medication and adoption of body postures/facial expressions which draw attention to the pain, e.g. grimacing, wincing, groaning. Such behaviours may produce their own reinforcements such as attention from concerned family members, relief from responsibilities and provision of habit-forming analgesic medication. Ultimately, the sufferer may cease to engage in any pleasurable activity of the kind associated with 'wellness', resulting in depression, anxiety and an increased awareness of pain. Thus, CBM focuses on increasing engagement in pleasurable activities, while disregarding pain behaviour.[22]

The subject of pain management is dealt with separately in this chapter, but it will be recognised that pain is frequently the foremost symptom in this group of disorders, therefore a brief overview of a relevant treatment approach is given here. Objectives for a CBM programme are suggested below, based on the work of Turk and Rudy:[23]

- combat demoralisation and defeatism
- foster the belief that the treatment really does work
- foster the belief that the patient is resourceful and competent and thus able to gain control over his or her problems
- teach patients to recognise and challenge maladaptive cognitive patterns
- teach a range of coping skills, both behavioural and psychological
- teach patients to attribute success to their own efforts
- facilitate maintenance and change on a long-term basis.

CBM course elements

A typical CBM course or programme for musculoskeletal/rheumatological disorders would include the following elements.

Education

- relevant health education which clarifies the facts about the disorder
- reconceptualising the pain experience, including the physical and psychosocial factors which reinforce the problem
- recognising the influence of factors such as muscle tension and posture in reinforcing pain
- developing self-mastery in relation to all aspects of the problem, e.g. symptoms and lifestyle.

Relaxation

- teaching appropriate muscle relaxation techniques[24]
- application of relaxation skills to real life situations.

Cognitive control

- recognition of maladaptive cognitive styles e.g. catastrophising
- challenging and modifying maladaptive cognitive styles
- teaching mental relaxation skills, e.g. visualisation, in order to manage pain.

Behavioural modification

- pain management/coping skills, e.g. activity pacing[25,26]
- scheduling pleasant activity
- goal-setting.

Finally, Keefe and Van Horn[8] have reviewed the issue of maintaining treatment gains in CBM interventions and emphasise the importance of relapse prevention. Accordingly, patients are asked to review previous set-backs in order to identify potentially high-risk situations. They are then assisted in developing contingency plans and strategies to prepare them for coping with likely problems and to prevent future relapse.

GENERAL MEDICAL DISORDERS

The conceptualisation of medical illness from a psychophysiological perspective

This perspective may include an almost infinite number of medical conditions. Such conditions may be precipitated, or aggravated, by psychosocial factors and their interaction with physiological systems. It is now becoming much more acceptable, from the theoretical point of view, to argue that all nominally 'physical' illnesses have a psychological/social component or factor to be taken into account. This may apply to the causes of the illness, the reasons preventing recovery, or its consequences for the individual's lifestyle.

Unfortunately, however, this opinion is frequently rejected by those who present with an illness complicated by psychosocial factors. Clinicians often meet with hostility when attempting to explore these aspects with their patients, as if it were insulting to suggest that the illness might be anything other than purely physical in nature. In view of the totally integrated and inseparable links between the mind and body, which are now beyond refutation, this attitude is, at best, out-dated. It must, of course, be recognised that enlightened attitudes are not universal amongst health care professionals, and they may be partly responsible for engendering retrogressive attitudes among those they attempt to help. Therefore, perhaps the most crucial task confronting health care professionals in this field is to assist clients in reconceptualising their illness. Further, treatment approaches should be holistic, involving educational, physiological, psychological and behavioural components in order to be fully effective. The cognitive-behavioural approach described here meets these criteria and comprises a truly comprehensive psychophysiological treatment regime.

The clinical group — its breadth and nature

Having stated that this clinical group may include an almost limitless number of conditions, there are certain disorders which crop up very commonly, or are particularly susceptible to the psychophysiological approach. Examples include:

- irritable bowel syndrome
- gastric/duodenal ulcer
- headache
- chronic fatigue syndrome
- disorders of sleep
- skin disorders.

In most of the disorders listed above, the level of physiological arousal is thought to exert a strong influence on symptoms and/or the disease process, e.g. irritable bowel syndrome, ulcer, headache. Behavioural or psychosocial features may also be important factors in others, e.g. chronic fatigue syndrome, disorders of sleep. Additionally, serious progressive or terminal illnesses such as multiple sclerosis and cancer frequently involve symptoms which can be eased by interventions such as relaxation training. The primary care team is very often the first port of call in these cases and it is posited that problems could be dealt with more effectively at this stage, thus preventing the escalation and complications, so often the ultimate outcome.

Three conditions have been selected here for the purpose of illustrating various ways in which the cognitive behaviour modification (CBM) approach may be applied. These are headache, disorders of sleep and chronic fatigue syndrome.

Headache

The difficulty of diagnosing and classifying headache symptomatology is complex. The recent attempt by Hopkins[27] to provide a simpler classification for chronic recurrent headaches demonstrates this problem:

- common headache, e.g. tension headache, common migraine, non-specific headache
- headaches with focal neurological symptoms, e.g. classical migraine
- vascular headache, e.g. those induced by increases in blood pressure or cranial vasodilation

- headache in association with raised intracranial pressure, e.g. cerebral tumour
- exertional and coital headache
- cranial neuralgias
- anatomical distortions or variations in the skull and facial bones.

Much recent research has involved comparative studies attempting to distinguish which treatments are most effective for which type of headache.[2] Few studies have produced clear results so far, but two main conclusions are beginning to emerge:

- specific psychological treatments, e.g. cognitive therapy, biofeedback and relaxation have proved to be effective
- the psychological approaches are at least as effective as drug treatment.[28,29,30,31]

The cognitive–behavioural model of headache acknowledges the integral role of psychological factors in chronic headache disorders. This approach emphasises the way in which the individual construes events and his reactions to those events. This is in contrast to the traditional model in which the physiological arousal which may have brought about the headache symptoms is targeted. For example, an individual who tends to perceive events around them negatively will tend to react with more physiological arousal and is consequently more likely to develop symptoms such as headache. Thus, in the cognitive–behavioural approach, the underlying causes are tackled, rather than their consequences. Key elements in the cognitive–behavioural approach include:

- learning to identify and monitor sources of stress and anxiety
- learning to identify the role that cognitive style plays in determining reaction to stressors
- learning specific coping strategies.[32]

Tools and treatment procedures

Headache diaries The use of a daily headache diary has been held up as a 'gold standard' in the treatment of headache.[28] The self-report headache diary is of value both to inform the treatment process, and as an outcome measure. Headache diaries should contain:

- a headache rating scale
- a section for recording related cognitions
- a section for the client to record any stressful events which precede the onset of the headache, as well as associated behavioural responses.

Completion of the diary will allow identification of key stressors and the cognitive style/ behavioural strategies which may be reinforcing the headaches.

Salkovskis[33] has suggested an appropriate self-rating scale which can be used in the measurement of headache severity:

0 – No headache
1 – Low level, intermittent awareness only
2 – Pain can be ignored intermittently
3 – Painful but can continue to work
4 – Severe, difficult to concentrate
5 – Intense, incapacitating

Techniques The appropriate nterventions will usually be suggested by the information collected in each individual's headache diary. However, the following list gives examples of a range of techniques which may be appropriate elements of a treatment package for chronic headache problems:

- breathing retraining
- biofeedback
- muscle relaxation training
- applied/differential relaxation training
- visualisation
- autogenic training
- cognitive therapy
- dietary advice
- exercise therapy.

General stress management approaches such as goal-setting and time-management techniques should be an integral part of all packages.

Lifestyle re-evaluation may also be an important part of the treatment programme and this may include exploration of work-related problems or adjustment of the emphasis accorded to the different activities making up the individual's lifestyle (see p. 162).

Disorders of sleep

Insomnia may present in various different forms:[34]

- delayed sleep onset
- insufficient sleep duration
- inadequate sleep maintenance e.g. early-morning wakening
- irregular sleep pattern from night to night.

The results of disturbed or inadequate sleep may include:

- fatigue during the daytime
- poor concentration/problem solving
- frustration/irritability/anxiety
- depressed mood.

Clearly, chronic insomnia can have devastating effects on an individual's social, occupational, physical and psychological well-being. The attending desperation has led to the prescribing of hypnotic medication on a huge scale. In 1982 approximately 14 million prescriptions for hypnotics were issued in the UK.[35] All drugs used as hypnotics carry with them some degree of health risk and this is frequently substantial, e.g. overdose toxicity, dependence and side-effects. For example, in 1988, the committee on Safety of Medicines advised that benzodiazepine dependence was a major cause for concern and that prescribing levels must be reduced. A steady decline in benzodiazepine prescribing levels has resulted but still remains unacceptably high. Non-drug alternatives to the management of insomnia are strongly recommended in the interests of both health and long-term effectiveness.

Aetiology

The aetiology of insomnia is multifaceted and some of the major causes are:

- physical disorders, e.g. cardiovascular disease, snoring, restless legs syndrome, pain, musculoskeletal disorders, tinnitus, digestive disturbances, breathing problems
- physiological factors, e.g. autonomic arousal, late-night eating/exercise, low activity levels during the daytime
- pharmacological factors, e.g. caffeine, nicotine, alcohol, stimulant drugs and certain prescription drugs
- psychological factors, e.g. anxiety, depression, stress/stressful life events, nightmares, preoccupation with sleeping difficulty
- disrupted circadian rhythm, e.g. due to shift work/jet lag, delayed/advanced sleep phase syndrome
- environmental factors, e.g. noise, temperature, light, sleeping environment not conducive to sleep, bed partner snoring
- poor sleep hygiene/habits, e.g. irregular schedule, over-sleeping, naps during the daytime.

Non-drug interventions for sleep disorders

Non-drug treatment regimes may involve a number of elements and examples of these are listed below.[34,35,36,37,38] In order to make an appropriate selection from these elements thorough assessment is needed. Also, in order to inform the treatment approach in each individual case, the use of sleep diaries is essential. An example of a sleep diary and self-rating scale for the measurement of sleep quality has been given in a recent report by the National Medical Advisory Committee.[35]

Education — sleep cycles, function of sleep and its effects. Sleep hygiene/habits which encourage good quality sleep, e.g. avoiding daytime naps, stimulants.

Sleep stimulus control — utilising routine cues to establish the association of retiring to bed with sleep onset, getting up if still awake after 10–15 minutes.

Sleep restriction — limiting the amount of time spent in bed to the duration normally spent actually asleep. Initially, there may be partial sleep deprivation but this is thought to be a positive factor in re-establishing good sleep hygiene.

Chronotherapy — used in circadian rhythm disorders in which, for example, the individual feels sleepy during the daytime rather than at night. This approach involves successively delaying sleep by three hours each day until the desired bedtime is reached.

Relaxation training techniques — muscle relaxation, breathing techniques, biofeedback, meditation.

Cognitive therapy — to identify and challenge negative attitudes to the problem. Insomniacs frequently see themselves as helpless victims of the disorder. This approach may also involve cognitive techniques to reduce intrusive thoughts such as thought stopping and visualisation.

Finally, it should be noted that the incidence of insomnia increases with age[38,39] and is exacerbated due to the reduced sleep requirements among older adults. Sleeping lightly and waking early are normal features in this age group. However, expectations about how much sleep is actually needed may not adjust accordingly. Treatment regimes should emphasise education about sleep and realistic sleep requirements, re-establishing conducive sleep routines, increasing daytime exercise and cutting out daytime napping.

Chronic fatigue syndrome

Debate still rages about the causes and pathology underlying chronic fatigue syndrome (CFS). No definitive aetiology exists as yet, and there is a great deal of argument and preoccupation over whether the disease is of primarily psychological or physiological origin.[40,41,42] In some quarters, considerable sensitivity about this issue has been aroused.[42] In the writer's opinion, a more constructive approach is offered by the psychophysiological school of thought, particularly in view of the widespread uncertainty about the aetiology of CFS.

What is CFS?

The Leeds Fatigue Clinic, which has been carrying out a major study[41] of CFS, have recommended the following diagnostic criteria:

1. A characteristic history of generalised chronic, persisting or relapsing fatigue exacerbated by minor exercise, causing significant disruption of usual daily activities and of over 6 months' duration.
2. A normal physical examination (excluding lymphadenopathy, muscle tenderness or pharyngitis).
3. Negative investigation results to exclude other chronic diseases.' Additional symptomatology such as concentration impairment and depleted lymphocyte counts may present contiguously.

The psychophysiological approach to treatment

Therapeutic programmes based on the Cognitive Behavioural Modification (CBM) model have been found to be remarkably successful in helping sufferers to cope more positively with CFS.[40,42,43] A typical group-based therapeutic programme has been described by the Leeds Fatigue Clinic[41] and this is outlined below.

Session 1: Introduction — using group work techniques, members share and explore the experiences and problems of living with CFS.

Session 2: Graded activity — using goal-setting and carefully graded activity, members are encouraged to increase their activity levels gradually.

Session 3: Diet and exercise — members share their views and develop a sensible and practical approach to this aspect of treatment.

Session 4: Stress and relaxation — members are provided with information about the links between stress and physical status/health. Relaxation techniques are taught.

Session 5: Effects on the way we feel — includes education about the effects of emotions and thoughts upon lifestyle and self-esteem. Positive cognitive coping strategies are explored, based on the CBM approach.

Session 6: Effects on the way we think — focuses on cognitive performance skills such as memory and concentration. Strategies to overcome problems are explored.

Session 7: Coping with others — social difficulties, e.g. disrupted relationships and role loss are explored along with relevant coping strategies.

Session 8: Evaluation — review of progress and planning for future consolidation of skills.

PAIN MANAGEMENT

Self-management of chronic pain is most applicable to people who 'have high behavioural but low pathological elements'.[44] It is also increasingly accepted that this group of people benefit most from a multidisciplinary approach to pain management.

In order to gain benefit maximally from a self-management approach to chronic pain it is crucial that both therapist and sufferer have an understanding of the nature of chronic pain and the effects that it has on the individual's lifestyle. For this reason we will look firstly at chronic pain and its effects before going on to look at the areas for intervention.

CHANGES IN LIFESTYLE

A distinction must be made between acute pain and chronic pain. Acute pain has a useful role in protecting and allowing healing in an injured part of the body and will gradually resolve. Chronic pain, on the other hand, assumes an entirely different role. Chronic pain is described as pain lasting longer than 3–6 months, and for many sufferers the extent of the pain experienced is beyond that which would be expected as a result of the primary cause of the pain.[45]

The experience of unrelenting pain has been shown to affect several aspects of the sufferer's life. These commonly experienced lifestyle changes alter physical ability, psychological well-being and behaviour with a corresponding imbalance in rest, productivity and leisure.

Physically, reduced levels of activity are often found. This is usually the result of protective measures being taken to avoid aggravating the pain. The inactivity influences physical and psychological processes. Physical effects of ongoing inactivity associated with chronic pain are decreased muscle strength, poor posture, changes in blood circulation and increased muscle tension.

Psychologically, sufferers may experience reactive depression as a result of their limited activity, changes in their role in the family and society, and feelings of being no longer in control of their lives. Part of the 'chronic pain syndrome'[46] involves the pain experience being modified by learning and behavioural adaptation.[44] A fundamental component of the modified learning and adaptation process is related to the communication of pain or pain behaviour.

PAIN BEHAVIOUR

In simple terms, pain behaviour may be described as ways of communicating with others about pain. This may be done through verbal and non-verbal means. This behaviour is useful in acute pain, as it encourages those around to support the sufferer during the healing process. With chronic pain, the pain behaviour may become reinforced by environmental events, for instance, increased attention from family members, avoidance of previously disliked activities. However, their effectiveness as a means of communication eventually diminishes and results in maladaptive behaviour.

Sufferers commonly describe disguising their behaviour in certain circumstances and trying to behave 'normally'. This results in acceptance by associates, but causes anxiety and tension in the sufferer. Alternatively, exhibiting pain behaviour may cause the person to be isolated and excluded from social interactions. Thus, neither approach is effective for the chronic pain sufferer, and part of the pain management approach involves understanding pain behaviour in order for the individual to be able to control its effects.

THE PAIN GATE THEORY

The pain gate theory provides a useful conceptual framework for understanding the physiological and psychological components of the experience of pain and their interaction. It is well established that pain sensations are conducted to the brain via the spinal cord. Melzack and Wall[47,48] identify three systems in the dorsal horn of the spinal cord which are significant in conducting pain sensations. These are the substantia gelatinosa, the dorsal column fibres and the transmission (T) cells. The substantia gelatinosa is thought to provide the 'gate control mechanism', with the dorsal column also inhibiting pain transmission at the spinal cord level.

One of the major influences on the spinal gating mechanism is the relative amount of activity in large-diameter and small-diameter nerve fibres: activity in large fibres tends to inhibit transmission, i.e. close the gate, while small fibre activity tends to facilitate transmission, i.e. open the gate. Two main types of nerve fibres are described as having a role in the conduction of pain — A and C fibres. C fibres are thin, unmyelinated, slow-conducting and are associated with dull generalised pain. A fibres, which are thicker, well myelinated and fast-conducting are associated with sharp pain. A fibres are thought to be important in the modification and inhibition of pain transmission via the C fibres. It is theorised that by increasing activities that facilitate transmission in the dorsal columns, i.e. via the A fibres, it is possible to inhibit pain transmission in the substantia gelatinosa.

Certain factors have been shown to be effective in inhibiting the cells in the dorsal horn of the spinal cord, i.e. closing the 'gate'. These include relaxation, distraction, exercise and improved mobility, and cutaneous stimulation techniques such as transcutaneous nerve stimulation (TNS). On the other hand, factors such as stress, tension, thinking about pain, lack of exercise and immobility are thought to open the 'gate' thereby allowing increased experience of pain. Therefore, pain management programmes will aim to address these areas of importance. In conjunction with this there are thought to be various chemical reactions which influence the pain experience. Endorphins, for example, which are thought to be associated with a sense of well-being, are among the pain-suppressing chemicals found. Endorphins are known to be released during activities such as relaxation and exercise. Therefore, the promotion of these factors is central to pain management.

FACTORS THAT INFLUENCE THE PERCEPTION OF PAIN

A healthy and happy lifestyle is held to be associated with lower perceived pain levels.[6] Attitudes and behaviours which increase perceived pain include the following:

- negative attitude to pain, i.e. 'awfulising' the pain (cultural influences may affect this factor)[7]
- taking on illness behaviours, e.g. general inactivity, not getting dressed, having no daily routine, 'pampering the pain'
- withdrawing from others and lack of participation in enjoyable activities
- taking no exercise
- poor diet
- low self-regard, negative self-talk
- adopting self-punitive attitudes, self-denial
- continually talking about and focusing on the pain
- focusing on activities which the individual is no longer able to do.

INTERACTION BETWEEN PAIN, ACTIVITY, THOUGHTS AND FEELINGS

Chronic pain sufferers may feel that they lack control over their lives and that everything they do is influenced by their experience of pain on a day-to-day basis. They may feel that there is little hope, as conventional medicine may have failed to relieve the pain. This can result in the sufferer becoming trapped in a downward spiral. At some point sufferers may attempt to take conscious and positive action towards regaining control, or they may take no action, resulting in a general loss of control over their lives (see Fig. 16.1).

GAINING CONTROL IN SPITE OF THE PAIN

Having looked broadly at the effects of chronic pain, the focus will now move to the process of regaining control in spite of the pain. Particular attention will be paid to the implementation of

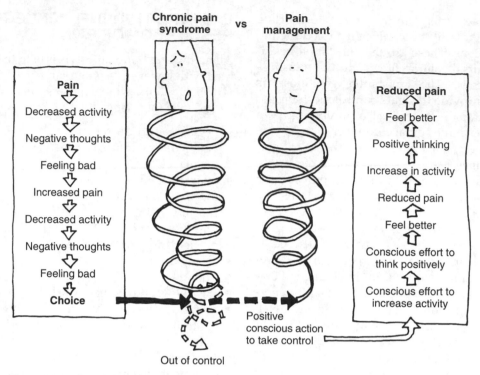

Figure 16.1 Chronic pain syndrome vs pain management.

interventions which have been found to be effective in chronic pain management.

Pain may very easily take over the sufferer's life leaving him or her feeling powerless. As therapists we aim to help people with chronic pain to gain insight into the way they are managing their lives and to make the positive changes needed in order to regain control. In practice, however, it is not so easy to achieve this grand goal.

The remaining part of this section looks at some of the main areas in which therapists can work with pain sufferers. These areas are:

1. Lifestyle balance
2. Personal management:
   - goal-setting
   - prioritising
   - time management
   - pacing.
3. Adaptation of the environment
4. Relaxation
5. Physical management:
   - exercise
   - diet
   - rest
   - sleep.

Lifestyle balance

As mentioned previously, chronic pain sufferers commonly experience changes in their lifestyle brought about by an imbalance in rest, productivity and leisure. On analysing how pain sufferers spend their time and energy it often emerges that they either:

- do very little and become stuck in the 'take it easy trap'[49]

or

- they become very busy, putting all their energy into one area of their lives, often because they feel obligated to do so; they seldom enjoy what they are doing and feel swamped by the demands of their perceived duty to that area, e.g. work, family.

It is therefore important to explore how individuals spend their time and energy and assist them in generating ideas about aspects they need to change or improve about their lifestyle. Useful areas to consider are:

- work and career
- financial situation
- physical well-being: exercise, diet, relaxation
- relationships, time for/with others
- education
- creative and cultural
- self and personal growth
- leisure and hobbies.

Lifestyle balancing does not merely involve putting equal amounts of time into each area, but rather, developing the recognition that all areas are important. For example, if someone is giving all their time and energy to work, the answer is not simply to reduce their work hours. Instead, they may need to involve themselves in a more varied range of pursuits — physical, creative, social and cultural.

Once the lifestyle aspects which the individual needs and wants to change have been identified, the way in which these changes will be achieved is then explored.

Personal management: goal-setting, prioritisation, time management, pacing

Changes in lifestyle associated with chronic pain result in the individual having less time and energy available for participating in a variety of activities. In order to maximise time and energy resources, a process of goal-setting in conjunction with prioritisation is necessary.

Pain management involves setting long-term goals which then need to be broken down into realistic short-term goals to facilitate their achievement. Prioritisation involves making decisions about which activities are most important to each individual.

Time management and pacing help to put the goals into action. It is necessary to plan ahead in order to accommodate the priority activities into the daily timetable. Identification and elimina-

tion of favourite time wasters can help to free up extra time. Priority setting also helps to inform choices about what to allocate time to. Identifying the individual's most productive time of day may also be useful in ensuring that the most is made out of each day.[51]

Pacing, a particularly important element of pain management, involves setting reasonable time limits for the chosen activities and attempting to keep within these on a daily basis despite fluctuations in the level of pain experienced. This is necessary in order to break the common activity cycle of overactivity on one day and consequent suffering for a few days after. It is also necessary to ensure that demanding activities are spaced out evenly during each day or week. Special events also need to be planned for.

In order to illustrate application of these concepts an example is given here using the long-term goal of walking children to school. Assuming that the individual is able to walk for 5 minutes on a 'bad' day and 10 minutes on a 'good' day, a time limit for walking is set at 7 minutes (about midway between the minimum and maximum time limit). In order to achieve this, the individual may drive most of the way to the school, parking a short distance from the school so that the walk from the car to the school and back would take seven minutes. This is practised every day until the individual becomes comfortable with the task at that level, and is ready to increase the time walked. However, this activity has to be planned for alongside other activities to be done in the same day, so it may be easier to achieve this in the morning. For example, when the individual could return home and rest for a short period while it is quiet, rather than in the afternoon, when the children are home from school. Pain management involves understanding these concepts and learning how to apply them to daily living.

Adaptation of the environment

The social and physical environment may play a significant part in the experience of pain. The social environment has been discussed in relation to pain behaviours, therefore the focus will now be on the physical environment. The principle of maintaining a good posture is central to interaction in the physical environment. This means that seating needs to be appropriate to enable the person to achieve a good posture in sitting; this also applies to sleeping positions.

Lifting needs careful consideration so as to eliminate heavy lifting and excessive or incorrect bending; laundry, for example, is often loaded downwards and heavy, wet washing then picked up from the floor. Simple alteration to the height of the support on which a laundry basket is placed can eliminate unnecessary strain. There are many practical solutions to common problems which can be addressed by applying the above principles.

Relaxation

Pain and tension go together and teaching people to relax with their pain rather than tense against it is crucial. This is frequently a difficult matter because sufferers tend to resist movement, so holding onto the tension. They may also feel that if they let go they risk losing control. Relaxation can involve a release of emotions as well as muscle tension and if people can learn to relax with their pain it can be reduced.

Posture is as important a part of relaxation as it is of pain management. Laura Mitchell's relaxation method[52] (see Chapter 8) teaches both posture and relaxation. This technique is easy to learn and adapt to activity and may also serve as a good starting point for other relaxation techniques, e.g. visualisation.

Each person is different and the therapist needs to find the relaxation method that suits individual needs. Techniques such as Laura Mitchell's simple relaxation,[52] basic autogenic training[53] and self-hypnosis[53] (see Chapters 8 and 9) are particularly good in pain-management applications because they do not require any focus on tension or tensing activities. Instead, a comfortable relaxed posture is recommended in conjunction with a positive state of mind.

Physical management

General physical well-being is important in pain management and the following areas should be considered:

- exercise
- diet
- rest
- sleep.

The exercise aspect is the only one expanded upon here because pain management involves a different approach to exercise. Most people who participate in exercise programmes probably expect to be told exactly how many of each exercise they are expected to do. Pain management differs in that individuals are encouraged to be in control of the exercise programme, setting their own individual goals for the number of each exercise to be completed, and when to do it. However, individuals should still be given overall professional guidance as to goal-setting and pacing in relation to exercise as with other activities. Therefore, exercise levels should be set at a realistic level, which can be achieved on a daily basis, in order to gain the longer-term benefits of the exercise regime.

CONCLUSION

This section has given a broad overview of pain management. Primarily it involves self-management, that is, assisting sufferers to gain a greater understanding of their pain and its effects, increasing both perceived and actual control of symptoms and lifestyle. Although many of the concepts involved in the management of pain are based on similar principles to anxiety management, an understanding of the specific nature of chronic pain is vital for therapists in this field.

CARDIAC REHABILITATION

INTRODUCTION

Less than 30 years ago in this country, a three-week period of bed rest was usual practice following a heart attack. Since then, great strides have been made in developing treatment strategies to address the detrimental effects of myocardial infarction (MI) on an individual's physical and psychological health. Early attempts focused on helping the patient adapt to future disability, but as knowledge about the detrimental effects (physical and psychological) of prolonged bed rest increased and the very positive benefits[54] of exercise, were more widely acknowledged, emphasis shifted away from ideas of disability and towards reconditioning. The past 30 years have seen a growth in cardiac rehabilitation programmes, particularly in the western world. Accompanying this growth has been recognition of the need for cardiac rehabilitation to include other factors such as education, risk-factor modification and stress management.

The World Health Organization[55] defines cardiac rehabilitation as

... the sum of activities required to influence favourably the underlying cause of the disease, as well as the best possible physical, mental and social conditions, so that they may, by their own efforts, preserve, or resume when lost, as normal a place as possible in the community. Rehabilitation cannot be regarded as an isolated form of therapy but must be integrated with the whole treatment of which it forms only one facet.

Thus, cardiac rehabilitation is a process which commences at the point of diagnosis and continues indefinitely (see Fig. 16.2). It is one which can adapt to the changing needs of individuals, at whatever point they may enter, e.g. following admission to hospital with an MI, via the GP or clinic with angina, or when re-referred due to a change in physical or psychological health or social circumstances. In order best to meet these needs and to influence positively the underlying cause of the disease and the physical, mental and social factors, a comprehensive multidisciplinary team effort is the preferred approach.

PSYCHOLOGICAL ASPECTS

This section will focus on:

- the psychosocial aspects of coronary heart disease (CHD)
- how stress management approaches may be used as part of a cardiac rehabilitation programme.

The diagnosis of CHD (either in the form of acute attack such as MI or angina) has grave

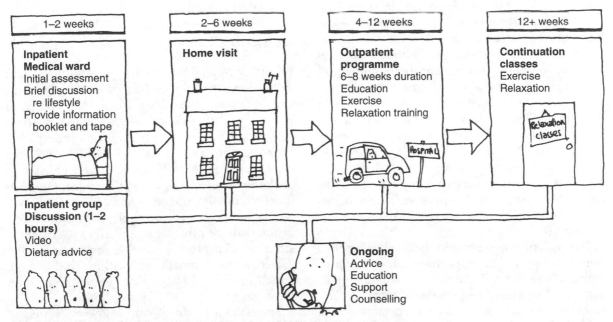

Figure 16.2   An example of a hospital-based cardiac rehabilitation programme.

psychological consequences. Anxiety,[56] fear, depression and loss of confidence are frequently documented traumas which result from the sudden, unexpected occurrence of the cardiac event.[57,58] Much of what is currently known about the psychological and social aspects of CHD results from research on middle-aged western males following MI and the growth of cardiac rehabilitation to encompass the needs of elderly people, women, people from ethnic minorities and those suffering from angina pectoris means that further research is needed before this knowledge can be generalised.

Immediately following MI patients typically deny what has happened to them.[59] 'Appropriate' denial of this kind serves to protect patients from the life-threatening nature of their situation, but it can prove harmful if it persists (e.g. the patient who denies having had an MI and continues to smoke or lift heavy items). After the initial denial, as the patient acknowledges recent events, a period of anxiety and depression may follow. Anxiety and depression are normal reactions to a traumatic life event and are experienced by about one third of patients following MI.[60] Patients who have a severe psychological reaction to MI may fail to resume normal activities of daily life, return to work,[61] or return to sexual function.[62] Indeed they are less likely to make and maintain the lifestyle changes promoted in rehabilitation. Without help they may adjust poorly and become increasingly preoccupied with their physical symptoms.[63] There is evidence to suggest that approximately one third of patients who receive no rehabilitation following MI are clinically anxious or depressed a year later.[64,65] The incidence of depression among patients recovering from MI is high. Whilst it resolves rapidly in many patients, others suffer from major depression[57] which has been linked with increased risk of mortality following MI.[66]

The patient is not alone in their suffering after a major cardiac event; partners are often profoundly affected.[67] They may experience guilt, anger and a sense of responsibility for their partner's present condition and future health.

Guilt, as experienced by the patient, may be caused by the rehabilitation team, who, in their attempts to identify risk factors, contribute to the patient's feelings that they must have done something wrong.[68] Johnson and Morse[68] examined the process of adjustment experienced by people following a heart attack. They found that patients varied in their adjustment following MI and identified four stages through which the patient struggles to regain a sense of personal control. These are defending oneself against threatened loss of control, coming to terms with the MI, re-establishing a sense of control and, finally, adjustment.

An awareness of how an individual is likely to react psychologically following MI can help the therapist focus treatment on the main areas of difficulty. The British Association for Cardiac Rehabilitation Guidelines[69] emphasise some key points for consideration when planning psychological intervention and suggest goals aimed at increasing quality of life and the prevention of secondary problems.

One important purpose of cardiac rehabilitation is to encourage the client to make lifestyle changes by modifying cardiac risk factors such as diet, smoking and stress. Stress reduction is an important part of psychological intervention in cardiac rehabilitation.

STRESS

In cardiac rehabilitation stress is best understood in relation to the biopsychosocial model of health and disease[70] (see Fig. 16.3). According to Engel,[70] nature is ordered in a hierarchical continuum with the individual at the highest level of an organismic hierarchy (which includes atoms, molecules, cells, tissues and organs), and at the lowest level of a social hierarchy (which includes family, society and nation). Each system is both a part and a whole in constant interaction with the others. Engel defines psychologic stress as 'all processes whether originating in the external environment or within the person, which impose a demand or requirement upon the organism'.

Psychological stress can trigger a series of physiological changes that in turn increase

Systems hierarchy
Levels of organisation

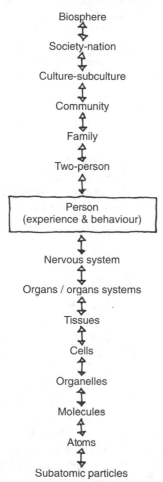

Biosphere

Society-nation

Culture-subculture

Community

Family

Two-person

Person
(experience & behaviour)

Nervous system

Organs / organs systems

Tissues

Cells

Organelles

Molecules

Atoms

Subatomic particles

Figure 16.3   The biopsychosocial model of health and disease.[70] Reproduced with kind permission of the American Psychiatric Association.

myocardial oxygen consumption (MVo$_2$) and lead to ischaemia.[71,72,73] Stimulation of the sympathetic nervous system triggers the release of epinephrine and norepinephrine into the circulation, resulting in quickening of the heart rate, a rise in blood pressure and vasoconstriction of the coronary arteries. The release of catecholemines and cortisol increase platelet aggregability, blood glucose and lipid levels. It is possible that in this way chronic stress may increase cardiovascular risk factors and expose the cardiovascular system in the presence of underlying CHD.

PSYCHOSOCIAL TREATMENT STRATEGIES IN CHD

The role of stress management

Individuals differ in the amount of support they need. Some require skilled help on an individual basis whilst the needs of others may be met in the group setting characteristic of outpatient programmes.

In addition to psychosocial support, education is essential. Teaching the patient to recognise 'fight or flight' as a natural response to anxiety can allay fears that any minor exertion or over-excitement will prove fatal. Learning about the relaxation response, its role in auto-immune stability and the need to practise provides a self-help tool. Helping the affected person to view what has happened as an opportunity for change may help to prevent self-blame and the tendency to regard the indicated lifestyle changes as unwelcome or draconian. Affirmations for health and well-being can be used to detract from the negative thought patterns which reinforce illness behaviour.[74]

The patient may also be introduced to complementary therapies — such as aromatherapy, massage, yoga and shiatsu — to help reduce arousal. Inviting a complementary therapist to speak as part of an outpatient programme or at an introductory session, establishes a link outside the hospital setting which continues after the course has been completed. Providing patients with natural tips to help them sleep — e.g. avoiding stimulating foods and drinks, such as chocolate, tomatoes, and coffee; taking regular exercise or restricting alcohol intake before bedtime — can prove invaluable. Other coping strategies for stressful situations such as learning how to be assertive and how to say 'no' are dealt with in Client Pack 7.

The way this information is imparted, and by whom, will depend on the way the cardiac rehabilitation is organised. Outpatient programmes provide the ideal opportunity for patient education and for experimentation with different techniques. However, it is usually 4–6 weeks after the MI, or slightly longer in the case of surgery, before the patient attends. It is helpful to provide some information whilst patients are still in hospital, or during a visit to their home immediately after discharge. This can be provided in an easy to follow written format, giving patients something to refer to in the early days and weeks. Teaching simple relaxation techniques and supporting these with a tape can also be helpful, providing patients are given the opportunity to ask questions and to make contact with the therapist if they are experiencing difficulties in mastering the skills.

At a time when patients are being asked to make essential lifestyle changes which require motivation and discipline, they may be especially vulnerable to maladaptive coping strategies which formed part of their previously chosen lifestyle e.g. smoking.

Body–mind interventions

There is an increasing awareness amongst health care professionals about the complex nature of the human organism and how body–mind interactions can have significant effects on health. Horwitz and colleagues[75] investigated the relationship between medication adherence and mortality after an MI in 2175 participants in the Beta Blockade Heart Attack Trial. They found that those who did not adhere well to prescribed medication regimes (i.e. took less than 75% of the prescribed medication) were 2.6 times more likely to die within a year of follow-up than good adherers. Poor adherers had an increased risk of death whether they took beta-blockers or a placebo. This suggests that those who did not adhere well had an increased incidence of mortality irrespective of whether the medication contained an active ingredient or not. Belief in the act of taking medication may have been a critical factor. Similarly, in planning intervention for prevention and recovery the therapist should consider the patient's values and beliefs. A key role of the therapist is to *empower* the patient to engage more actively in their own healing process/recovery.

Cardiac rehabilitation is well placed to integrate mind–body (psychophysiological) interventions such as relaxation, imagery, meditation, therapeutic yoga and complementary therapies into its programmes. Such techniques, which elicit the relaxation response, can play an important role in addressing the harmful effects of the fight or flight response and other cardiac risk factors such as high blood pressure, smoking and cholesterol.[76,77,78,79,80,81] The physiological changes brought about by the relaxation response (decreased oxygen consumption, heart rate, respiratory rate and levels of arterial blood lactate)[82,83] have a favourable impact on myocardial oxygen supply and demand. Thus, psychological changes involving reduced anxiety and hostility are also likely to exert a beneficial influence on the physiological problems commonly found in people with heart disease.[84]

Relaxation techniques

Van Dixhoorn and colleagues[85] demonstrated the improved effectiveness of exercise training when used in conjunction with relaxation and an enhanced physical and psychological outcome. This enhancing effect has also been shown by others.[86] Ornish[87] combined visualisation, meditation and relaxation exercises with moderate exercise and a vegetarian diet. He reported that after one year it is possible to reverse CHD. He noted a positive relationship between the time spent meditating and the amount of disease reversal. Smaller studies have looked at the use of relaxation training in femoral angiography,[88] heart surgery,[89] coronary care units and the treatment of angina pectoris[90] with encouraging results. However, larger randomised controlled trials are needed to distinguish the effects of relaxation from other rehabilitation efforts.

Not only is the relaxation response used to counteract the effects of stress and to address other cardiac risk factors but, equally, it can be used as a tool to empower the individual and to restore balance. Recognition is growing concerning the roles of the right and left cerebral hemispheres and their respective influence on memory, creativity, learning, problem-solving and stress reduction.[91] Understanding the brain's basic functions and applying techniques based on these functions can resource the natural capacity for learning and encourage mental and physical harmony.

Nash[92] suggests the need for stress management strategies to be directed away from reinforcement of left-brained functions such as organising, time-planning, goal-setting and prioritising (which may have contributed to the patient's condition) and towards right cerebral hemisphere strategies. These strategies involve an increased awareness of one's bodily and emotional reactions and developing intuition. Such strategies include using abdominal breathing, deep relaxation, meditation and visualisation in order to mobilise the parasympathetic nervous system. According to Nash, the peer group setting involved in cardiac rehabilitation programmes lends itself to these strategies, and shared experiences add concrete validity and reinforce independent practice.

CONCLUSION

People with heart disease suffer from a complexity of physical, psychological, emotional and social problems. Their needs differ in severity. In answer to this, cardiac rehabilitation has developed as a multidimensional approach that includes exercise training, education about health and lifestyle issues, stress management and counselling. This section has considered only one aspect of cardiac rehabilitation — the psychophysiological. With reference to theoretical material, it has touched upon some problems that may be experienced by the patient following MI and considered how stress management strategies might be helpful in addressing these.

REFERENCES

1 Lipsitt D R 1991 Can we really teach psychosomatic medicine? A review of successes and failures. Psychotherapy and Psychosomatics 56(1–2):102–111

2 Salkovskis P M 1992 Somatic problems. In: Hawton K, Salkovskis P M, Kirk J, Clark D M (eds) Cognitive behaviour therapy for psychiatric problems — a practical guide. Oxford Medical Publications, Oxford

3 Creed F, Mayou R, Hopkins A (eds) 1992 Medical symptoms not explained by organic disease. The Royal College of Psychiatrists and the Royal College of Physicians of London, London

4 Partridge C 1990 Psychological factors in recovery from physical disability. In: Hegna T, Sueram M (eds) Psychological and psychosomatic problems. Churchill Livingstone, Edinburgh

5 Lehrer P M, Woolfolk R L (eds) 1993 Principles and practice of stress management, 2nd edn. The Guilford Press, New York

6 Hellman C J, Budd M, Borysenko J, McClelland D C, Benson H 1990 A study of the effectiveness of two group behavioral interventions for patients with psychosomatic complaints. Behavioral Medicine 16(4):165–173

7 Strong J, Ashton R, Chant D, Cramond T 1994 An investigation of the dimensions of chronic low back pain: the patient's perspective. British Journal of Occupational Therapy 57(6):204–208

8 Keefe F J, Van Horn Y 1993 Cognitive–behavioral treatment of rheumatoid arthritis pain. Arthritis Care and Research 6(4):213–222

9 The Clinical Standards Advisory Group 1994 Report on back pain. HMSO, London

10 Health and Safety Executive 1995 Good health is good business — an introduction to managing health risks at work (musculoskeletal disorders). HSE Books, Suffolk

11 Brown G K 1990 A causal analysis of chronic pain and depression. Journal of Abnormal Psychology 99:127–137

12 Raspe H H, Rehfisch H P 1990 Entzundliche rheumatische Erkrankungen. In: Basler H D, Franz C, Kroner-Herwig B, Rehfisch H P, Seemann H (eds) Psychologische Schmerztherapie. Springer, Berlin/Heidelberg/New York, pp 328–374

13 Rudy T E, Kerns R D, Turk D C 1988 Chronic pain and depression: towards a cognitive–behavioral mediation model. Pain 35:129–140

14 Weiser S, Cedraschi C 1992 Psycho-social issues in the prevention of chronic low back pain — a literature review. Baillière's Clinical Rheumatology 6(3):657–684

15 Block A R, Kremer E, Gaylor M 1980 Behavioral treatments of chronic pain: the spouse as a discriminative cue for pain behavior. Pain 9:243–252

16 Anderson L P, Rehm L P 1984 The relationship between strategies of coping and perception of pain in three chronic pain groups. Journal of Clinical Psychology 40:1170–1177

17 Flor H, Kerns R D, Turk D C 1987(b) The role of spouse reinforcement, perceived pain, and activity levels of chronic pain patients. Journal of Psychosomatic Research 31:251–259

18 Parker J C, Iverson G L, Smarr K L, Stucky-Ropp R C 1993 Cognitive–behavioural approaches to pain management in rheumatoid arthritis. Arthritis Care and Research 6(4):207–212

19 Turner J A, Jensen M P 1993 Efficacy of cognitive therapy for chronic low back pain. Pain 52(2):169–177

20 Nicholas M K, Wilson P H, Goyen J 1992 Comparison of

cognitive–behavioral group treatment and an alternative non-psychological treatment for chronic low back pain. Pain 48(3):339–347

21 Caudill M, Schnable R, Zuttermeister P, Benson H, Friedman R 1991 Decreased clinic use by chronic pain patients: response to behavioral medicine intervention. Clinical Journal of Pain 7(4):305–310

22 Basler H D 1993 Group treatment for pain and discomfort. Patient Education and Counselling 20:167–175

23 Turk D C, Rudy T E 1988 A cognitive–behavioral perspective on chronic pain: beyond the scalpel and syringe. In: Tollison C D (ed) Handbook of chronic pain management. Williams and Wilkins, Baltimore, pp 222–236

24 Jackson T 1991 An evaluation of the Mitchell method of simple physiological relaxation for women with rheumatoid arthritis. British Journal of Occupational Therapy 54(3):105–107

25 Hafner C 1995 Getting the better of pain. Therapy Weekly May 18:7

26 O'Hara P 1995 Points to consider: pain management. Occupational Therapy News July:12

27 Hopkins A 1992 Management of chronic headache. In: Creed F, Mayou R, Hopkins A (eds) Medical symptoms not explained by organic disease. The Royal College of Psychiatrists and the Royal College of Physicians of London, London

28 Blanchard E B 1992 Psychological treatment of benign headache disorders. Journal of Consulting and Clinical Psychology 60(4):537–551

29 Holroyd K A, Nash J M, Pingel J K, Cordingley G E, Jerome A 1991 A comparison of pharmacological (amitryptyline HCL) and nonpharmacological (cognitive–behavioural) therapies for chronic tension headaches. Journal of Consulting and Clinical Psychology 59(3):387–393

30 Blanchard E B, Appelbaum K A, Nicholson N L 1990 A controlled evaluation of the addition of cognitive therapy to a home-based biofeedback and relaxation treatment of vascular headache. Headache 30(6):371–376

31 Blanchard E B, Appelbaum K A, Radnitz C L et al 1990 A controlled evaluation of the addition of thermal biofeedback and thermal biofeedback combined with cognitive therapy in the treatment of vascular headache. Journal of Consulting and Clinical Psychology 58(2):216–224

32 McCarron M S, Andrasik F 1987 Migraine and tension headaches. In: Michelson L, Ascher L M (eds) Anxiety and stress disorders — cognitive–behavioral assessment and treatment. Guilford Press, New York

33 Salkovskis P M 1992 Somatic problems. In: Hawton K, Salkovskis P M, Kirk J, Clark D M (eds) Cognitive behaviour therapy for psychiatric problems — a practical guide. Oxford Medical Publications, Oxford

34 Espie C A 1993 ABC of sleep disorders. Practical management of insomnia: behavioural cognitive techniques. British Medical Journal 306(6876):509–511

35 National Medical Advisory Committee 1994 The management of anxiety and insomnia. HMSO, Edinburgh

36 Bootzin R R, Perlis M L 1992 Nonpharmacologic treatments of insomnia. Journal of Clinical Psychiatry 53(6):37–41

37 Kennerley H 1995 Managing anxiety — a training manual, 2nd edn. Oxford Medical Publications, Oxford

38 Lader M, Smith T 1992 The medical management of insomnia in general practice. Round Table Series: no. 28. Royal Society of Medicine Services, London

39 Edinger J D, Hoelscher T J 1992 A cognitive behavioral therapy for sleep-maintenance insomnia in older adults. Psychology and Aging 7(2):282–289

40 Oliveck M 1994 OTs have ideal skills to combat CFS. Therapy Weekly, Dec 8

41 Pemberton S, Hatcher S, Stanley P, House A 1994 Chronic fatigue syndrome: A way forward. British Journal of Occupational Therapy 57(10):381–383

42 Stepney R 1996 Feeling tired and confused. The Independent 26 March

43 Sharpe M, Hawton K, Simkin S et al 1996 Cognitive behaviour therapy for the chronic fatigue syndrome: a randomised controlled trial. British Medical Journal (312):22–26

44 Hardy P, Hill P 1990 A multidisciplinary approach to pain management. British Journal of Hospital Medicine 43:45

45 Bonica J (ed) 1990 The management of pain, 2nd edn. Lea and Febiger, Philadelphia

46 Sternbach R 1987 Mastering pain — a twelve-step regimen for coping with chronic pain. Arlington Books, London

47 Melzack R, Wall P D 1970 Psychophysiology of pain. International Anaesthesiology Clinical Anaesthetics Neurophysiology 8(1):3

48 Melzack R, Wall P D 1982 The challenge of pain. Penguin, London

49 Peck Connie 1982 Controlling chronic pain. Fontana Collins, Glasgow

50 Niven N 1994 Health psychology: an introduction for nurses and other health care professionals, 2nd edn. Churchill Livingstone, Edinburgh

51 Tubesing D A 1981 Kicking your stress habits — a do-it-yourself guide for coping with stress. Whole Person Associates, Minnesota USA

52 Mitchell L 1977 Simple (physiological) relaxation. John Murray, London

53 Davis M, Robbins Eshelman E, McKay M 1983 The relaxation and stress reduction workbook, 2nd edn. New Harbinger Publications, Oakland USA

54 Hellerstein H K, Hornsten T R, Gardbarg A et al 1967 The influence of active conditioning upon subjects with coronary artery disease: cardiorespiratory changes during training in 67 patients. Canadian Medical Association Journal 96:758–759

55 World Health Organization 1993 Needs and action priorities in cardiac rehabilitation and secondary prevention in patients with coronary heart disease. WHO Technical Report Service 831. WHO Regional Office for Europe, Geneva

56 Cassem N H, Hackett T P 1977 Psychological aspects of myocardial infarction. Medical Clinics of North America 61:711–721

57 Shleifer S J, Macari-Hinson M M, Coyle D A et al 1989 The nature and course of depression following myocardial infarction. Archives of Internal Medicine 149:1785–1789

58 Kaye P A Dugard P 1972 Psychological reactions to a coronary care unit. Journal of Psychosomatic Research 16:437–447

59 Levine J, Warrenburg S, Kerns R, et al 1987 The role of denial in recovery from coronary heart disease. Journal of Psychosomatic Medicine 49:109–117

60 Schockern D D, Green D F, Worden T J, Hamison E E, Spielberger C D 1987 Effects of age on the relationship between anxiety and coronary artery disease. Psychosomatic Medicine 49:118–126

61 Cay E L, Vetter N, Phillip A, Duggard P 1973 Return to work after heart attack. Journal of Psychosomatic Research 17:231–243

62 Bloch A 1975 Sexual problems after myocardial infarction. American Heart Journal 90:536–537

63 Byrne D G, White H M, Butler K L 1981 Illness behaviour and outcome following survived myocardial infarction: a prospective study. Journal of Psychosomatic Research 25:97–107

64 Cay E L, Vetter N, Phillip A E 1972 Psychological status during recovery from an acute heart attack. Journal of Psychosomatic Research 16:425–435

65 Lloyd G G, Cawley R H 1982 Psychiatric morbidity after myocardial infarction. Quarterly Journal of Medicine 51:33–42

66 Frasure-Smith N, Lesperance F, Talajic M 1993 Depression following myocardial infarction. Impact on 6 month survival. Journal of the American Medical Association 270:1819–1825

67 Coyne J C, Smith D A F 1991 Couples coping with a myocardial infarction: a contextual perspective on wives' distress. Journal of Personality and Social Psychology 61:404–412

68 Johnson J L, Morse J M 1990 Regaining control: the process of adjustment after myocardial infarction. Heart and Lung 19:126–135

69 Coats A, McGee H, Stokes H, Thompson D 1995 BACR guidelines for cardiac rehabilitation. Blackwell Science, Oxford

70 Engel G L 1980 The clinical application of the biosychosocial model. The American Journal of Psychiatry 137(5):535–544

71 Medich C, Stuart E M, Deckro J P, Freidman R 1991 Psychophysiologic control mechanisms in ischaemic heart disease: the mind heart connection 5:10–26

72 Freeman L J, Nixon P G F 1985 Dynamic causes of angina pectoris. American Heart Journal 110:1087–1092

73 Rozanski A, Bairey C N, Krantz D S et al 1988 Mental stress and the induction of silent myocardial ischaemia in patients with coronary artery disease. New England Journal of Medicine 318:1005–1012

74 Hay L 1985 Heal your body: the mental causes for physical illness and the metaphysical way to overcome them. Heaven on Earth Books, London

75 Horwitz R I, Viscoli C M, Berkman L et al. 1990 Treatment adherence and risk of death after a myocardial infarction. Lancet 336:542–545

76 Patel C H 1973 Yoga and biofeedback in the management of hypertension. Lancet 11:1053–1055

77 Patel C, Carruthers M 1977 Coronary risk factor reduction through biofeedback-aided relaxation and meditation. Journal of the Royal College of General Practitioners 27:401–404

78 Patel C, Marmot M G, Terry D J 1981 Controlled trial of biofeedback aided behavioural methods in reducing mild hypertension. British Medical Journal 282:2005–2008

79 Patel C, Marmot M G, Terry D J, Carruthers M, Hunt B, Patel 1985 Trial of relaxation in reducing coronary risk: four year follow up. British Medical Journal 290:1103–1105

80 Patel C, North W R S 1975 Randomised controlled trial of yoga and biofeedback in management of hypertension. Lancet 19:93–95

81 Shoemaker J E, Tasto D L 1975 The effects of muscle relaxation on blood pressure of essential hypertensives. Behavioural Research and Therapy 13:29–43

82 Benson H 1975 The relaxation response. William-Morrow, New York, USA

83 Benson H, Beary J F, Carol M P 1974 The relaxation response. Psychiatry 37:37–46

84 Mayou R 1984 Prediction of emotion and social outcome after a heart attack. Journal of Psychosomatic Research 28:17–25

85 Van Dixhoorn J, Duivenvoorden H J, Pool J, Verhage G 1990 Psychic effects of physical training and relaxation therapy after myocardial infarction. Journal of Psychosomatic Research 34:327–337

86 Rovario S, Holmes D, Holmsten R 1984 Influence of a cardiac rehabilitation program on the cardiovascular, psychological and social functioning of cardiac patients. Journal of Behavioural Medicine 7:61–81

87 Ornish D, Brown S E, Sherwitz L W et al 1990 Can lifestyle changes reverse coronary heart disease? Lancet 336:129–132

88 Mandle C L, Domar A D, Harrington D P et al 1990 Relaxation response in femoral angiography. Radiology 174:737–739

89 Miller K M, Perry P A 1990 Relaxation technique and postoperative pain in patients undergoing cardiac surgery. Heart and Lung 19:136–146

90 Amarosa-Tupler B, Tapp J T, Carida R V 1989 Stress management through relaxation and imagery in the treatment of angina pectoris. Journal of Cardiopulmonary Rehabilitation 9:348–355

91 Lawlor M 1988 Inner track learning. Pilgrims Publications, Canterbury, England

92 Nash W 1992 Stress management and coronary rehabilitation — are soft strategies effective? Journal of the International Stress Management Association 9:10–14

17

Working with individuals

The original edition of this book focused mainly on the requirements of therapists working in group settings. However, many therapists work primarily with individual clients who frequently present with a combination of physical and psychological problems. This chapter, therefore, attempts to address the needs of therapists working in various clinical settings in formulating individualised anxiety management training (AMT) programmes.

WHEN IS INDIVIDUALISED AMT INDICATED?

Although AMT is clearly very appropriately and effectively applied in a group setting, there are many reasons why this approach might be contraindicated or precluded by circumstance. Typical examples of such cases are suggested in the following list:

Idiosyncratic/special needs. Those with marked hearing, speech or memory problems, behavioural problems / marked emotional lability.

Physical conditions. Complex / atypical physical conditions requiring a specialist approach. It is also frequently impractical for therapists working with dissimilar physical disorders to collect enough appropriate clients for sufficiently timely group training.

Community work. Again, although anxiety management groups are often successfully organised in community-based locations, individualised programmes are sometimes more appropriate and practical. This is especially true when goal-orientated exposure programmes are indicated, e.g. phobic desensitisation, resocialisation. In such cases, the therapist may need to start within the client's home, gradually enabling the client to move out into the community.

Pre-group training. It is sometimes necessary to provide some initial AMT in order to enable clients to attend a group. This is often the case when marked social anxiety or travel phobia is present.

Post-group follow-up. Even where clients have attended an entire anxiety management course within a group-based setting, individual follow-up sessions are highly recommended. Firstly, this is usually the most convenient and efficient way of collecting individualised treatment outcome data. Note also that treatment effects are often shown to have been consolidated at follow-up.[1] Secondly, some clients may report unresolved problems at the end of group-based courses which are best dealt with in a more focused context. Thirdly, many clients face the prospect of finishing a course of treatment more confidently when offered follow-up sessions, even on a strictly limited basis.

In-depth/longer term work. Some of the case histories in this chapter are illustrative of this application for relatively severe or enduring mental health problems. A more intensive and individualised approach, which can be delivered over a longer period of time, may be more realistic in such cases.

FORMULATING ANXIETY MANAGEMENT PROGRAMMES FOR INDIVIDUAL CLIENTS
Screening and selection

In the writer's opinion, the selection criteria for AMT is remarkably broad, provided that the approach used is adapted carefully to suit the needs of the client in question. Indeed, anxiety is a significant feature of most mental health problems. However, it is important to emphasise that some contraindications apply, particularly in relation to those clients suffering from acute psychiatric disorders. These are ennumerated in

Chapter 11 p. 99, and page 126 of Chapter 14. Linked to this issue, screening guidelines for referring agencies should be prepared, based on appropriate selection criteria and clearly stating any contraindicated conditions. Although there are certain exceptions, the flexible context of the individual treatment setting allows the therapist to tackle compounding problems that are often precluded in a group setting, e.g. excessive state anxiety, behavioural/memory problems.

However, it is essential that referrers and clients understand fully what they are being referred for. It is necessary to ensure that anxiety is actually a major feature in the client's problem history. Obtaining a full history at the outset helps to ensure treatment relevance and ultimate client commitment to the process.

Assessment

The individual treatment setting often allows for more comprehensive assessment and treatment evaluation procedures than is usually possible in group settings. Since anxiety is a multifactorial problem, it is recommended that several facets are measured, e.g. physiological, occupational, cognitive and psychosocial.[2] Chapter 13 in this book deals with assessment and evaluation in depth; therefore only an outline will be included here.

Some appropriate types of assessment include:

1. Structured interview schedules designed to identify:
   - the history of the problem, precipitating and maintaining factors
   - current functional deficits, lifestyle
   - current coping style
   - client's attitudes/beliefs about the problem
   - social circumstances
   - other treatments previous/current including medication.[3,4]

2. Behavioural assessments, e.g. shopping/travel assignments involving exposure to a feared situation.

3. Therapist observations: muscle tension

levels, posture, breathing habit, pulse and respiration rates.

4. Formal anxiety-testing tools, e.g. Spielberger's State-trait anxiety inventory.[5]

5. Self-rating scales/log books.

Goal-setting

Clear goals of treatment should always be formulated and agreed with the client. The client's goals should provide the framework which informs the treatment process and measures its ultimate success. It will be necessary to ensure that goals are:

- practical and specific
- clearly and simply defined
- relevant to client's problem
- realistic
- achievable.

They should be constantly referred to and refined during treatment and reviewed at the end.

Treatment process

The foundations of a productive therapeutic partnership between the client and therapist are laid down at this stage. Wherever appropriate, a written treatment contract is highly recommended. It is essential to make the treatment contract time limited, but set within a realistic time frame for the client concerned. This should be negotiated and agreed with each individual.

Treatment plans can be organised into goal-based modules so that when clients have achieved their initial goals they can progress to the remaining modules. Treatment phases frequently fall into the following basic modules, although not all of these will be appropriate for every client:

1. Physical anxiety management skills, e.g. rationale of fight/flight stress response, muscle relaxation, controlled breathing, differential relaxation.

2. Cognitive anxiety management skills, e.g. rationale and recognition of negative and irra-tional thoughts/beliefs, positive cognitive strategies, mental relaxation/rehearsal methods.

3. Application, e.g. goal-setting, problem-solving, panic management, practical assignments involving graded exposure.

4. Follow-up, e.g. work towards discharge, encouraging increasing self-reliant application of skills with decreasing supervision from therapist.

In practice, modules often overlap, especially in the initial/interim stages of treatment, but achievements relating to each module may still be reviewed separately as treatment progresses. Further improvements may continue to be demonstrated over time, and regular monitoring provides useful information for the therapist and, hopefully, a powerful spur for the client. The most vital component of the monitoring process should be done by the clients themselves. This includes completion of self-rating scales and diaries to record progress in relaxation practice and other personal assignments. When working on cognitive anxiety management skills, there will also be a need to give verbal and written assignments to collect the necessary information, e.g. diary of negative automatic thoughts. This material may then be used as the basis for subsequent sessions in which the therapist assists the client in identifying and challenging negative/irrational cognitive patterns. Finally, in order to encourage compliance and consolidate learning gained from homework assignments, each session should start with feedback from homework.

During the 'application' module, the ultimate goals of treatment will usually be the paramount consideration. Assignments involving exposure may frequently be required, e.g. shopping, social events, practising assertiveness skills. The beauty of the individual treatment-setting comes into its own at this stage in which a highly personalised plan can be developed and worked through at the client's own pace.

Discontinuing treatment

Follow-up sessions at increasingly widely spaced intervals with the client working on remaining goals comprises the final stage of the programme. This stage involves gradual reduction in support and supervision from the therapist. The primary goal is to enable clients to graduate to a stage where they are able to formulate their own strategies for dealing with problems and set-backs. The emphasis is therefore placed upon anticipation of likely difficulties, and long-term planning of effective coping responses. Kennerley[3] has termed this 'blueprinting'.

One common problem involves attempts on the client's part to draw out the treatment programme while failing to complete assignments or participate constructively. While avoiding a judgemental approach towards the client's difficulties, expectations of the client must be clear at the outset and kept at the forefront of the treatment process. The therapist should adopt a supportive and creative approach in assisting clients to recognise the obstacles to progress and tackle avoidance.

The decision to discontinue treatment will also be made easier if it is based on objective data and is goal-related. The following questions will need to be asked:

- Has the client achieved none/too few of their goals?
- Has the client achieved all/most of their goals?

In either of the above cases, it is counter-productive for clients to continue aimlessly in the same treatment situation. Where treatment has been fully or partially successful, they should be helped to move rapidly forwards to treatment termination. Failure in treatment is frequently linked to consistent default in attendance or non-completion of homework assignments. Where this occurs, alternative approaches which may suit the client's needs more effectively should be explored. Also see Chapter 15: 'Troubleshooting — some common problems'.

Finally, it may be useful for the therapist treating clients in individual settings to consider ways in which positive aspects of group working, e.g. peer support, feedback and identification, can be compensated for, perhaps through involving friends/relatives and support groups.

CASE HISTORIES

The following illustrative examples have been informed by the writer's own clinical experience in order to demonstrate some of the diverse ways in which anxiety management techniques might be applied and responded to in clinical practice.

Case one — Patricia

Background

Patricia was referred from an acute admission ward where she was diagnosed with a depressive illness complicated by phobic anxiety. Patricia was 55 years of age and this was her first presentation with a mental health problem. Until her breakdown, Patricia had a long history of having coped with a very demanding lifestyle as a single parent with a full-time job as an office manager. She was the sole breadwinner and, over the years, had gradually lost all her social support resources through bereavement and the breakdown of a close relationship with a friend. When her daughter started to reach adulthood and there were attempts to make her redundant from her job, Patricia's major roles in life were seriously threatened. At this stage she started to become depressed and anxious, engaging in social withdrawal and avoidance behaviour.

Treatment plan

The aims of the anxiety management component of the total treatment plan were as follows:

1. Provide basic information about the physiology and psychology of stress reaction.
2. Teach muscle-relaxation skills.
3. Teach correct breathing skills, including techniques to manage hyperventilation in panic situations, e.g. shopping.
4. Teach mental relaxation methods, e.g. Benson's relaxation response.
5. Enable Patricia to identify and challenge self-defeating behaviour and attitudes, e.g. avoidance, social withdrawal, self-denigratory beliefs.
6. Set personal assignments based on Patricia's own goals. These included:

- shopping tasks of increasing challenge levels
- sorting out her personal possessions and tackling household chores
- setting up interviews with her employers to discuss plans for her future
- making contact with former friends and seeking new social outlets
- exploring alternative occupational outlets, e.g. voluntary work.

In addition to AMT, Patricia's treatment plan also included creative therapy groups to enable her to explore and confront various issues associated with the major theme of loss in her life. She also attended some bodywork activities to help her to release muscle tension and increase energy levels. Social and supportive therapy groups were also included to increase her confidence and encourage interaction in social settings.

Progress in treatment

Phase one: Patricia worked hard to learn the new techniques although she encountered great difficulty in disciplining herself to practise relaxation techniques at first. She displayed a tendency to withdraw into her bedroom for days at a time, avoiding social contact and tackling household tasks which had by now become well overdue. She also complained of deep-seated muscle rigidity and pain around the neck and shoulders. On palpation, these areas were extremely tense and Patricia had made little progress in relaxing them. However, she was beginning to have some success in general muscle relaxation and in applying breathing techniques to control episodes of panic which she experienced when shopping.

Phase two: Patricia had commenced the programme with very poor self-esteem. She felt rejected and ill-used by her employers and, without a productive and satisfying role in the workplace, she saw herself as being worthless. She learnt to recognise and challenge some of her negative automatic thoughts and to develop positive cognitions to sustain her when confronting feared situations. She also spent some time working on irrational and self-defeating aspects of her core belief system, e.g. 'In order to be a worthwhile person, I must be totally successful at work'.

Phase three: In line with her personal goals, she also started to reduce social withdrawal and avoidance behaviour. Periods spent in bed during the daytime gradually reduced — although this behaviour tended to recur at times of increased stress, e.g. interviews with employers. Patricia also began to establish new social contacts and started to look into the possibility of doing some voluntary work.

Outcome

The foregoing phases of treatment lasted over a period of one year from her first presentation as an in-patient on an acute psychiatric ward. During follow-up she was supported through the painful process of agreeing redundancy terms with her former employers. She also managed to establish herself in voluntary work. Shortly afterwards her depressive illness apparently resolved and Patricia was discharged at her own request, having achieved all her personal goals and showing consistently low anxiety scores on self-rating scales. In the therapist's opinion there were some deeper underlying issues which had not been fully dealt with, particularly concerning relationships and social support structures. However, Patricia had learned a range of coping skills enabling her to deal with stressful situations and had gained a positive outlook on the future.

Case two — Kevin

Background

Kevin was referred for anxiety management through the out-patient clinic of an acute psychiatric unit. He was 22 years of age and had been diagnosed as suffering from an acute anxiety disorder. This was his first presentation to a mental health service.

Kevin was an insulin-dependent diabetic and described a precipitating event involving a hypoglycaemic episode which had occurred rather dramatically during a meeting at work. He had felt extremely humiliated and helpless following this event. His dread of a recurrence gradually increased to such an extent that he started to suffer from panic attacks while at work. At the time he commenced treatment he had been unable to go to work for several weeks. Kevin lived with his parents and described his social circumstances as supportive.

Treatment plan

Kevin requested that the treatment period be brief, in order to facilitate his return to work at the earliest possible date. His anxiety was beginning to be compounded by realistic worries over the negative effect his extended sick leave might have on his prospects at work.

1. Provide rationale for physical and psychological symptoms experienced, focusing in particular on panic and hyperventilation.
2. Teach muscle-tension reduction and correct breathing techniques, reinforced by intensive personal practice programme.
3. Provide regular feedback on progress from therapist's observations and personal progress graph derived from self-rating scales.
4. Assist Kevin in identifying and challenging negative automatic thoughts which precipitate the panic episodes.
5. Teach mental relaxation skills, e.g., meditation-based / visualisation. Use visualisation skills to prepare for stressful situations associated with returning to work.
6. Set and carry out targets relating to the goal of returning to full-time work, for example:

- visit work to discuss plans with line manager
- go in and work on low-stress tasks for half a day
- work half-days for an entire week on low-stress tasks
- work full week taking on only low-stress tasks
- work full week taking on increasingly challenging tasks.

Progress in treatment

Phase one: Kevin was initially reluctant to attend for treatment and was very conscious of the stigma he felt was involved in accepting help for his problem. He failed to attend the first two appointments. However, once started, he quickly grasped the principles involved in anxiety management and was assiduous in practising relaxation skills at home.

Phase two: Kevin was anxious to recommence work as soon as possible but still felt uncertain about his ability to cope with his anxiety at work. Practical targets were agreed allowing him to make a gradual return to work while still attending anxiety management sessions to consolidate his skills and provide support during this stressful phase.

Phase three: Kevin was able to return to part-time work after a period of three weeks in treatment. In the event, he jumped several hurdles at once by achieving some targets faster than expected. He did not experience any further episodes of panic at work and reported being able to recognise when his anxiety levels were beginning to escalate. At such points he used his relaxation skills successfully to reduce arousal at an early stage.

Outcome

Kevin returned to full-time work after a period of six weeks. He had achieved all goals and targets set and demonstrated consistently low anxiety scores. Treatment was discontinued at his own request and he refused follow-up. Although Kevin had eventually accepted treatment and used the opportunity extremely well, he was keen to return to his normal lifestyle as soon as possible. However, he retained links with the out-patient clinic on a long-term follow-up basis.

Case three — Irene

Background

Irene presented through the out-patient clinic of a psychiatric unit with a history of chronic anxiety, psychosomatic pain and panic attacks. Irene was 52 years of age and her husband had recently retired. She found his being around the house during the day difficult to adjust to, although she reported that their relationship was basically supportive. Their only child had married and emigrated two years previously. There were no grandchildren.

Irene described herself as having a rather timid nature and experienced problems in asserting herself. She saw herself as being a poor 'coper'. Irene tended to avoid social contacts as much as possible and dreaded occasions which involved her having to visit family relations. She was frequently troubled by pain in her legs, neck and shoulders, and was beset with fear that this might be due to some underlying illness of a serious nature. Her panic attacks were associated with hyperventilation and a long-standing habit of shallow, rapid breathing.

Treatment plan

1. Provide education about the effects of anxiety on bodily reactions, e.g. association between panic symptoms and hyperventilation, and between pain and muscle tension.

2. Teach muscle relaxation and correct breathing techniques and agree personal practice regime.

3. Teach applied and differential relaxation skills, e.g. active and emergency relaxation, breathing control techniques.

4. Discuss how negative automatic thoughts and core beliefs associated with poor self-esteem may contribute to anxiety symptoms.

5. Assist Irene in identifying and challenging her own negative thoughts and core beliefs, e.g. 'I can't cope'/'I'm a failure'.

6. Enable Irene to set and tackle realistic goals concerned with feared situations such as driving and socialising. The choice of goals to emphasise the inclusion of more personally enriching activities into her lifestyle.

Treatment progress

Phase one: Irene readily grasped the main principles of anxiety management but experienced difficulty in applying them in practice. Irene had a long-standing habit of shallow breathing which quickly gave way to hyperventilation and panic in response to minor stressors. High levels of muscular tension were also identified at various sites. These sites corresponded to areas which Irene had associated with pain, e.g. abdomen, neck and shoulders, legs. Intensive muscle-relaxation training and breathing re-education was then given, over a period of 3–4 months.

Irene was also introduced to the concepts associated with negative thinking and anxiety at this time and began to recognise some of her self-defeating cognitive patterns.

Phase two: Despite assiduous practice, Irene took a relatively long time to master muscle relaxation and correct breathing. Although she initially felt disheartened by this, she started to accept the inevitability of set-backs and learned to view herself more rationally and less harshly on her 'bad days'. She was beginning to develop her own ways of challenging her automatic assumptions when facing difficulties. Instead of the constant refrain of 'I can't cope', she started to remind herself of the coping skills she had mastered and perceive daily stressors in a more realistic and proportionate manner.

Phase three: Irene began to achieve more success in controlling her arousal state at times of stress. Her self-ratings began to show a much deeper level of relaxation following home practice sessions and the frequency of panic attacks began to reduce. However, she still suffered from some residual muscle tension in certain areas, e.g. abdomen and legs. Irene started to face previously threatening events with more equanimity and planned some targets, e.g. visits to relatives/entertaining, which she had been putting off for some time.

During this phase, although not all the problems Irene had originally presented with were completely resolved, it was recognised that she now needed to move forward more independently. The focus therefore shifted onto a follow-up regime in which Irene formulated practical goals concerned with improving her general quality of life and carried them out between sessions.

Outcome

The space between meetings with the therapist was gradually increased until her final discharge around nine months after her first presentation. At treatment termination, Irene had achieved almost all her goals and, most importantly, had gained a more positive perspective on herself and her life. It was recognised that Irene had had to attempt to change long-standing patterns of behaviour and emotional reaction. While Irene was still essentially the same person, finding many ordinary situations challenging, she now had a more positive set of skills and attitudes with which to help her face these struggles.

Case four — Matthew

Background

Matthew was 23 years of age when he was referred for anxiety management training, having been given a diagnosis of schizophrenia five years previously. Matthew's condition was adequately controlled by medication and there were no active psychotic features at the time of referral. He had suffered his first psychotic episode while studying for a computer sciences degree, which he eventually completed successfully. Since then, anxiety about facing interview situations and using public transport, had contributed to his subsequent difficulties in obtaining employment. He was living at home with his parents and reported this situation to be reasonably free from conflict.

Treatment plan

1. Provide education about the effects of anxiety on bodily reactions.

2. Teach muscle relaxation and correct breathing techniques and agree personal practice regime.

3. Teach applied and differential relaxation skills, e.g. active and emergency relaxation, breathing control techniques.

4. Assist Matthew in identifying and challenging negative and irrational thinking patterns associated with his anxiety.

5. Agree and implement exposure plan for tackling fear of using public transport.

6. Focus on social-skills training for general and specific application within interview and work situations.

7. Teach goal-setting and problem-solving techniques in order to plan and implement a realistic and systematic approach to job-seeking.

Treatment progress

Phase one: Matthew experienced great difficulty in committing himself to treatment during this stage. He frequently missed appointments and failed to complete homework assignments and practice relaxation techniques independently. He had become extremely demotivated and hopeless about his future prospects. It was recognised that longer-term work would be required in Matthew's case. He was encouraged to persist with home practice and to set small, achievable targets. A strong emphasis was placed on monitoring and providing feedback on his progress through the use of graphs, charts and diaries/log books.

Phase two: During this phase treatment emphasis was placed upon testing and reinforcing Matthew's understanding of the skills he was attempting to learn. The CBM approach[3,4] was utilised in order to assist him in working on some of the irrational belief systems which were contributing to his anxiety. At this stage he was also referred to a social-skills training group as an adjunct to individual work. Matthew's motivation and skill in applying anxiety management techniques was beginning to improve and he was now using all forms of public transport independently.

Phase three: The work now shifted onto application of skills for social and work-related situations. Matthew was assisted in formulating realistic targets and goals, and a clear time frame in which to implement them. His goals included exploring further training opportunities and broadening his social and leisure outlets. He also visited job advisory services to look into available options. Sessions were now more widely spaced with the emphasis on Matthew carrying out the work and reporting back. Some set-backs did occur at this stage, in which Matthew turned up at the session having failed to carry out agreed assignments. His reasons for default were discussed fully in a non-judgemental manner and alternative assignments were negotiated.

Outcome

Nine months after his first presentation for treatment Matthew was ready to interview for jobs, although at a less competitive level than he had been aiming at previously. He was encouraged to look on his first few interviews as opportunities to practise his skills. In the event, he was successful at his second interview. He required some additional follow-up support during his first few months in the new job when he experienced increased anxiety levels. Matthew was discharged for continuing support by the community mental health worker.

REFERENCES

1 Deffenbacher J, Suinn R 1982 The self-control of anxiety. In: Karoly P, Kanger F (eds) Self-management and behavioural change. Pergamon Press, New York
2 Payne R A 1995 Relaxation techniques — a practical handbook for the health care professional. Churchill Livingstone, Edinburgh
3 Kennerley H 1995 Managing anxiety — a training manual, 2nd edn. Oxford Medical Publications, Oxford
4 Hawton K, Saldovskis P M, Kirk J, Clark D M (eds) 1989 Cognitive behaviour therapy for psychiatric problems — a practical guide. Oxford Medical Publications, Oxford
5 Spielberger C D 1983 Manual for the state-trait anxiety inventory (Form Y). Consulting Psychologists Press, California

18

Working with older people

Alice Mackenzie
(Stress and anxiety among older people)

Juliet Vinçon
(The use of T'ai Chi as an anxiety-reduction technique for elderly people)

STRESS AND ANXIETY AMONG OLDER PEOPLE

INTRODUCTION

This chapter is concerned with exploring how stress affects older people, and suggesting strategies for its management. Issues related to anxiety disorders experienced by older people are discussed, followed by a look at the incidence and prevalence of anxiety disorders among this client group. The final section describes how T'ai Chi can be used as a therapeutic activity with this client group.

Firstly, it is necessary to define what is meant by 'older people'. It is recognised that there is a risk in defining any group of people by age alone. Older people are not a homogeneous group. There are many social, psychological and biological differences that affect the ageing process and the experience of ageing. But, for the purposes of this chapter, those defined as older people are aged 65 years and over. This is still the age most often used administratively for planning services for older people, primarily because 65 years is still seen as the standard retirement age. It is also recognised that there are differences related to age within this large group of older people; those aged over 75 years who require community support services often have different needs compared to older people under 75 years of age.[1,2]

Anxiety as a normal human response to stress[3] and as a clinical disorder has been defined elsewhere in this book. However, anxiety may affect older people in special ways,[4,5] to which we will now turn our attention.

STRESS AND COPING AMONG OLDER PEOPLE

Given the paucity of studies relating to stress in older people it is impossible to conclude whether or not coping abilities change with age. However, a number of variables appear to have a particular influence on stress in older people, including:

- differences in stressful events
- ongoing strains and coping
- differences in the rate of biological ageing
- psychosocial factors
- demographic factors.

Added to the above, most studies are cross-sectional and do not give any sense of continuity.[6,7] To understand psychological stress and ageing, stressful events and ongoing strains need to be explored within the context of the individual's overall life experience and the individual's ageing process. The personal meaning that stressful events and ongoing strains hold for individuals and groups of people need to be understood in the context of their overall life; their values, beliefs and cultural background.[7]

Life events

Life events associated with old age often involve actual loss and changes related to loss. Common events are:

- retirement
- economic changes
- multiple bereavements
- changes in the family structure
- changes in health status
- onset of chronic illness leading to a decrease in abilities to perform activities of daily living
- loss of home.

These events are often perceived negatively by society at large leading to the stereotyping of older people and the stigmatising of old age. Generalisations about how older people define

and cope with stressful events commonly result. Some of the above events are experienced by older people as sources of stress, but it is worth noting that in some studies older people have reported higher rates of life satisfaction and psychological well-being when compared to younger people. These differences could be due to stoical attitudes peculiar to the recent and current generation of older people. Alternatively they could be due to a number of factors including lower health expectations, or to developmental change occurring as people age associated with an increase in resilience, or to changes in cognitive appraisal when faced with difficult situations.[7,8,9]

Life events and meanings attached to events can change as the person ages. Younger and older people can be equally fearful of future losses but the type of loss feared may be different. For example, a 68-year-old man is not so likely to face redundancy, but is more likely to face the onset of a life-threatening and possibly debilitating health problem such as a heart disease. Suggested sources of stress among older people include:

- fear of crime
- financial insecurity
- poor health leading to decreases in self-esteem and social isolation
- caring for a spouse or relative
- being a burden to their family
- giving up one's home and moving into a nursing home.[5,8,9,10,11]

In a small qualitative study[12] older people saw loss of health, loss of function and loss of independence in activities of daily living as inevitable results of the ageing process. From these perceptions arose concerns about their future, which appeared to be a source of stress. But rather than passively accepting what they saw as an inevitable decline, this group of older people used proactive, creative and varied approaches to their anticipated losses. It has been suggested that in order to manage the uncertainty of the future associated with old age, older people deny worrisome and possibly despairing feelings, preparing instead to keep active and busy.[8,13]

Loss and bereavement

Considering how common the experience of loss is for older people, the prevalence rate for mental illness among older people following bereavement is relatively low. In general, results from studies looking at changes in psychological well-being following bereavement are equivocal. It is recognised that psychological upheavals and difficulties occur immediately after a bereavement, but only a few older people appear to have significant difficulties coping two years post-bereavement. Mortality may increase during the first six months of bereavement, but then it gradually drops as the period after bereavement is extended. Within these rates there are gender differences.

How people cope with bereavement and other losses is a complex issue influenced by many variables. But overall it appears that older people cope well with loss events and are able to use strategies to help them come to terms with and minimise the feelings of loss.[10,14,15] Within this generalisation there are differences. Depression may occur after an experience of loss in old age if an earlier loss experience has been unresolved; the loss experienced in old age may reawaken unresolved feelings associated with the earlier loss.[8,9,12]

Ongoing strains

Ongoing strains related to physical health problems, financial strain, fear of crime and social isolation can affect an elderly person's psychological well-being. Older people who experience economic stresses and ill health together are likely to experience more stress-related symptoms than those experiencing just one of these problems. Ongoing stress may be experienced by those older people who, because of health problems, have become dependent on an adult child or another significant family member. The changes in the relationship may re-awaken earlier conflicts, or the elderly person may feel uncomfortable about the reversal of roles.[5,8,9,16,17,18]

In relation to fears of crime, it is not clear whether this is a chronic strain or a stress event associated with being old. A fear of crime can be influenced by the level of criminal activity in the local community, and by the level of media attention given to criminal activity.[18]

Changes in health status

Changes in health status rate high as stressful events among older people. In the UK the rates of older people reporting long-standing illnesses increase with age. Changes in physical health can lead to:

- pain
- restrictions in lifestyle
- loss of functional independence
- loss or change of role
- the person becoming housebound leading to social isolation
- changes in accommodation.

Any one of the above factors or a combination of them can contribute to an increased experience of stress and possible anxiety.[9,16,17,19]

Many studies identify perceived health status and impairment in activities of daily living to be strong predictors of life satisfaction and psychological well-being. A decrease in physical health may contribute to the person becoming housebound and consequently socially isolated, contributing to a decrease in the person's psychological well-being. Subtle changes in an elderly person's health status leading to lifestyle changes may precipitate the onset of anxiety or agoraphobia. A typical example is that of an elderly person developing an illness affecting their heart which leads to feelings of insecurity and anxiety. These feelings are compounded by the attendant physiological symptoms of anxiety, prompting the individual to visit a doctor. The doctor may, inadvertently, reinforce the person's anxiety further by concentrating on the physical disease, i.e. the heart disease. In this example, it is easy to understand why the individual might respond by restricting their activity to the extent that they become housebound.[4,16,20,21,22]

Although health worries are frequently associated with older people the degrees of worry are not so consistent. In her study on age, health-related stress and coping strategies, Aldwin[17] found a positive and significant association between age and health: health problems were the most frequently identified recent stressful event among older people. However, they did not rate the actual stressfulness of these events as being particularly high. These results were also confirmed in another similar study.[9]

In understanding the effects of stress, life events, loss, health changes and ongoing strains it is necessary to look at what older people themselves define as stressful events, and the internal and external resources they have. Examples of internal resources are:

- motivation
- self-esteem
- personality traits
- health status
- health expectations
- life experience
- values and belief system.

Examples of external resources are:

- the person's physical environment
- economic status
- marital status
- social networks.[6,7,8]

Personal resources will now be considered further in relation to social support and coping strategies.

Social support

The role of social support as a personal resource is complex, but it is acknowledged that an elderly person's psychological well-being can be influenced by the strength of their social network. Epidemiological studies carried out in America with older people have shown a significant relationship between increased risk of mortality and morbidity, and low levels of social support. Other studies cited have shown that recovery has been facilitated by introducing social support as part of rehabilitation programmes. In one study a significant association was found between the strength of social ties and

rates of depressed mood; the fewer social ties people have the higher their depressed mood scores. It is suggested that low levels of social support can be influenced by chronic financial strain and a fear of crime; financial strain can engender feelings of distrust, which in turn leads to social isolation. Conversely social support, if it is defined as emotional support, can help in the reduction of economic strain and increase the person's mastery of coping. Socialisation has also been identified as a helpful coping strategy among elderly widows.[6,10,15,16,18]

Social support and social networks can have different meanings; social network does not necessarily mean the same as social support.

Support comes when people's engagement with one another extends to a level of involvement and concern, not when they merely touch at the surface of each other's lives ... the final step depends on the quality of the relations one is able to find within the network.[6] (p. 340)

Coping strategies

Different cohorts may demonstrate different types of coping strategies; these differences will be due to historical factors, cognitive appraisal of the events, resources available, cultural and educational variations.

The outcome of a stressful event or ongoing strain will be affected by the type of coping strategy used and resources available. In a study of 90 elderly women with osteoarthritis, the coping strategies used by the individuals in the sample were measured in relation to their life satisfaction. Emotive, palliative and confrontative coping strategies were measured using the Jalowiec Coping Scale. After controlling for the socioeconomic status of individuals, a positive relationship was found between the use of these coping strategies and life satisfaction; overall the coping strategies selected by this group had a positive effect on their life satisfaction. Those who used emotive coping strategies appeared to have lower rates of life satisfaction.[20]

In Gass's study[15] of elderly widows, helpful and unhelpful coping strategies were identified. Helpful strategies were: keeping busy, participating in social groups, learning new skills, reviewing their spouse's death, recalling happy memories, religion and prayers. Unhelpful strategies were taking medication or alcohol, blaming self, sleeping more, using fantasy and 'bargaining with God'.[15]

Internal and external resources will influence the effectiveness of the coping strategies used.[8,15,20,23] For example, in one study,[23] a relationship was found between economic status and the type of coping strategies used. Those in the lower socioeconomic status groups used active behavioural coping strategies, such as making a plan of action and following it through, in response to a stressful event. People in the higher socioeconomic groups were more likely to use cognitive coping strategies to change their perception of stressful situations, for example, attempting to look on the positive side of a situation.

One way of understanding coping strategies used is to look at the strategies in relation to the older person's experience. Sometimes it is assumed that older people automatically lose their sense of autonomy because of environmental and physical limitations. But studies on age and coping suggest the opposite; in general older people are not 'passive copers'[17] (p. 175). Aldwin,[17] using a modified version of Folkman and Lazarus's Ways of Coping Scale, focused on two coping strategies: instrumental coping and escapism with 228 self-selected community-living adults between the ages of 18 and 78. She found age was not related to the efficacy of coping. The older adults perceived they had less control and responsibility for the stressful event (the most frequent event being a health problem), but the results showed a negative association between age and escapism; the older adults were as likely to use instrumental action as a coping strategy as the younger adults.

The suggestion is that older adults will have had many years of facing stresses, losses and frustrations from which they will have gained coping experience. Many older people will have learned through their life experience which coping strategies were ineffective and which were effective in enabling them to cope more successfully with difficult situations. Or, alternatively, older people may have learned to avoid difficulties through learned helplessness behaviour, thereby restricting their activities.[9,17]

We have explored several sources of stress that have particular meaning to older people, and therefore may cause anxiety. Assuming anxiety disorder to be one of the negative outcomes of stressful events it is now necessary to look at anxiety among older people.

ANXIETY DISORDERS AMONG OLDER PEOPLE

An elderly person will experience and demonstrate similar symptoms of anxiety as those experienced by younger adults. Differences in symptom emphasis in the elderly are often associated with cognitive and bodily symptoms. Thus, a lack of concentration or difficulties in recall due to anxiety, may lead to the erroneous assumption that the individual is cognitively impaired. Similarly, bodily symptoms of arousal may be interpreted by the elderly person as evidence of a life-threatening illness.[4,5]

There are three suggestions about why older people are more likely to complain of bodily symptoms. One is that doctors may have less interest in the mental state of an elderly person. Secondly, because of the biological changes associated with ageing, the elderly person's body is more likely to cause them to worry about their body. Physiological changes can easily become the focii of fears of ill health and decline. Or the person may have a physical illness as well as an anxiety disorder. Hypochondriasis and physical illness are not necessarily mutually exclusive.[5,24]

Incidence and prevalence of anxiety in older people

Self-reported perceptions of general health difficulties appear to increase with age, but compared to musculoskeletal problems, hearing and eyesight difficulties, mental health disorders seem to be under-reported.[19] Not many epidemiological studies of anxiety and related disorders among older people have been carried out and prevalence estimates vary across these studies. This variability is due to the different survey methods used, the lack of standardised methods of collecting data, and differences in how anxiety in later life has been defined and classified.[25,26,27,28]

Longitudinal studies show a decrease in the prevalence of anxiety, depression and obsessive–compulsive neuroses.[29] GP consultation rates show a decrease in consultations by older people with anxiety disorders. Data up to 1986 shows an overall age-related increase in admissions to psychiatric hospitals, but of these admissions, anxiety disorders account for only a small number of the in-patient and out-patient admissions. It is also known that older people are among the heaviest users of anxiolytic drugs.[19,25,27]

A review of epidemiological studies of anxiety disorders in the elderly from 1970 onwards show specific anxiety disorders to be less common in elderly people compared to younger adults, but the rates of generalised anxiety and depression in old age is similar to that of younger people. Compared to other phobic disorders which present for the first time during later life, agoraphobia is significantly higher.[27]

Two particular studies carried out in the UK amongst community-living older people have found similar results. Firstly, a large proportion of the samples were found to be psychiatrically well. Of those with a psychiatric disorder a high proportion were found to have either generalised anxiety or phobic disorders. In one of these studies a prevalence rate of 3.7% was found for generalised anxiety, no association was found between cognitive impairment and generalised anxiety, but those with high generalised anxiety scores had higher dependency scores.[25]

In a study with nursing home residents a strong association was found between the incidence and prevalence of anxiety and increased functional and cognitive impairment.[26]

Co-morbidity

Co-morbidity is when two disorders coexist such as anxiety and depression.

Although studies on co-morbidity among older people are limited, the prevalence of the coexistence of anxiety and depression is thought to be similar to that of younger age-groups. Lindesay et al[25] found a significant association between generalised anxiety and depression. Of those with a phobic disorder, a third were also depressed. Whether depression starts before anxiety or vice versa is unclear and not easy to disentangle. Likewise, the co-morbidity of physical illness and anxiety: Lindesay[22] found an association between cardiovascular and respiratory symptoms and phobic disorder, and onset of phobic disorder was associated with recent episodes of physical illness.[22,25,27]

Phobic disorders

In the Guys/Age Concern study[25] phobic disorder was one of the most frequent disorders in the elderly population; the rates were highest amongst women in the 65–74 age-group. Amongst those with phobias, the prevalence rate for agoraphobia was 7.8%, significantly more common than for the other phobias. The total prevalence rate for phobias was 10.0%. Those with agoraphobia had significantly higher dependency scores.[22,25]

Compared to other phobias, the onset of agoraphobia appears to occur later on in life and its onset seems to be related to a recent episode of physical illness or a life-threatening event. In one study, over half of those with agoraphobia experienced the onset after the age of 65, and the commonest cause was related to an episode of physical illness such as a myocardial infarction, a fracture, cerebral vascular accident, sudden visual impairment or surgery. In a few cases the person had experienced other types of traumatic event, such as a mugging or a fall at home.[21,25,27]

Overall it may appear that anxiety disorders decline with age, but there may be several reasons for challenging this impression. Anxiety disorders in older people may not be identified and properly diagnosed by doctors. Alternatively the lifestyles of older people may enable them to avoid contact with stressors, or psychological reactions to stressors may change. Some older people may also be embarrassed about presenting with a mental health problem.[5,29,30]

Professionals themselves may have an assumption that an elderly person's 'disabling fear' is normal and reasonable for their age, so when an elderly person presents at a clinic or hospital, their phobic disorder may not be identified. Older people can be appropriately careful of dangers in their environment; it would not be correct to assume that a reduction in an elderly person's activity is just because they are old or have a physical illness. Reduced activity related to phobic avoidance may be an important cause of older people being housebound.[21,25] It is important not to dismiss the disabling effect of anxiety symptoms on an elderly person and their quality of life.[24] We have all met older people in different health care settings who are distressed and disabled in activities of daily living by their anxiety symptoms. As suggested by Lindesay et al,[25] there is no evidence supporting the fact that a chronic fear with 'disabling ... avoidance is a normal and inevitable outcome of the ageing process' (p. 326).

In the clinical setting a strong relationship can be observed between anxiety disorders and the amount of hospital and social services care 'given' to older people. The decision as to whether an elderly person can manage at home and what support they need to help them manage will be influenced by their abilities to perform activities of daily living; debilitating anxiety may well affect their capacity to perform these activities.[22,25]

ASSESSMENT AND INTERVENTION

Approaches to assessment

A range of factors need to be included when assessing an elderly person prior to anxiety management training, relaxation therapy and other anxiety-reduction interventions. Some broad suggestions are given below which can be applied to older people seen in different settings and/or requiring different types of stress reduction/anxiety management programmes.

Establish the possible cause(s) of the anxiety

It is essential to know whether the elderly person is anxious because they have a physical illness, or they have a physical illness with symptoms very similar to those of an anxiety disorder. Secondly, it should be established whether the anxiety is being caused by an intolerance to drug(s) they are taking. Certain 'over the counter' drugs can cause anxiety; or the elderly person's tolerance to certain stimulants such as caffeine may have decreased. Does the anxiety disorder coexist with a chronic physical illness? In a study of 220 elderly out-patients with a diagnosis of anxiety, two-thirds of the sample were found to have a chronic physical illness as well. These physical investigations should be done swiftly and thoroughly.[4,5,24]

The following questions should also be asked:

1. Has the elderly person recently experienced a stressful event?

2. Are they experiencing ongoing strains or a build up of several stressors?

For example:

- Have they recently developed a physical illness?
- Has a significant person in their family recently died?
- Have they recently moved accommodation away from their familiar community and environment?

3. If the client has recently experienced a stressful event(s), what does the event mean to the client?

How long has the elderly person experienced anxiety?

It is suggested that life-long anxiety disorders in older people are much more difficult to change and resolve compared to sudden-onset anxiety disorders.[5] This is not to say that elderly people who have experienced anxiety throughout their lives would not benefit from some kind of anxiety management, but it is important that the goals you and the client set are realistic, and resolve compared to sudden-onset anxiety disorders.[5] This is not to say that elderly people who have experienced anxiety throughout their lives would not benefit from some kind of anxiety management, but it is important that the goals you and the client set are realistic, time-limited and planned in accordance with the client's history.[31]

What external resources does the client have?

The kind of questions that might be asked in relation to the client's external resources include the following:

- What is the person's socioeconomic status?
- Are they experiencing ongoing financial strain?
- How much social support does the client have?
- Have they experienced changes in their interpersonal relationships?
- What does their social support network mean to them?

What internal resources does the client have?

Examples of internal resources include the person's physical health, self-esteem and motivation.

- Do they have a chronic illness which they are worried about or which is undermining their independence?
- Have they recently experienced changes in their hearing and visual abilities?
- How do they experience their locus of control?

Apparent lack of motivation may be due to the person's sense of helplessness and poor self-esteem; both these factors can affect their ability to develop a sense of control over their anxiety and sources of stress. What coping strategies are they using or have used in the past? Identify coping strategies that have been helpful and those that have been unhelpful.[3,15,20]

Is the client cognitively impaired as a result of one of the dementias?

It is often clear when the client has some cognitive impairment, but this is not always the case. It is important to differentiate between apparent cognitive impairment which is a result of a lack of concentration, and that which is a result of the early stages of one of the dementias. A good medical history and clear diagnosis should assist you in this, but observations arising from other assessments will be of value. Relevant tests such as The Clifton Assessment Procedures for the Elderly (mental ability section),[32] the Abbreviated Mental Test[33] or the Mini-Mental State Examination,[34] may help to diagnose any ongoing cognitive impairment.

Establish clear and defined goals with the client

These will vary from client to client, depending on their individual needs and abilities. For example, the client who is living independently in the community will require goals based on what they themselves identify as their difficulties and what outcomes they want. Reaching this point may not be easy. Clients may present their needs in vague and broad terms, or they may attribute their feelings to a physical illness. In some cases clients may be reluctant to disclose their problems. The therapist will need to establish a rapport with the client and gently but firmly facilitate them in defining how their anxiety is affecting their activities. What activities are they not able to do because of their anxiety? Of those, which do they want to be able to do? Where the client's anxiety coexists with a physical illness, the therapist's best approach is to acknowledge the client's pains, fears and worries related to the physical illness. Once a rapport has developed, the client can be invited to join a simple exercise and relaxation group in preparation for an anxiety management programme.

Related approaches such as a T'ai Chi group may also be appropriate for those with a combination of physical and anxiety problems. This will enable the therapist and the client to find out if relaxation techniques are likely to be of value to the client. Where there are a number of clients been standardised on an elderly population; thus there is a need to look for measures appropriate to older people. However, for assessment and evaluation in general, see Chapter 13.

Use of anxiety management programmes with older people

Anxiety management programmes for older people living independently, without cognitive impairment, and where anxiety is the primary problem, would be similar to programmes used with other age-groups. An example of a basic anxiety management programme can be found in Chapter 11. In general, helping the older person to practise different methods of relaxation, develop a regular routine of daily activity, and link coping strategies to activities that are stressful, will be key elements. Homework assignments may be used to facilitate this process.[3,5,35] But, there are some points of particular pertinence to older people which the author believes require special attention; these are discussed below.

Physical illness, fears of declining health

Given that health worries rate fairly high in the elderly population it would be valuable to provide some group-based education and focused discussion on the following topics:

1. How our bodies change with age, the differences between physiological changes that occur as a result of stress and those that occur because of the ageing process. This would need to be done sensitively and yet firmly given the realistic fears that an elderly person may have, especially if they have a chronic illness such as cardiac disease or emphysema. A health professional with specialist knowledge in cardiac/respiratory disorders may have a particular contribution to make.
2. The ageing process. What does getting older mean to clients? For example, possible changes in health, activities and social roles.

3. Healthy behaviours; how to maintain physical and mental health through meaningful activity.
4. Developing patterns of daily activity, finding ways of adapting activity (social and self-care) while maintaining the desired quality of life; this can assist in the reduction of helplessness.[5]

The author suggests these discussions are planned and time-limited, set within the boundaries of the overall anxiety management programme. The above themes are best planned over several sessions, allowing clients the opportunity gradually to express negative thoughts and worrisome feelings about ageing as well as positive aspects of their lives. Well planned and clearly focused sessions will help the therapist not to collude with the clients' possible views that making changes are impossible and of no use. This can easily occur when clients' hold strong negative views about themselves, and respond with feelings of helplessness to the experience of getting older. Such a discussion is best carried out in a setting which can facilitate support between group members.[3,31,35]

Social isolation

What meaningful social supports can be established to buffer the clients' stresses and help them manage their anxiety in the long term? If possible this should be incorporated into the programme right at the beginning. Finding out about community and volunteer groups can be set as homework.[35] The author knows of one support group that developed naturally at the end of an anxiety management course for older people. The group meets regularly in the community in one of the client's homes, with minimal support from an occupational therapist.

Changes in learning processes

Learning continues to take place as we age but at a slower rate. It has been found that older people can 'be more focused and determined than their youthful counterparts, ... able to accomplish significant education goals'[36] (p. 67). But there are factors that can undermine or assist older people learning new things. Unfamiliar learning environments, quick, pressurised learning situations can undermine an elderly person's ability to learn. Older people need time to learn new techniques and information; learning will be easier if materials and information are presented in a 'clutter-free' manner and repeated clearly. Cognitive mediators, such as meaningful visual images can help the learning process. Learning will be easier if the person can associate the new material being presented with an experience or situation that is familiar to them.[31,36]

The therapist needs to take care not to patronise; although a person's learning processes change with age their intellectual capacities do not necessarily deteriorate unless the person has a dementia. Clinical practice shows that some clients want to maintain their intellectual abilities. Participating in an anxiety management course can support this, but the therapist will need to differentiate between the client intellectualising their anxiety and the client who wants to maintain their intellectual abilities as well as learning to manage their anxiety.

Hearing difficulties

Gradual hearing loss is part of the ageing process, but can be exacerbated by noise pollution. A particular hearing difficulty among older people is that of discriminating differences in the physical stimulation of tone, especially discerning higher tones. In a conversation it may be more difficult for an older person to hear words of higher pitch. These changes may have implications for the person's current levels of anxiety, and may bring about changes in their inter-personal behaviour. Hearing difficulties should also be considered when running anxiety management and relaxation therapy groups.[36] A session on hearing difficulties and how to cope with them may be helpful if a number of clients in a group have hearing difficulties. A speech and language therapist may be able to contribute to such a session.

It is acknowledged that it is not advisable to present relaxation in a totally quiet area; clients need to learn to manage their anxiety in real-life situations, and these will often include noise.[3] But with elderly clients the therapist needs to choose locations that have minimal noise interference. It is important to be aware of the difficulties the clients may have in hearing the instructions, teaching material and any discussion. The group and teaching presentation should be adapted accordingly, e.g. by adjusting factors such as proximity, volume and tone of voice.

Changes in visual acuity

Changes in vision are complex, and certainly not all older people suffer from glaucoma and cataracts. But overall visual acuity does decrease with age. Poor visual acuity will occur especially where the lighting is poor or where the background and the detail is poorly contrasted. This will have implications for how educational material is presented to older clients. Hand-outs and transparencies need to be clearly printed in large type.

Working with clients who have a chronic physical illness

Part of the therapist's assessment should have included an assessment of the client's ability to carry out activities of daily living; it is important for the client and therapist to know how restricted the client is by their physical illness and how restricted they are by their anxiety. Then, a graded programme, similar to the one over the page is advocated.

Working with clients who are excessively preoccupied by their physical status

There are numerous reasons why some clients become so focused on their physical pains and complaints. It should be recognised that the physiological changes related to the biological ageing process may be distressing. If a client has a life-threatening illness they may feel very frightened, but be unable to articulate their fears. The stigma attached to mental illness among the present generation of older people may make it easier for older people to talk, instead, about their physical complaints. The stoical 'stiff upper lip' characteristic of some older people may also inhibit them in talking about their fears and worries.[4,8,24]

Where a preoccupation with physical symptoms is acting as a defence mechanism, this needs to be respected but not colluded with. Not easy! If a person is holding fast to their physical symptoms and pains the following is suggested. First, the team or others involved in the care of the client need to be in agreement as to how to respond to the client. Second, the therapist needs to build a rapport, acknowledging the client's pain and distress. It is vital to remember that these pains and worries are very real to the client. It may be appropriate to adapt an anxiety-management programme, giving more time to health education, especially if there are several clients with similar difficulties. The author suggests that a suitable programme might include the following aspects:

1. A regular exercise and relaxation session with some simple education on 'how our bodies work', and what happens if a person becomes anxious.
2. The Mitchell relaxation or contrast relaxation done sitting in chairs with some visual imagery based on the person's pleasant memories, e.g. visiting a favourite garden or park.
3. Encouraging the clients to share the experience at the end of the relaxation.

A programme such as this is aimed at increasing the person's self-esteem, giving the client a positive experience of relaxation.

A T'ai Chi group can also be a useful addition to such a programme, especially for clients attending a day hospital or a community group. The authors believe T'ai Chi has physiological, social and psychological benefits for older people with anxiety. It may also help reinforce health promotion initiatives, enabling clients to become aware of their bodies and their health, in a fun and relaxed environment. The final section of this chapter is devoted to the application of T'ai Chi as an anxiety-reduction technique in elderly people.

Working with clients who have cognitive impairment

Anxiety can be particularly marked in clients who are in the early stages of dementia,[24] and agitated behaviours are common in this condition. Agitated behaviours can occur as a result of increased stress:

when the number of stressors or the intensity of stressors increases, dysfunctional (agitation) behaviors occur ... interventions or environments that would lessen stress should decrease the occurrence of agitation behaviours[37] (p. 34).

A variety of psychosocial and environmental interventions can help reduce agitation among people who suffer from dementia. Two particular media are suggested; one is music, the other is hand massage or therapeutic touch. Music, if appropriately selected to individual client's tastes, perhaps based on information from family or friends, can have a positive effect on agitated behaviours.[38]

Hand massage using hand cream or oil or therapeutic touch can have a relaxing effect on clients who have agitated behaviour. In one study an increase in relaxed behaviours and a reduced pulse rate were observed after hand massage and therapeutic touch.[37] With both these media it is essential that the therapist knows their client and presents the activity to the client in a quiet and familiar environment, and in a non-threatening manner. It is important that the therapist adapts and adjusts the intervention in response to the client's non-verbal and verbal behaviours which may well be expressing satisfaction or dissatisfaction with the intervention.

CONCLUSION

Elderly clients will vary in their experiences of stress, anxiety and coping strategies. It is important that, as therapists, we give them opportunities to use and benefit from anxiety management and stress-reduction techniques. Therapists should strive to be creative and adaptable in their approaches to working with older people, realising and recognising the unique and meaningful experiences of each elderly person they encounter.

THE USE OF T'AI CHI AS AN ANXIETY-REDUCTION TECHNIQUE IN ELDERLY PEOPLE

THE BACKGROUND AND HISTORY OF T'AI CHI

A Chinese proverb says:

A journey of a thousand miles starts with one small step.

T'ai Chi is a dynamic system of balanced movement practised for its benefits of relaxation, health and peace of mind. It has been chosen for particular emphasis here in order to illustrate its potential in reducing anxiety and improving general health in elderly people.

Throughout China, thousands of men and women of all ages take to the parks early in the morning for their daily T'ai Chi exercise to prepare their minds and bodies for the day ahead. This ancient health practice has its origins in China but is now widely practised throughout the western hemisphere. The movements involved are slow yet powerful, emphasising body awareness and relaxation. Each movement has a symbolic representation — some derived from martial arts, others derived from ancient Taoist images of nature — and they have names such as 'white crane spreads wings', 'hands wave like passing clouds', 'step forward and punch'. These systems of therapeutic exercise are characterised by slow and gentle movements encouraging receptivity, i.e. heightened awareness of the body's internal and external movements. Traditionally, in China, T'ai Chi is an exercise specifically suited for older people. T'ai Chi is an exercise and an art.

Origins

Historical records of Chinese exercises date back 4000 years. Regulated body exercises and special breathing techniques were said to be used to cure disease. In 1979 a silk book dating from the Han Dynasty (206BC to AD24) was discovered, known as the Dao Ying Xing Qi Fa (Method of Inducing Free Flow of Chi). It bears drawings of men and women in exercise positions similar to T'ai Chi

exercises still widely practised today.[39] The founder of T'ai Chi is thought to be Chang San Feng, a 12th century Taoist monk. He is said to have been inspired to develop T'ai Chi after witnessing an inconclusive battle between a snake and a crane. Chang observed how the responsive loose and circular movements of the snake were an excellent way to avoid the sharp stabbing actions of the crane's beak. From this it is thought he recognised the principles of T'ai Chi, in particular that force does not have to be met with force, and that strength can be found in softness.

The Chinese medical model

In the Chinese medical model good health is a matter of balancing the chi, the life force or vital energy of the body, which flows in meridians or pathways throughout the body. Chinese doctors believe that the chi can be improved and enhanced. As T'ai Chi improves circulation in general, it helps to ensure the chi does not get blocked. T'ai Chi, like acupuncture and acupressure, is a preventive way of ensuring harmony of the chi in the body. The highest goals of Chinese medicine are the prevention of disease and the maintenance of good health. Legend has it that in ancient times the Chinese physician was paid only when his patients were well. The aim was to avoid the use of curative acupuncture needles.

T'ai Chi as a movement system

T'ai Chi consists of a series of postures woven together into a specific continuous flowing sequence or 'form'. There are many different T'ai Chi forms with stylistic variations. But what they all have in common is their attention to detail and precision while appearing to be effortless. Classical T'ai Chi forms can take up to half an hour to practise and up to two years to learn. Some forms are hundreds of years old and have been passed down through the generations from teacher to pupil.

Health exercises

In addition to T'ai Chi, there are numerous sets

of Chinese health exercises such as the Eight Brocades or the 'Eighteen Stance Method' of 'T'ai Chi-Chi Kung'. These offer a suitable introduction to this way of exercising for older people because they can be adapted to sitting or standing, and they do not involve stepping and changes of direction.

WHAT IS UNIQUE ABOUT T'AI CHI?

The body is moved in a relaxed way without using any force. The person is encouraged to develop a root. This is done by letting go or releasing muscle tension through the length of the body into the feet and into the ground. If the exercises are done sitting down, as is often the case with elderly people, the person is encouraged to root through the pelvis into the chair. This lowering of the centre of gravity improves balance.

Other principles of T'ai Chi are as follows:

1. Relaxation — the whole body becomes relaxed (but not collapsed), especially the chest, shoulders and elbows.
2. Moving with centre — centring means focusing your mind on the 'tan t'ien', the centre of energy in the abdomen a few inches below the navel. This Chinese focal point corresponds closely to the body's centre of gravity and stability.
3. Correct posture — i.e. erect lengthened spine, pulled up from the crown of the head.
4. Slow and even movements.
5. Coordination of the whole body — the body aims to move as a complete unit. The movements of the extremities, e.g. the hands, reflect movements of the torso.
6. Breathing — breathing should be natural, deep, abdominal breathing. The abdomen expands with inhalation and flattens with exhalation to create deep and slow breathing. Some T'ai Chi teachers emphasise that the breathing should coordinate the body movements. For example, inhale when pulling back, exhale when striking. This can be useful in the beginning, but in practice, if the movements are done at an even tempo, using the body in a relaxed manner, the breathing takes care of itself. The body movements themselves encourage deeper breathing.
7. Concentration — mental concentration and focus is required. Consequently both the body and mind are working during practice.

T'AI CHI IN BRITAIN AS A THERAPEUTIC EXERCISE

T'ai Chi crept west following the sixties as a generation of seekers began looking to the east in their search for peace and self-actualisation. Just as it has become possible to take a class in yoga at adult education centres, it has in recent years become possible to find classes in T'ai Chi.

With the growing interest in this gentle adaptable exercise, several studies have taken place looking at the possible therapeutic benefits. With the uptake of complementary therapies in recent years in the UK, T'ai Chi could well become another therapeutic option. The fact that T'ai Chi continues to be used by millions of people throughout the world as a daily medicine / therapy suggests that some special value is felt by those who practise it.

T'ai Chi can be used in the symptomatic treatment of stress, and as part of a rehabilitation programme. It directly counters the symptoms of stress by:

- teaching a relaxed posture which helps counter increased muscle tension and stiffness in the neck, shoulders and back
- encouraging slow, deep abdominal breathing in order to counter the rapid short breathing accompanying feelings of panic
- encouraging concentration on the precise movements helps to combat worry and preoccupation with past or future events.

BENEFITS OF T'AI CHI FOR OLDER PEOPLE

Physiological benefits

The slow and gentle movements help maintain and improve flexibility of the joints, range of movement and muscle tone. No jerky, overextended movements are used; instead the person is taught to work within their own limitations and 'make friends' with their body.

There is a relatively high incidence of falls among older people, leading to anxiety and subsequent reduction in activity. It is suggested that T'ai Chi, which helps to improve coordination and balance, may help in the prevention of falls and consequent reductions in activity. According to a recent study sponsored by the National Institute on Aging, old people who exercise are less likely to have a fall and if they do they are less likely to hurt themselves. Eight separate studies using different types of exercise ranging from T'ai Chi to weight training were carried out by the institute's researchers. These studies showed that exercise in general reduced the likelihood of falling by about 10%. If the exercise involved balance training, the risk of falling was reduced by 17%. T'ai Chi was one of the best exercises and reduced falls by 37%.[40]

It is also posited that T'ai Chi can improve the health of the circulatory and respiratory systems. Mild exercise seems to have a beneficial effect on the immune system, particularly for older people. Sharp and Parry-Billings[41] described a Chinese study by Sun Xusheng et al which involved 30 healthy men and women aged 60 or more who regularly participated in T'ai-Chi, together with 30 control subjects, matched for age and sex. The T'ai Chi subjects were shown to have significantly increased numbers of active 'T' cells in their blood (approximately 40%).

Psychological benefits

T'ai Chi relaxes both body and mind. The exercises have accompanying images which the mind is actively engaged in translating into movements. The beauty and simplicity of the movements are thought to be therapeutic in themselves. T'ai Chi exercise can help a person feel relaxed and centred, as well as facilitating concentration and attention. The clients are encouraged to engage as fully as possible by focusing on the images involved so that concentration is improved. If the mind wanders, movements often waiver thus giving immediate feedback.

Management of stress

T'ai Chi teacher, Lawrence Galante,[42] taught T'ai Chi to a group of staff and psychiatric patients in America, during the seventies. The hypothesis behind the project was that T'ai Chi, with its emphasis on relaxation through body awareness, could provide a non-threatening method for clients to relearn basic trust in their bodies. Through T'ai Chi the clients were provided with a practical internal experience that could improve the quality of their lives. 'As the client's ability to experience the relaxed, centered state grew, so did their awareness of themselves when they were not in that state'. Galante suggests that this exercise provided good material for discussions on the management of stress.[42] (p. 73) Although this study was carried out with younger adults there is no reason to suggest that this principle cannot be applied to older people.

Social benefits

T'ai Chi is a group activity thereby encouraging socialisation. Working in pairs for part of the class introduces an element of fun and socialisation. Responding to others without words focuses the attention onto the body but also demands awareness of another person; thus students of T'ai Chi remain aware of themselves and, at the same time, aware of others.

WORKING WITH T'AI CHI
Adapting T'ai Chi to the hospital setting

If T'ai Chi is to be taken up as a therapeutic activity a teacher trained in T'ai Chi is needed. To work with older people in hospital it is necessary to find an experienced T'ai Chi teacher who is also aware of the special needs of elderly people. The ideal situation is for the T'ai Chi teacher to work with the hospital team, thus ensuring the appropriate selecton of clients, communication about the clients' needs and support for the T'ai Chi teacher.

Aims of a T'ai Chi group

- to improve body awareness and concentration
- to improve self-esteem
- to learn about and improve balance and coordination
- to develop group cohesion through non-verbal interaction
- to provide an educational experience about a new physical art
- to provide a complementary regime to more vigorous exercise.

Class content

In the clinical context involving elderly people, T'ai Chi classes must often be adapted to suit the needs of a group who find standing too tiring. One formula suggested by the author involves an extensive warm-up, usually sitting down, working with T'ai Chi principles of centring, increasing awareness of the body, and focusing on the breath. This is followed by standing and moving sequences, and, most importantly, working in pairs.

CONCLUDING REFLECTIONS

The underlying philosophical ideas such as finding strength in softness have appealed to some of the clients. Although the movements come from another culture, crossover is possible because the dignity and peacefulness of the precise movements may have universal appeal. Some of the Chinese images may be presented alongside more familiar images facilitating acceptance and understanding.

For others the visualisation of bringing the breath down to the lower abdomen/tan-t'ien helps to quieten the breathing and the mind.

Although the class is essentially non-verbal, the support of the group is experienced through shared activity and the challenge of learning a new skill.

REFERENCES

1 Tinker A 1992 Older people in modern society, 3rd edn. Longman, London
2 Coleman P, Bond J 1990 Ageing in the twentieth century. In: Bond J, Coleman P (eds) Ageing in society. An introduction to social gerontology. Sage Publications, London
3 Keable D 1989 The management of anxiety. A manual for therapists. Churchill Livingstone, Edinburgh
4 Pitt B 1982 Psychogeriatrics: An introduction to the psychiatry of old age. Churchill Livingstone, Edinburgh
5 Finlay-Jones 1986 Anxiety states in the elderly. In: Murphy E (ed) Affective disorders in the elderly. Churchill Livingstone, Edinburgh
6 Pearlin L I, Leiberman M A 1981 The stress process. Journal of Health and Social Behaviour 22:337–356
7 Lazarus R S, DeLongis A 1983 Psychological stress and coping in aging. American Psychologist 38(3):245–254
8 Coleman P 1990 Adjustment in later life. In: Bond J, Coleman P (eds) Ageing in society. An introduction to social gerontology. Sage, London
9 Powers C B, Wisocki P A, Whitbourne S K 1992 Age differences and correlates of worrying in young and elderly adults. The Gerontologist 32(1):82–88
10 Rowe J W, Khan R L 1987 Human aging: usual and successful. In: Cox H (ed) Annual editions: aging. The Dushkin Publishing Group, Connecticut
11 McPherson B D 1990 Aging as a social process. An introduction to individual and population aging. Butterworths, Toronto
12 Moneyham L, Scott C B 1995 Anticipatory coping in the elderly. Journal of Gerontological Nursing 21(7):23–28
13 Erikson E H, Erikson J M, Kivnick H Q 1986 Vital involvement in old age: the experience of old age in our time. Norton, New York
14 Matthews A M 1991 Widowhood in later life. Butterworths, Toronto
15 Gas K A 1987 Coping strategies of widows. Journal of Gerontological Nursing 13(8):29–33
16 Turnbull J M 1989 Anxiety and physical illness in the elderly. Journal of Clinical Psychiatry 50(11):40–45
17 Aldwin C M 1991 Does age affect the stress and coping process? Implications of age differences in perceived control. Journal of Gerontology: psychological sciences 46(4):174–180
18 Krause N 1991 Stress and isolation from close ties in later life. Journal of Gerontology: social sciences 46(4):183–194
19 Department of Health 1992 The health of older people: an epidemiological overview. HMSO, Volume 1
20 Down-Wamboldt B 1991 Coping with life satisfaction in elderly women with osteoarthritis. Journal of Advanced Nursing 16:1328–1335
21 Luchins D J, Rose R P 1989 Late-life onset of panic disorder with agoraphobia in three patients. American Journal of Psychiatry 146:920–921
22 Lindesay J 1991 Phobic disorders in the elderly. British Journal of Psychiatry 159:531–541
23 Spritzer A, Yoram B-T, Golander H 1995 The moderating

effect of demographic variables on coping effectiveness. Journal of Advanced Nursing 22:578–585

24 Weiss K J 1994 Management of anxiety and depression syndromes in the elderly. Journal of Clinical Psychiatry 55(2):5–11

25 Lindesay J, Briggs K, Murphy E 1989 The Guys/Age Concern survey: prevalence rates of cognitive impairment, depression and anxiety in an urban elderly community. British Journal of Psychiatry 155:317–329

26 Parmelee P A, Katz I R, Lawton M P 1993 Anxiety and its association with depression among institutionalized elderly. The American Journal of Geriatric Psychiatry 1(1):46–57

27 Flint A J 1994 Epidemiology and comorbidity of anxiety disorders in the elderly. American Journal of Psychiatry 151(5):640–649

28 Surtees P G 1995 In the shadow of adversity: the evolution and resolution of anxiety and depressive disorder. British Journal of Psychiatry 166:583–594

29 Eastwood R, Corbin S 1985 Epidemiology of mental disorders. In: Arie T (ed) Recent advances in psychogeriatrics. Churchill Livingstone, Edinburgh

30 Copeland J R M, Dewey M E, Wood N, Searle R, Davidson I A, McWilliam C 1987 Range of mental illness among the elderly in the community. Prevalence in Liverpool using the GMS-AGECAT package. British Journal of Psychiatry 150:815–823

31 Garfinkel R 1979 Brief behavior therapy with an elderly patient. Journal of Geriatric Psychiatry 12(1):101–109

32 Pattie A H, Gilleard C J 1979 The Clifton assessment procedures for the elderly. Hodder & Stoughton

33 Research unit of the Royal College of Physicians and the British Geriatrics Society 1992 Standardised assessment scales for older people. The Royal College of Physicians of London and The British Geriatrics Society

34 Folstein M F, Folstein S E, McHugh P R 1975 Mini-Mental state: a practical method for grading the cognitive state of patients for the clinician. Journal of Psychiatric Research 12:189–198

35 Blair S 1990 The elderly. In: Creek J (ed) Occupational therapy and mental health. Churchill Livingstone, Edinburgh

36 Stokes G 1991 On being old. The psychology of later life. Falmer Press, London

37 Snyder M, Egan E C, Burns K R 1995 Interventions for decreasing agitation behaviors in persons with dementia. Journal of Gerontological Nursing 21(7):34–40

38 Gerdner L A, Swanson E A 1993 Effects of individualised music on confused and agitated elderly patients. Archives of Psychiatric Nursing VII(5):284–291

39 Chuen L K 1991 The way of energy: mastering the Chinese art of internal strength with chi kung exercise. Gaia, London, UK

40 Province M A, Hadley E C, Hornbrook M C 1995 The effects of exercise on falls in elderly patients. Journal of American Medical Association 273(17)

41 Sharp C, Parry-Billings M 1992 Can exercise damage your health? Athletes who train hard seem unusually prone to illness. But the complexities of the immune system make it difficult to understand why. New Scientist 135(1834):33

42 Galante L 1989 T'ai Chi. The supreme ultimate. Weiser, New York

19

Working in community settings

Jenny Coleman

As we near the end of the 20th century there is an increasing pressure in all aspects of health care to treat only the acutely ill in hospital settings and to provide all other services elsewhere. This 'elsewhere' is called the community, a varied and disparate place. For the therapist the core elements of anxiety management practice in the community are identical to those in hospital or clinic settings. There are, however, some significant differences in context and emphasis which need to be considered, and some practical issues to address.

Community work can mean working within the primary health care team, running anxiety management groups in a variety of community settings, becoming involved in health education and preventative work, or working in a teaching/consultative way with other service providers or carers.

WORKING WITH THE PRIMARY HEALTH CARE TEAM

Working as part of the primary health care team is, in many ways, the ideal situation for the anxiety-management therapist. Here the interrelationship between mind and body, physical and psychological health is most evident, and the therapist whose work spans the whole has both much to offer and a constantly challenging and exciting field in which to practise.

With the Department of Health's current policy of encouraging secondary mental health services to concentrate on those with serious and enduring mental health problems, often interpreted as those who suffer from psychotic illness, the care of people suffering from anxiety will remain with the general practitioner to an even greater extent than before.

In this transitional period the anxiety-management therapist who receives referrals from medical sources will continue to receive those referrals both from in- and out-patient mental health services and from the primary health care team. In the future it is likely that the major source of referrals will be direct from primary health care.

This change of context from psychiatric unit to general practice is likely to have a significant and generally positive effect on work with those who present with anxiety states. It will also introduce new groups of clients, those whose anxiety is part of a medical or surgical condition, those who are experiencing stressful life events and those who could benefit from advice and guidance in the adoption of more healthy lifestyles.

Working in primary health care — getting started

Each general practitioner or group of practitioners is a small independent business. This is true for both fundholders and for non-fundholders. In view of this, working arrangements should be clarified separately with each practice. It should not be assumed that because a system works well in Dr. Bloggs' surgery that it will necessarily work in Dr. Jones' surgery. Therapists who work as part of a larger organisation, a Health Trust for example, will find that some part of their organisation — variously called Business Planning, Contracting, or Marketing — has developed links with local primary health care. It is essential for therapists to work in close collaboration with the people in these departments who have knowledge and skills concerning the contracting process. Some therapists have found that significant parts of a contract have been agreed by others before they are involved. This can cause difficulties. It is advisable to ensure that therapists are involved at the earliest point possible in the contracting process. Independent therapists,

or those without specialist contracting departments, will need to pay particular attention to the following aspects.

1. Clarity about the nature and scope of the services to be offered, including interventions to be used, what difficulties they are appropriate for, the amount of time available.
2. Identify any groups of people to whom it will not be possible to offer a service and agree procedures for referring back or on to other professionals.
3. Most surgeries prefer to develop a personal relationship with an identified therapist or small team of therapists. That therapist or therapists should make personal contact with all the doctors or other staff likely to refer patients. Time spent developing communication at this stage will be amply justified later. As new staff join the surgery, the therapist should make it his or her business to get to know them and to ensure that they understand how an anxiety management service can fit into the general picture of provision for the patients. Some written information can be helpful here.

THE PRESENTATION OF ANXIETY IN PRIMARY HEALTH CARE

Mental health

The prevalence of anxiety disorders in the population at large has been estimated at between 4% and 8%.[1] It has been calculated that of these about half suffer from general anxiety disorders, many of which require long-term management. A general practitioner with the national average list of between 2100 and 2300 patients is likely to have 80–85 patients at any one time whose primary diagnosis is anxiety. In addition to those who fulfil diagnostic criteria for one of the clinical anxiety disorders, many more people experience transient, but recurrent anxiety symptoms which cause them considerable distress and significant functional disruption. The care of both these groups of patients is likely to be undertaken by their general practitioner. Anxiety symptoms are often a feature of other chronic psychiatric disorders and the general practitioner, who manages the ongoing care of the majority of these patients, is often presented with these difficulties.

The management of anxiety states, once frequently treated with benzodiazepines, has become more problematic for the general practitioner. New pharmacological treatments have been proposed and clearly have their place. However, Jane Da Roza Davis and Michael Gelder,[2] in their recent review of anxiety states and their management, conclude that there is increasing evidence to indicate that many acute anxiety states can be treated more satisfactorily without drugs, or by a combination of medical and psychological treatments. Such careful management of cases of recent onset may prevent some of the problems that arise with more chronic conditions. This approach is also frequently more acceptable to the patients. General practitioners are generally well aware of current management advice, but lack the time or the specific expertise necessary.

Physical health

The role of anxiety and the stress reaction in the development or aggravation of many physical disorders is well recognised, as is the considerable psychological stress which usually accompanies physical illness. This is most likely when a condition is chronic or life threatening and affects not only the immediate patient but other members of the family. The primary health care team is the central, and for some people the only, medical support in these situations.

Life events

Members of the primary health care team often become involved with ordinary families during stressful life events. This may include birth and the integration of the baby into the family, illness and disability, and death and the process of dying. Even in situations where their presence is not indicated on medical grounds many people regard doctors as the most obvious source of help. One study[3] found that the family doctor

was the most frequent source of help, after close family or friends, to whom people said they would turn when facing a personal difficulty or emotional problem. This involvement gives primary health workers a key role in monitoring and mediating distress. An important part of the work of the anxiety-management therapist is helping all members of the primary health care team support the patient in these situations and helping them to identify when to involve the therapist more directly.

Preventative work and health education

This is an area of work which is increasingly being seen as part of the work of the primary health care team. Here too the anxiety-management therapist has a part to play providing specific stress management courses or contributing to programmes on Looking after your Heart, Stopping Smoking, Healthy Retirement, Preparation for Parenthood and so on.

ENVIRONMENTAL FACTORS — SOME PRACTICAL CONSIDERATIONS

The physical space within which therapy is undertaken has an appreciable impact on the work. This is as true within the primary health care setting as everywhere else. The therapist's responsibility to the patient includes ensuring that the environment within which the work is carried out is as conducive to successful therapy as possible. The following comments relate to work undertaken at the surgery. Consideration of the issues raised in working in patients' homes is covered separately.

Some therapists are regarded as an integrated part of the team and enjoy equal rights in laying claim to working space; some are regarded as visitors and have to employ much tact and diplomacy in negotiating space. Primary health care teams and their facilities vary enormously, but the belief that there is not enough space for the work that needs to be done appears universal. So whether the therapist's approach is 'tactful' or 'terrier' she should be clear about her requirements for the work, both the ideal and the minimum necessary, and be prepared to argue her case. Requirements will differ according to whether the therapist is working with individuals or with groups. For work with individuals, which includes the possibility of an occasional family member or fellow health professional joining the sessions, experience has shown the following small list to be essential:

- a large enough space for three chairs and a desk or table
- privacy: a place free from interruption and where conversation can not be overheard; this would also mean a reasonably quiet place
- sufficient warmth, light, ventilation, etc.

The things that would be nice to have, in addition, include:

- the same place for each meeting
- a pleasant and welcoming environment which is not overly medical, i.e. free of desks overflowing with medical equipment; pleasant pictures rather than a poster of the dissection of the eye
- a clock placed where it may be easily seen by both parties
- a working space for the writing up of notes and records.

While by no means universal, an increasing number of primary health care settings contain larger rooms within which group work can be carried out. For work with groups the essentials would be:

- a room that is large enough to accommodate the group comfortably
- sufficient similar chairs for all group members
- space for some presentation equipment — at the very least a suitable wall for putting up visual aid posters or for overhead projection
- privacy — as for individual sessions
- sufficient warmth, light, ventilation, etc.

Additional features which would benefit the group include:

- a space that is a comfortable size for the

optimum group size of 8–12 members including group leader(s) — neither too squashed nor so spacious that it feels alienating
- a pleasant environment — as for individual sessions
- space for coats, bags, etc.

TREATMENT COMPONENTS OF COMMUNITY WORK IN PRIMARY HEALTH CARE

Assessment

Each piece of work begins with an assessment process. The assessment of the patient's situation and difficulties by the therapist is the same process in the community as in every other setting and is amply covered in the chapter on assessment (Ch. 13). The assessment of the therapist by the patient in order to make a judgement about the potential help which could be provided before deciding whether to engage in therapy, also takes place in every other setting, but is perhaps more obvious to the therapist when working in the community. Away from the social pressures of the hospital or clinic setting patients seem to feel more able to exercise choice. The therapist's ability to engage the patient in a working partnership, the foundation-stone of all work, is therefore highlighted. A very positive aspect of this situation is that, once achieved, the open commitment of the patient to the work can produce significant change at a speed which can be surprising to those who are used to working within institutions.

Interventions

The exact components of an anxiety-management strategy are as varied as the people who employ them. Important parts of the package are:

Information and education This is arguably the most significant intervention of all.

Strategies to reduce the physiological consequences of stress

1. Relaxation techniques — chosen with the patient to address particular needs and situations.

2. Exercise and physical activity — for many people an excellent short-term method of alleviating stress. Taking up regular physical exercise, particularly if it can also be social in nature, contributes to people's continued physical and mental health. It is also often more likely to be maintained than relaxation exercises and emphasises normal activities.

3. Psychoactive drugs — whilst acknowledging the justified hesitation about drugs, carefully chosen in conjunction with the doctor, appropriate medication can provide a short respite period for the patient during which other strategies can be formulated to change either the anxiety-provoking situation or the patient's reaction to it.

Strategies to address the way a patient thinks about a stressful situation

1. Consideration of beliefs and goals — this may involve identifying dysfunctional beliefs or unrealistic goals and working with the patient to re-examine them and consider which remain true and important for him or her.

2. Development of a realistic appraisal of the situation and of the strategies which could be utilised to change it, together with their cost implications for the individual.

Strategies to increase the resources available to the patient in dealing with the stressful situation

1. Consideration of skills or knowledge needed — this could involve the therapist either in teaching skills or in identifying with the patient where the relevant skills/knowledge can be obtained.

2. Accessing resources — some resources are supplied by other people or agencies and help may be needed either to develop a network of such resources or to use resources which are already available but which the patient has difficulty in utilising. For example, the man made redundant who is prevented by his beliefs about male roles from accepting the support which his wife could give him, both emotionally and financially.

Number and frequency of sessions

As in all therapeutic work the aim should be to provide the minimum intervention necessary to allow the patient to make and maintain helpful change.

When working with individuals, if an anxiety management approach is to prove helpful, significant improvement is usually obvious to both patient and therapist by the third meeting. If no improvement is noted by the fifth meeting then an alternative strategy should be considered. For most patients a treatment contract of five to eight sessions is appropriate.

As much of the treatment is carried out by the patient practising techniques, attempting changes or monitoring situations between meetings with the therapist, space has to be left for these processes. Meetings should take place no less than one week apart and, as the work progresses, meetings can usefully be spaced out to once every two weeks or once a month. A final or review meeting at least a month after the previous one is usually helpful.

A 'standard package' of anxiety management offered to an individual patient in their GP's surgery might therefore be:

- one assessment meeting
- one treatment session a week later
- two further treatment sessions at fortnightly intervals
- one treatment session one month later
- one review meeting six weeks later.

In this case the total number of sessions would be six with a total duration of 15 weeks.

CASE STUDIES

Some illustrative case studies will indicate the scope of the work which can be done with individual patients.

Harry

Harry was a builder who had suffered a spinal injury when he fell from some scaffolding. His fracture was at C7 and, although he was confined to a wheelchair he was a fit young man and had made a good physical recovery. He had been discharged from the spinal injury unit but needed to attend the physiotherapy department for regular treatment and monitoring to prevent the development of contractions. This he was failing to do. Harry's doctor suspected that his anxiety about leaving home in his wheelchair was responsible.

As he was reluctant to venture out, an appointment was made with Harry for a home visit. The assessment process was spread over two visits and during the course of this it became clear that Harry had suffered from considerable social anxiety long before his accident. There were also unresolved issues relating to his accident, leaving Harry with the feeling that his shock, anger and grief at the dramatic change in his life had been ignored by the medical team. He believed that they only considered his physical state, and this also applied to his family who were determinedly cheerful and positive, allowing no space for negative feelings.

A package was devised with Harry which included some initial education about the physiological effects of anxiety and the teaching of strategies to overcome those effects. Using these strategies Harry and the therapist agreed a series of 'challenges', ventures into the outside world which gradually introduced him to varied social situations and which included making and keeping appointments with the physiotherapy department. The meetings which monitored these challenges were also used for consideration of the family expectations and rules with which Harry approached his world, and to allow space for him to ventilate his feelings about the new role which he had been forced to adopt since his accident. Although Harry's wife did not join in any of these meetings, the couple used them as a focus for opening up discussion between them and both benefited from the opportunity to share their feelings and ideas.

Harry and the therapist met for a total of twelve meetings, including the two initial assessment meetings. During the early stages of treatment they met weekly, gradually spacing the meetings out to every other week and finally to one a month, the entire contact having a duration of just over six months. At the end of this time Harry was not only regularly attending the Physiotherapy department, he was able to undertake, without undue anxiety, many social tasks which he had avoided or dreaded since childhood.

Aruna

Aruna was an accountant and business woman whose business life was demanding and satisfying. She was also a member of a large extended family, a wife, and mother of two school-age children. She suffered from bouts of pain and digestive difficulties which after extensive investigation had been diagnosed as irritable bowel syndrome (IBS).

Aruna and the therapist met at the surgery. It was soon evident that although Aruna recognised that her very busy lifestyle was contributing to her difficulties, she was unable, or unwilling, to make any real changes in her current life patterns. Therapy concentrated therefore on providing her with some strategies which could be used to ameliorate the stresses she would continue to face. Her right to decide what changes she would make was acknowledged.

The role of stress in her condition was explained. Simple and brief relaxation techniques were taught. Together Aruna and the therapist considered her life pattern and opportunities for buffer activities were identified. She was encouraged to plan ahead as much as possible and avoid taking on too many demanding activities at any one time.

Aruna and the therapist met on five occasions at the surgery. These meetings were spaced over the relatively long period of four months because of Aruna's busy lifestyle.

Aruna continued to suffer bouts of IBS and to need medication on a regular basis. However, she felt that she was now able to reduce the frequency and intensity of these attacks by the use of stress management strategies. She had gained an increased sense of control over her own condition which considerably reduced the distress she experienced.

Margaret

Margaret was 20 and lived with her sister in a shared flat. They had moved to London from their home just outside Manchester just over a year earlier. Margaret's older sister, who was employed by a large banking institution, had the opportunity of transferring and Margaret had decided to move with her. She had found a job and for the first few months all had gone well, but then one of the women she worked with was violently mugged on the way home. Everyone in the office was upset and shocked by this and the following day, a Friday, Margaret (clutching her bag tightly) hurried home and found that her heart was racing and her breathing difficult by the time she arrived. Over the weekend she felt fine and gave the matter little thought but on the way home on Monday she experienced a panic attack as she waited for the bus. In the days following, several more occurred, two so severe that she had attended the casualty department of the local hospital. Her sister, initially sympathetic, was becoming exasperated by her constant need for companionship and reassurance, and Margaret herself was terrified that she would be admitted to a psychiatric ward.

Margaret met the therapist at her doctor's surgery. Her concern that she would be found to be 'having a breakdown' raised her anxiety levels to the point where she was beginning to hyperventilate as she entered the surgery. The symptoms, triggered by hyperventilation (including dizziness, tingling around the mouth, and a feeling of distance from reality), were growing and therefore causing a further escalation in her anxiety levels. The therapist's first task clearly was to help her to regain control. A simple strategy, commonly known as the 'Paper Bag Technique' was immediately taught to her.

Hyperventilation, which is characterised by a brief inbreath and a forceful outbreath, washes an excessive amount of carbon dioxide from the blood. The resulting changes in blood acidity levels lead to the unpleasant symptoms mentioned. These symptoms provoke anxiety and further hyperventilation. To counter this the sufferer is instructed to cover the mouth and nose, classically with a paper bag, in Margaret's case with cupped hands. The sufferer is then instructed to breathe, as calmly as possible, into the bag and then to re-inhale the air in the bag. This air, richer in carbon dioxide than the general atmosphere, restores the levels in the blood to more normal levels and the hyperventilation cycle is blocked. Margaret did as she was told and somewhat to her surprise found that it worked. A careful explanation of *why* it worked was then given to her. This set the scene for the rest of the work. Her symptoms and their causes were examined and normalised. Margaret set about the task of controlling her symptoms using a combination of relaxation techniques and positive and reassuring thoughts. She was able to move rapidly to the position where anxiety symptoms produced not the terrifying fear that she was going mad, but accurate identification and control. After four meetings she felt confident enough to continue independently.

Note: Although it is interesting to speculate about why the mugging of a colleague was so disturbing to Margaret, and what might be present in her own history or psychopathology to contribute to her reaction, such questions were not part of the agenda which Margaret brought to the sessions and investigation of them could have undermined still further her own confidence in her ability to control her life.

SKILLS NEEDED BY THE THERAPIST WORKING IN PRIMARY HEALTH CARE

Education and training

The treatment of anxiety is not the preserve of any one profession. Just as the symptoms and aetiology of the condition are best understood from an holistic perspective, so the background of therapists vary and many different disciplines have contributed to effective treatments. The need for a thorough knowledge of both physiology and psychology is clear. This knowledge is not quickly acquired and the growing level of demand for anxiety management interventions together with the shortage of many of the professionals with relevant background knowledge could lead to a worrying situation in which underqualified people apply simplistic models which address only the needs of those who are least distressed and where potentially serious symptoms are overlooked. It is the responsibility both of the therapist and of the employing body to ensure that this does not occur.

The basic education of a potential therapist should include:

- anatomy, physiology, medicine and surgery
- psychology and psychiatry
- specific anxiety-management education and training.

Anatomy, physiology, medicine and surgery

People seen in primary health care settings may have been seen first by a general practitioner who should identify and investigate any primary physical problems. This is not universal, however, and the 'eight minutes per patient' norm for GPs plus the well-known phenomenon of the patient omitting to reveal important facts to the doctor at first interview, contribute to the firm belief that therapists working in this area should have a sound basis of knowledge of physiology and medicine, sufficient to allow them to identify signs that warrant further investigation.

A case example, known to the author, which illustrates potential difficulties is that of a man referred by his GP for help with panic attacks. During the course of the assessment interview — considerably longer than the one the doctor had been able to allow him — he said that he was not aware of any precipitating factors, but that he did know when he was going to have an attack because he smelt a funny smell just beforehand. Alerted by this the therapist questioned him further and discovered that after an 'attack' he slept for some time and that one of his sisters had suffered from epilepsy. He was referred back to his GP with the tactful suggestion that a neurological investigation might be indicated. Professions that are likely to provide this basic knowledge include nursing, occupational therapy and physiotherapy.

Psychology and psychiatry

Again the level of knowledge should both be sufficient to underpin and inform the work which is undertaken and to allow the therapist to identify areas outside his or her competence which require investigation by specialists. In addition to psychologists and psychiatrists the professions which will provide this basic knowledge include psychiatric nursing, some specialist social work and occupational therapy.

Specific anxiety management education and training

This should include the physiology of anxiety, assessment, the selection and implementation of appropriate treatment interventions, skills for working with groups and with individuals. In short all the skills which are covered in this book plus some experience of implementing them, in a setting where initially the support and supervision of other experienced therapists is readily available, and where increasing autonomy can be developed.

Assessment skills

Specific task-related skills for community work

Organisational skills When working in a wide variety of places away from an office base, good organisation is essential. The therapist must be prepared for a wide range of demands, and, as much of the work undertaken is supported by written or taped information given to patients, this involves ensuring that a sufficient stock and range of these materials is carried.

The therapist also needs to have sufficient office supplies available to be able to write to a fellow health professional or a patient without returning to base first. These would include:

- headed note-paper
- carbon paper
- envelopes and stamps.

This both saves time in communicating and makes good use of any time which becomes available should a patient be unable to keep an appointment.

Skills in the selection or writing of information sheets The primary use of written materials is to reinforce and supplement information given during sessions and to support home practice. It is important, therefore, that this information speaks with the voice of the therapist. This can be achieved either by the therapist selecting material which is congruent with his or her own approach and basing sessions around it, or by preparing handouts which use phrases and concepts which the therapist has found to be particularly helpful in conveying information and therefore uses frequently during sessions. As experience grows, therapists tend to develop their own style of delivery and the benefit of custom written handouts increases. Similar information often needs to be available in different formats to suit the needs of patients with different ability or desire to comprehend the theoretical concepts behind the approach. There is also a need for information to be available in a range of languages, appropriate to the population of the area. This is more evident when the use which is made of the handout by many patients in explaining to their families their difficulties and the treatment they are receiving is considered. For most therapists this will mean the involvement of others in obtaining translations.

Communication skills

Communication with the patient

Important as it is for the therapist to understand the theoretical concepts underpinning the work and the interventions which flow from these concepts, this understanding will count for nothing if it cannot be conveyed to the patient in a way which enables him or her to improve the situation. For any communication to take place we know that the parties involved have to both speak and listen. First ensure that you and the patient can hear and understand each other. This may mean arranging for a translator or signer to be available. Having addressed the language question there are several key elements to consider in working towards good communication.

1. The engendering of confidence — the patient has to believe that the therapist knows what he or she is talking about and has something to offer and is therefore worth listening to. In primary health care a great deal of credibility is obtained by the setting and the fact that most referrals involve the doctor. To build on this credibility therapists must be organised and professional in the initial assessment interview, be clearly comfortable in their own knowledge of theoretical concepts and aware of the initial impression their own non-verbal communication is making on the patient. This includes the clothes worn. Unfair as it may seem, many patients appear to find it easier to accept information and advice from relatively conservatively dressed therapists.

2. Information should be given in a form which is understandable to the patient. Time and encouragement should be given for the patient to ask questions and to relate the information to their own situation.

3. Therapists must ensure that they are alert to the unique situation which each patient brings to the work and modify the interventions accordingly.

Communication with other professionals

Communication with the rest of the primary health team is also of great importance. When first starting to work with a GP practice it is essential to agree communication strategies which are acceptable to all involved. These should cover:

- referral
- information on work being undertaken
- discharge information
- information on the volume and nature of the work for the purposes of monitoring the contractual agreement
- quality monitoring information.

Communication with reception staff needs particular attention. A good relationship with the people who run the reception desk can be crucial to success in working in primary health care. This can be facilitated by:

1. Always letting the reception staff know when the therapist expects to be at the practice and which patients are due to be seen.
2. If there is no specifically designated room it is worth spending time explaining to reception staff, who usually organise such things, what type of room is preferred for the therapist's purposes.
3. When the therapist or a patient has to cancel an appointment the practice reception staff should always be informed.
4. When appointments have to be cancelled agree how and by whom the patient will be informed.
5. Make sure that appointment booking arrangements are clear. Retaining control of bookings is usually preferable, then the need for subsequent appointments at planned intervals can be allowed for. If the practice insists on making appointments on the therapist's behalf, a conservative blocking out process should be agreed.
6. Finally, it is advisable for the therapist to carry their own 'Room Engaged' sign with them. This avoids some, but not all, of the incidences of other staff interrupting your treatment sessions.

Networking knowledge and ability

Therapists should be aware of, and develop links with, a wide range of services which could be helpful to their patients. Some of these services will be specialised but most are part of the ordinary social infrastructure of communities. Bringing these services to the knowledge of the patient and, where necessary, supporting the patient in accessing them can become a significant part of the treatment package. Relevant services will include:

- specialist mental health services
- local authority services — housing, education, social services — how and where they are accessed
- sports and leisure facilities
- voluntary and self-help groups

- adult education facilities
- social and community groups.

A small range of information leaflets can be carried or, if space permits, kept at the surgery. This should include information about public transport links.

ANXIETY MANAGEMENT WORK IN PATIENTS' HOMES

Therapists who work in the community, whether they receive referrals from the mental health services or from primary care, are often asked to see patients in their own homes. There are benefits and disadvantages to working in a patient's home and these should be considered carefully before undertaking such work.

The benefits

1. The patient's home is usually available without complex negotiations.
2. The patient may feel more relaxed and at ease at home.
3. Assessment may be more complete if patients are seen in their own environment.
4. Other members of the family, children or adult dependents may be more easily accommodated.
5. For some patients who are unable to leave their homes it becomes the only place possible to start any work.

The disadvantages

1. Interruptions can be more frequent in a patient's home and when they do occur are less easily controlled by the therapist.
2. Patient confidentiality can be harder to maintain when visiting people at home. Many patients are concerned about explaining the visit of a professional, complete with large bag containing handouts etc. to family or neighbours.
3. The business-like atmosphere of the treatment session is often more difficult to create or sustain in a patient's home.

4. The opportunity to discuss anxieties and fears in a neutral space, which allows a psychological break on leaving the treatment room, and avoids the risk of polluting the home space, can be very important for some patients.
5. The safety of the therapist, not just in the particular home but in the area, should be considered.
6. Travel time and distance between patients adds to costs and may reduce the number of people who can be seen.

RUNNING ANXIETY MANAGEMENT GROUPS IN COMMUNITY SETTINGS

For many people the benefits of group work to address their anxiety is significant and group work is the treatment of choice. An acknowledged difficulty in all anxiety management work has always been that of helping patients to take their skills out of the treatment setting and into their everyday life. Placing the skill training in the community and out of a hospital or clinic setting can contribute to the successful transfer of skills. It also normalises the experience of anxiety, helping to designate it as a condition which the individual can understand and control rather than one which a doctor must treat.

Sources of referral

The therapist will need to be constantly proactive in seeking referrals to a community-based anxiety management group. The process starts at least two months before the anticipated start date of the group with information being sent to all who might wish to refer, giving information about the group and the referral process. This long timescale is necessary to allow for the collection of referrals and the individual assessment of potential group members.

Referrals to such a group can come from general practitioners or from the secondary mental health services. Successful groups can contain people from both sources provided that the range in severity of symptoms is not too wide. They can also incorporate people whose reaction to stress is affecting either their psychological or physical health. Other variables, gender, age, ethnicity, social and economic background should be considered in forming a stress management group. The usual rules of group dynamics apply. Members must be able to recognise enough similarities between themselves and others to form a group. This does not mean complete homogeneity. One isolated individual, particularly one who is different in two dimensions such as the lone young man within a group of older women, may affect the group process deleteriously. A well-balanced mix adds to the richness of experience available to the group.

The assessment process and content of an anxiety management course remains standard. The differences are concerned with the context.

What's in a name?

The use of the title 'Stress Management Course' has been found to be more successful in the community. Stress is a situation we all experience and are happy to admit to, indeed there is almost a pride in being under stress with its associations with highly paid business people. A course to learn to manage stress has an educational/personal development sound to it which is often more acceptable to participants and to the owners of community venues.

Finding a venue

Allow a considerable amount of time to find and negotiate a suitable venue. With luck, the local voluntary services council will have a list of rooms for hire, if not the therapist will have to investigate personally the facilities available at community centres, adult education venues, church halls and libraries. There is no substitute for going out and visiting all rooms and halls in the area which might be suitable. Do not rely on the opinion of others, who probably have only a hazy idea about the suitability of a room.

There are a number of points to consider in relation to the venue.

1. A venue will need to be of a suitable size

and have appropriate facilities. Again consider the minimum needed:

- a room that is large enough to accommodate the group comfortably
- sufficient similar chairs for all group members
- space for some presentation equipment — at the very least a suitable wall for putting up visual aid posters or for overhead projection
- privacy
- sufficient warmth, light, ventilation, etc.

And then consider the additional facilities which would contribute to your own or the group members' comfort:

- sufficient and accessible electric sockets
- a reception or waiting area
- toilets on site
- presentation equipment provided.

Access to the venue is of great importance:

- are there good public transport links?
- is there a car park?
- how accessible is the venue for those with mobility difficulties?

2. What else is the venue used for? An adult education facility or a community centre with many other activities going on can be a positive advantage in encouraging group members to increase their use of local facilities. Beware of an adult education setting which mainly caters for 17–20 year olds. Many older participants can feel profoundly alienated and awkward in such an environment.

3. Clarify insurance responsibilities and billing arrangements.

4. Check access arrangements to the room:

- Who has a key to let the therapist and group in?
- Is their telephone number known to the therapist?
- Does the key-holder have the therapists address and telephone number?
- What alternative arrangements are there if the key-holder has flu or is on leave?
- If there is no reception/waiting area, can the room be opened before the group starting time to allow group members who arrive early to wait out of the rain?

4. Presentation equipment is sometimes available in venues. However this is variable and when it is available tends to be charged at alarming rates. It is advisable for therapists to have their own portable flip chart stand and pad together with a selection of pens. A portable overhead projector is helpful, and of course handouts, written material, plain paper and pens for group members is essential.

5. Don't forget the 'Room Engaged' notice for the door and, for the first meeting of the group, some signs indicating where the group is being held.

6. Time-keeping. If the room does not have a clock consider bringing one with you, large enough so that all can see it.

7. Relaxation equipment. If the course includes practising relaxation techniques while lying on the floor you may wish to ask group members to bring a mat, rug or sleeping bag with them. Be prepared to supply some for members who have nothing suitable or who cannot transport them.

8. Tape recorder. If taped music or relaxation instructions are to be used, bring both the tapes and a player. If there are no suitable electric sockets available ensure that the player can use batteries.

9. Make sure all verbal agreements are confirmed in writing.

10. Inter-group communication. Ensure that group members know how they can convey necessary messages to the therapist, and not to the venue, in between group meetings. Plan how and by whom the group could be informed if a meeting has to be cancelled at short notice — for example if the therapist is ill.

Stress management courses such as these are infinitely portable and with minor modification to address particular group concerns can be run for specific groups such as teachers, housing department staff, carers' groups. In these circumstances it is likely that the venue would be arranged or provided by the organisation concerned, but the therapist should still check that the minimum facilities are provided.

THE THERAPIST AS A RESOURCE FOR OTHER SERVICE PROVIDERS AND CARERS

In addition to direct work with individuals or groups of patients the community-based anxiety management therapist can achieve much by working with other service providers, either to enhance and support their work with patients, or to address with them their own need to manage their stress. This applies both to professionals and to the clients' carers. Examples include:

- health education and health promotion initiatives
- joint working in specialised areas e.g. drug and alcohol

- training programmes for health and care staff
- staff stress management training.

CONCLUSION

With a very few exceptions the community is the setting in which anxiety-provoking situations are encountered, and it is in the community that they have to be faced and overcome. The logic which suggests that the community is the ideal setting for anxiety management training is irresistible. The scope of the work is enormous and the therapist's contribution greatly needed and increasingly valued.

REFERENCES

1 Weissman M M, Leaf P J, Holzer C E, Merikangas K R 1985 The epidemiology of anxiety disorders: a highlight of recent evidence. Psychopharmacology Bulletin 21(3):538–541
2 Da Roza Davis J, Gelder M 1991 Long term management of anxiety states. International Review of Psychiatry 3(1):5–17
3 Barker C, Pistrang N, Shapiro D A, Shaw I 1990 Coping and help seeking in the UK adult population. British Journal of Clinical Psychology 29:271–285

20

Understanding and surviving occupational stress and burnout

Gill Westland

INTRODUCTION

Occupational stress is being recognised increasingly across a range of jobs. Long hours, fear of redundancy, lack of confidence, changing workplace practices, greater use of information technology and perpetual re-organisation — as often as once every six months — are factors contributing to the likelihood of work stress continuing.[1] Society's sensitivity to stress issues has also sharpened. This growing public awareness has two aspects. Firstly, there is the belief that trauma and stress can be ameliorated with stress management and counselling. Secondly, job stress can be the subject of litigation. Legal claims against employers concerning job stress are accumulating, and can include the areas of sexual harassment and bullying. John Walker, a social worker, successfully argued in November 1994 in the High Court that his employers, Northumberland County Council, were responsible for his two nervous breakdowns. Chris Johnstone, a senior house officer, who alleged that his mental health problems were caused by long hours and pressure of work eventually made an out-of-court settlement.[2] Walker's case implies that public sector bodies should not ignore complaints about pressure of work from fewer staff working longer and harder simply because there are limited financial resources to deal with stressors.[2]

It is incumbent on organisations to consider job stress for their own legal protection, to minimise the high costs of lost working days and to enhance the health and well-being of the organisation. The Institute of Management estimates that stress accounts for 50 to 60 million lost working days annually, costing the UK £7 billion.[3]

Job stress and the caring professions

Within the caring professions, job stress research has focused on nursing, medicine, ambulance/paramedics, social workers and dentists. Occupational therapy, physiotherapy and speech therapy need more investigation. Sutherland and Cooper[4] argue for an understanding of stress within all health care professions because of their important place in society and the impact that they have on others.

THEORIES OF OCCUPATIONAL STRESS

Occupational stress theory is based on general research and thinking about stress and anxiety outlined in Chapters 1–5 of this book. A summary of occupational stress theories is given below.

The response-based model — the unconscious response of an individual to a disruptive environment. The individual experiences stress and predominantly physiological responses are explored.

The stimulus-based model — an accumulation of job stressors.

The transactional/interactional model — this is the most popular model and incorporates the above models. Stress arises from an interaction between an individual and the environment in which there is an appraisal of threat (primary appraisal), followed by a secondary appraisal of resources to cope. Stress occurs when external and internal demand is appraised as more than the person's resources.

The person–environment fit model — this is connected to the transactional/interactional model:

... the interaction of objective variables in the environment and objective variables in the person affect corresponding interactions between subjective properties of the environment and subjective properties of the person to influence strain and health.[5]

The fit or misfit between the individual and environmental variables is studied. The model is criticised for regarding the relationships as stable and static.[6]

Psychotherapeutic models — the theory for these models is drawn from psychodynamic psychotherapy, analytical psychology, humanistic and integrative psychotherapies to understand job stress. Stress and anxiety at work arise when an individual's ego defences are undermined and uncomfortable, unconscious material is trying to emerge. Intense work pressures coupled with significant events can re-stimulate defended areas from childhood. When this happens individual and organisational factors may be studied. For example, the institution's inherent defences may be breaking down and no longer providing a container for anxiety. Emphasis in this model is placed on understanding the unconscious meaning of behaviours and their function for the individual and the organisation. See for example Menzies[7] and Skynner.[8]

WHAT ARE THE SYMPTOMS OF OCCUPATIONAL STRESS?

Job stress can be categorised as psychological, physical and behavioural with obvious overlaps between categories.

Psychological symptoms

Psychological symptoms include job dissatisfaction; boredom; frustration; isolation; resentment; difficulties with concentration, memory, problem-solving and decision-making; depression; and anxiety. Some of these are problems in themselves which can worsen job stress.

Physical symptoms

Stressors activate changes in hormonal and chemical defence systems of the body giving rise to a range of symptoms, e.g. sense of fullness in the head, aches and pains. Prolonged changes in the immune system and hormonal functioning are thought to be precursors of illness. Job stress and cardiovascular disease are linked.[4] Gastrointestinal conditions are established as linked with job stress; and skin diseases, allergies, migraine and headaches, sleep disturbance and respiratory disease are also mentioned in studies of job stress.[9]

Behavioural symptoms

Individual behavioural symptoms include increased drug and alcohol use, increased smoking, overeating or undereating, avoidance of work, aggression to and/or withdrawal from family or colleagues, rigidity in attitudes and resistance to change.

In the organisation symptoms include absenteeism, leaving the job, accident proneness and loss of productivity. Group phenomena such as scapegoating, splitting, blaming, evasion of responsibility and failures in completing assigned tasks emerge in the sick organisation.[8]

OCCUPATIONAL STRESS AND BURNOUT

Definition of burnout

Occupational stress literature has traditionally been based on research in industry, whilst 'burnout' literature arose in the mid-1970s from research in the human service sector. Initially these were separate areas of study, but there is now some cross-fertilisation.

The term 'burnout' was used by Maslach[10] to define a particular form of job stress found in professional carers such as nurses, doctors, social workers and probation officers. It is a response to the emotional strain of dealing with human beings. Burnout is also defined as the result of ongoing job stress without resolution.

Theoretical perspectives on burnout

As in occupational stress the dominant model used is the transactional one.

Boadella[11] has an interpersonal explanation for the exhaustion and lack of energy experienced by psychotherapists at the end of the day. Drawing on Jung and Reich, he describes the therapist's love, care and warmth (the core or true self) going towards a client. When the therapist experiences exhaustion, it is because the core is meeting the 'character defence', the secondary layer of the client. This layer is similar to Jung's concept of 'shadow', it is 'the mixed up layer full of confusion, tension, anxiety, stress'. If the core of the therapist could meet the core of the client there would be no exhaustion. Farber and Heifetz[12] found that psychotherapists believed burnout was due to the lack of mutual attentiveness, and the giving inherent in the therapeutic relationship. Therapeutic relationships demand a balance of involvement and concerned detachment. Overinvolvement is significant in burnout and with it goes diminished job satisfaction.[13]

Several models of psychotherapy now accept that professional carers often have childhood difficulties which, unconsciously, the carer is trying to resolve. Often carers unconsciously choose to work with clients who have problems related to their own. If these unacknowledged problems are not made conscious and faced squarely then carers are likely to use their relationships with clients to deny their own problematic feelings and preserve a semblance of adult competence. Meanwhile, the clients carry the problems for both parties. As carers project their unknown needs from childhood onto their clients, the clients become dependent and do not get their needs met. Carers end up working harder and harder to meet the supposed client need and get less satisfaction from work. Schlapobersky writes: 'This spiral underlies the exhaustion found amongst many in these fields and may be the root of many forms of 'burnout' and work-related stress'.[8]

Garden,[14] writing from a Jungian perspective, sees carers as mostly Jung's feeling types: people who are warm, sympathetic, aware of how others feel, trusting and enjoy pleasing people. She sees burnout as a positive disintegration of the individual who has become overidentified with the feeling function. Burnout serves a homeostatic function as the individual creates a new equilibrium, part of the individuation process. She calls for more, specific study of personal, unconscious characteristics in burnout research.

Symptoms of burnout

Symptoms of burnout overlap with those of job stress. Physical and emotional exhaustion, reduced personal accomplishment, low self-esteem and depersonalisation are pervasive. Depersonalisation leads to the objectification of clients to a greater extent than professionalism demands.[10] Staff may take refuge in professional roles. Clark[15] has commented on the therapeutic limits of strictly defining oneself according to role. Treatments may tend to be stereotyped according to diagnosis, rather than tailor-made for the individual. This dehumanising approach to patients can lead to callous and abusive practices. Medication may be over-used and physical restraint used unnecessarily. Margison[16] writes of stressed psychiatrists giving priority to pharmacology, use of the organic illness paradigm, diagnosis and use of technical procedures to limit personal distress. Failing to listen to patients and understand their perspective can provoke anger and violence, which superficially justifies the measures being used, and provokes a further vicious cycle of crisis management.

Burned-out providers tend to avoid patients, taking longer over non-patient tasks, lengthening lunch breaks and shortening the working day by arriving late and leaving early. Frequently those affected leave the job or the profession altogether. Turnover of staff as frequently as one to two years can become organisationally institutionalised. Commonly carers move from people-work to administration or technical work.

Organisationally, the quality of service may be in decline and staff morale low even though statistically the organisation may be performing well. Departments will relate in a hostile, distrustful manner and bureaucratic territory and red tape becomes more tightly defined and guarded. Extra-organisational conflict also increases.[17]

INDIVIDUAL VARIABLES THAT INFLUENCE OCCUPATIONAL STRESS AND BURNOUT

The following variables are considered to be important influences on job stress and burnout:

- personality characteristics
- general characteristics
- social support
- coping ability
- life events and home/work interface
- stress survival factors.

Personality characteristics

Personality characteristics will prevent, or predispose towards, job stress, but all care workers are at risk.[10] Freudenberger[18] describes three personality types vulnerable to burnout:

- 'the dedicated worker' who takes on extra commitments on top of a caseload
- 'the over committed worker' who lives to work and has no time for a social life
- 'the authoritarian worker' who believes only he or she can do the job.

The Type A personality, who is aggressively driven by time, a pressure to achieve and compete is vulnerable to heart disease.[19] Sinatra and Lowen[20] suggest that the Type A personality overworks to compensate for a broken heart. Parental love was based on performance or satisfying the image the parent had of the child rather than being unconditional. So in adulthood the Type A personality strives to gain the love they never got in childhood. In spite of success the individual is never satisfied and needs to continue to strive. The Type A personality is vulnerable to work stress because of high levels of frustration from work stressors, and less ability to deal with job stress effectively. Colleagues tend, for example, to be seen as competitors rather than potential sources of support.

Sometimes there is a misfit between a person and the job situation. Introverts, for example, have a higher level of cortical activity than extroverts, and so are more highly aroused and are thought to tolerate less stimulation than extroverts. Introverts tend to withdraw when stressed and benefit from clear role definition. Extroverts adapt more easily to changes.[4,21] High neuroticism is linked with high activity in the visceral brain, particularly the hypothalamus and sympathetic nervous system. Neurotics and neurotic-introverts are most susceptible to work stresses.[21]

Maslach[10] found that people who were poor at limit-setting, unable to assert themselves and exert control over situations were susceptible to burnout. Those lacking confidence and ambition; those who are reserved and conventional are also at risk.

Rotter[22] described a continuum of those individuals who feel able to control events (internal locus of control) and those who feel controlled by events (external locus of control). Those with an internal locus of control deal more successfully with pressure.

General characteristics

Gender and ethnicity

Job stress affects men and women. However, since the majority of therapists are women, it is important to look at specific job stressors for women. Dual career families juggle with home and work commitments with few role models. Professional women with pre-school children have frequent conflict between home and work commitments, and conflict spills over from one area to another. Women at management level have pressures from sex stereotyping and socialisation.[4] Minority groups have additional stresses from prejudice encountered and role models may be lacking leading to confusion and conflict.[23]

Age and length of experience

Maslach[10] found younger workers more at risk than older ones. Sweeney et al[24] found that occupational therapists who had been qualified longer tended to score lower on job stress in the dimensions of rewards and recognition and patient contact. However, the sample was relatively small and from one health district and should be interpreted with caution. Tyler and Cushway[25] found that senior nurses perceive more job stressors, but have a wide range and frequent use of adaptive coping skills which seem to guard them from the negative psycho-logical effects of stress. Mid-life is a vulnerable period for men and women as their roles change. Pre-retirement and retirement are also potentially stressful times.

Social support

Burnout is least for married carers with children. Single people fare worst.[10] The family can provide support, which buffers stressors.[23] Apart from family support, supportive social networks can offer individuals closeness, a sense of well-being and the stability of belonging to a group. Support has been shown to have a significant buffering effect on burnout.[13] Health workers who received reassurance from supervisors fared better in terms of occupational stress than others.[26]

Coping ability

Coping with stressors involves appraising the situation and reacting in an adaptive or maladaptive way. One way of coping would be to build one's defences and deny that there is a problem. This may be a short term way of coping in response to a crisis, but maladaptive if it is the only way of dealing with stress, since it effectively denies reality.[5] Lazarus and Folkman[27] look at problem-focused coping to moderate the problem, and emotion-focused coping to manage the emotional consequences of stressors. Both the resources available for coping and reactions as ways of coping should be considered. Coping can involve changing the personal meaning of the stressor, or altering the relationship between oneself and the stressor. An example would be developing a personal life so that work became a part rather than one's whole life.

Life events and home/work interface

Work stress will be affected by what other stressors are being experienced concurrently. It is extremely difficult to separate work and other stressors; however, both work and home factors need to be considered in relation to work stress.

Stress survival factors

The 'Hardy Personality' is able to maintain health in the face of stress. These individuals are committed to what they are doing; they feel in control and know they are able to influence events. They see challenge as normal, and are therefore more able to cope.[28] Pelletier[29] has studied individuals who have achieved beyond the norm in adverse circumstances, whom he calls 'transcenders'. They have characteristics in common with the Hardy Personality and seem to be able to draw on inner strength in the face of trauma. Delbecq and Friedlander[30] found that a high survivor group of executives coped with stress and avoided burnout by clearly structuring time. They worked long hours, but work and leisure were separate with no work going home. Home was a place of refuge and relaxation. Their spouses organised most of the domestic domain and were also their confidantes. They were clear in communications with their spouse. This was not taken for granted and they gave time to their spouse for romance and expressed their deep appreciation. They were physically fit and paid heed to fitness. They scheduled mini breaks and holidays after busy periods and when their energy was felt to be running low. Their work involved a sense of mission and with it a passion which was infectious.

WORK-SETTING VARIABLES THAT INFLUENCE OCCUPATIONAL STRESS

Work-setting variables are one aspect to examine in a comprehensive approach to job stress. These may include:

- role characteristics
- job characteristics
- interpersonal relationships
- organisational structure
- management practices.

Role characteristics

Role ambiguity

Role ambiguity arises from unclear job objectives and responsibilities, often through poor communications. For example, lack of professional identity was experienced as a stressor for occupational therapists in one study.[24] It is usual to experience role ambiguity in a new job; many jobs will contain some ambiguities and most organisations have less defined areas.[31] The uncertainty and lack of predictability is stressful.

Role conflict

Role conflict occurs when there are conflicting demands or instructions, where the individual has to do things which are not seen as part of the job, or perhaps where there are ethical conflicts. Complying with one set of demands makes it impossible, difficult or uncomfortable to do another. Another variant of role conflict is that of clinical demands conflicting with administrative ones.

Overload or underload

Overload may be quantitative, when too many behaviours are expected in a given time; or qualitative, when behaviours which are too difficult are expected.[32] Role underload occurs when a person is in a role that is constraining, there are not enough demands, or the person has skills not being used.

Job characteristics

Some occupations carry more intrinsic stress than others but certain characteristics of work seem to generalise.

Lack of control, long hours and shift work

Lack of control of the pace of work set by a team or machine is stressful, and repetitive jobs tend to provoke stress symptoms through boredom and frustration. New technology can create pressure as individuals have to adapt continually.[23]

Working long hours can be detrimental to health and commuting to work can add the strain of being stuck in traffic on congested roads, as well as lengthening the working day.

Shift work affects physical and mental efficiency, and motivation. If shifts involve night-work, sleep patterns get disrupted and can cut people off from social and family life.[23]

Risk and danger

Working in an environment with constant or intermittent danger or with expectation of danger is stressful, due to constant high arousal. However, there appears to be adaptation in some high-risk jobs such as the armed forces, police and fire service.[23]

Working conditions

Stressful physical conditions include over- or under-heating, noxious smells, poor hygiene, inadequate or unsuitable lighting, poor ventilation, noise, vibration and furniture design. Building design can also affect relationships for better or worse.[4]

Interpersonal relationships

Relationships with people are generally more stressful than relationships with tasks and have been linked with cardiovascular disease.

Relationships with colleagues

Cohesive work groups are best able to cope with stress.[33] For managers, the lack of a peer group can lead to isolation and lack of support. Levinson[34] has described the 'abrasive personality' who is difficult to work with because she ignores the interpersonal aspects of working relationships, putting achievement to the fore. Peers can also exert group pressures to conform to a particular way of working, which can conflict with individual desires.[32]

Relationships with supervisors

The leader(s) in an organisation exerts the most influence on work relationships. Supervisors who allow employees to participate in decision-making and give opportunities for two-way communication will mitigate against job stress. However, individuals also have different leadership needs, and tasks and situations will demand different styles of leadership. Leadership is needed for both task direction and support. There is some evidence that in stressful jobs employees' performance is enhanced by strong task direction. Stressful interactions with superiors seem to be universal.[31] This is related both to the real power that they have, and transferential aspects brought to the relationship. Women can be subject to misuse of power by male supervisors in the form of sexual harassment. A woman can also be supported by a male supervisor, but her competence used by him for his own advancement rather than hers.[23]

Relationships with subordinates

Leaders can be stressed by subordinates. Middle managers are vulnerable to stressors in their position between ground-floor workers and higher management. They often feel an absence of power and yet have to carry out decisions made at higher levels and face the direct consequences of these. Technical employees promoted to managerial responsibility for people on the basis of their technical ability can experience problems. Managers expected to manage in a participatory style can experience conflicts between different demands.[23]

Relationships with clients

The more contact there is with clients, the more reports of high levels of emotional exhaustion.[10] Sweeney et al[24] found patients' lack of motivation to get well was a significant stressor in this area.

Organisational structure

Decentralised organisations are less stressful to workers because of opportunities to participate in decisions, which gives greater sense of autonomy, control and meaning to work.[23]

Sudden change, job security and job transitions

Sudden change at work as in relocation, and job

transitions such as maternity leave, returning to part-time work, clinical rotation within a department, changing jobs or position in the organisation, are potentially stressful. Redundancy is stressful. Also, lack of, or perceived lack of job security, as well as coping with the loss of former colleagues can be stressful.[23]

Position in the organisation

Workers at lower levels in organisations report more stress. The variables are quantitative and qualitative workload, lack of career progression, poor supervisory relationships and role conflicts. Employees who work at the boundaries of organisational groupings — for example, those with clinical and managerial responsibility, senior managers relating inwardly and externally — report conflict.

Culture of the organisation

The culture of an organisation is shaped by the personalities at top-level management. For example, autocrats create a climate of fear; managers who engage in power manipulations and political intrigue can pressurise subordinates with demands and expectations.[31] However, all organisational members play a part in creating the culture. 'Downsizing' and budget-cutting can lead to job insecurity, competition between employees and unrealistic deadlines creating a stressful work culture. Handy[35] found that nurses had little real communication with psychiatrists, and this was mirrored in the nurses' avoidance of contact with patients.

Territory

Work territory is the personal space that an employee works in. Some workers feel isolated if there are not others around, and other workers can feel crowded by their colleagues.[23]

Management practices

The way that employees are managed will impact on their experience of work stress.

Induction practices and training

New workers appear to experience lower levels of stress if they have a good socialisation experience in the beginning. Experiencing oneself as trained to do the job can mitigate against stress.

Career development

Under- and over-promotion, status incongruence and thwarted ambition can be stressors.[23] Lack of job security, and actual or believed obsolescence can cause anxiety and frustration.[31] Career development stresses are a problem particularly in mid-life, especially for men, even if the person is successful. Simultaneously, in mid-life occurs recognition of one's mortality, and the goals which have/have not been achieved. Work can become a focal point for these feelings. The anticipation of retirement can be stressful for the older worker and concurrently there can be more dissatisfaction at work.

Feedback on performance and rewards

Lack of feedback and vague or critical feedback are stressful. Performance appraisal can be stressful for supervisor and supervisee. Matteson and Ivancevich[31] suggest performance feedback should be an open, two-way process to minimise anxiety. This enables both participants to be better informed about each other. Lack of supervisor or colleague feedback is likely to be more significant for carers where their client group does not give much feedback. For example, in rehabilitation work the carer's effectiveness is frequently only apparent when rehabilitation is absent. The absence of rewards can be demoralising. Rewards can include promotion, increased remuneration, privileges, perks and recognition of competence.

INTERVENTIONS
Approaches and levels

Much less is known about what is most effective in terms of interventions for job stress than its causes and results. Therapists should not forget that stress is part of life and intervention at any level is to establish an optimum level of stress or stimulation for peak performance.[32] Interventions are frequently considered at the individual or organisational level; Handy[35] discusses interventions at a societal level, and wants acknowledgement that some stressors are cultural and societal. Her study of psychiatric nurses discusses contradictions highlighted by critical psychiatry, arising out of the function of psychiatry within society. For example, psychiatry is both a form of social control and therapeutic care. She cites a societal-level intervention, a national movement in Italy, 'Psichiatria Democratica', which had equivocal results, but intended to replace traditional psychiatric care with genuine community care.

Carroll and White[17] have an ecological model for the analysis of burnout, which could be used for different levels of intervention. This would amount to an holistic model. They see all levels as dynamic and interacting with each other and impacting to varying degrees on the whole system. The levels are:

- the person
- the department — the smallest unit of organised work (microsystem)
- the institution/organisation — the collection of smaller units (mesosystem)
- non-work systems, e.g. family, other organisations (exosystem)
- societal/cultural/world-wide level — (macrosystem).

Quick and Quick[32] divide interventions into primary, secondary and tertiary ones. Primary interventions are aimed at slowing or stopping stress; secondary ones at detecting and treating it; and tertiary ones at alleviating discomfort and restoring function. They can be made at individual or organisational level, or both.

Interventions can be directed at stressor, response or symptom. Lazarus and Folkman[27] direct intervention at problem-solving — equivalent to stressor intervention — or emotion focused — equivalent to response. Lazarus[6] suggests a transactional approach which takes the individual and the work environment as a single unit of analysis, and matches individual and environment. Interventions can prevent, buffer, combat or enable coping, or dealing with stress.

Interventions are theory-biased and approaches will appeal to different individuals from their own predelictions and biases. It is possible to combine approaches and levels of intervention, but intervention is a complex area. Job stress is a dynamic, ongoing process, so interventions need to be considered in a process-oriented manner.

Diagnosis

Before interventions are made, a diagnosis should be formulated and then interventions selected accordingly.

INDIVIDUAL INTERVENTIONS

Quick and Quick[32] warn of individual interventions which are a sop and do not deal with necessary structural change. Individual intervention should be individualised because job stress is highly individualised. By giving choice to the individual, participation and motivation will be enhanced, and the person's internal resources will be activated. Therapists tend to have a raft of resources but lose sight of them when distressed.

Tubesing and Tubesing[36] see burnout as affecting the whole person and have a whole person approach to intervention. Solutions may be found in every dimension of life. This is in spite of symptoms being mostly in one area. For example, symptoms in the physical domain do not necessarily call for physical interventions. They see as fundamental the activation of 'internal wisdom' both to diagnose the problem and to discover ways for the individual to self-regulate and heal him or herself. They warn against quick, 'off the shelf', consumerist solutions. Pelletier[29] points out that living a healthy life is no guarantee of health. Health is fundamentally an inner quality.

Information-seeking

Therapists need to be aware of current research into job stress and burnout, to identify symptoms of stress in themselves and know basic ways of dealing with problems. Some authors think this should be part of training, others think theory can only be understood from the practical experience of doing caring work.

Self-awareness

Therapists may eschew self-awareness for protective reasons. Often, a stimulus, such as a personal crisis will be needed to develop self-awareness. Self-awareness involves monitoring oneself to:

- recognise personal signs and symptoms of stress
- identify stressors
- assess resources for coping with and preventing stress (deficits and abilities), both adaptive and maladaptive
- discover blocks to vitality and well-being.

Tubesing and Tubesing[36] regard burnout as a crisis of personal energy and advocate understanding of energy conservation and replenishment. Most therapists will need to discover an optimum energy economy, i.e. what energy they have, what depletes it and what increases it.

Diaries and self-assessment scales used for patients may be used for self-monitoring and various books include self-assessment measures. But, the first step is to put time aside on a regular basis, and throughout the working day, for self-monitoring.

Pre-conscious and unconscious phenomena often manifest in bodily terms, so body awareness monitoring during the work day can be particularly illuminating. Changes in breathing patterns, physical sensations such as pressure or tightness in the head, coupled with analysis of activity, thoughts, feelings and reactions to situations can identify precisely stressor points in the day.[37] The theory of the Vasomotoric Cycle[38] can be used for self-assessment. Vasomotoric Cycle theory is based in physiology and embraces energy concepts. Cycles occur constantly. The organism is constantly making adjustments for equilibrium and self-regulation. The need for adjustment arises out of the various stimuli impacting on it. A brief cycle would be an inbreath followed by an outbreath. Many cycles occur concurrently. Cycles can also be looked at over longer periods, e.g. a day, month, year or longer. The cycle has four stages:

Charging (tensing) — the organism has been stimulated internally or externally to prepare for action/expression. This is equivalent to a stimulus provoking the flight/fight response. Sympathetic nervous system activity predominates. For example, noticing it is nearly time to deliver a speech.

Expression/action — for example, standing and delivering the speech. It can involve subtle movements, talking, breathing out, etc. Parasympathetic nervous system activity begins to become dominant.

Winding down — the speech has been delivered and received well. There is a further, gradual discharge of bodily tensions as the person chats to friends about his or her achievement.

Deep relaxation/recuperation — resting in preparation for the next cycle, for example going home, thinking over the talk, relaxing in a bath and going to bed.

See Figure 20.1, the vasomotoric cycle.

For optimum health it is important to complete each stage. Most people, unfortunately, through a variety of past and present circumstances do

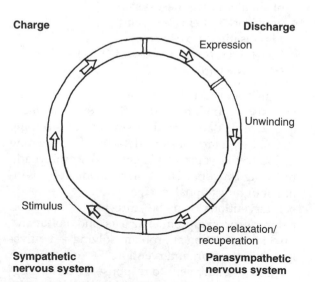

Figure 20.1 A diagrammatic representation of the vasomotoric cycle based on Boyesen.[38]

not complete cycles fully. This is where vitality is lost or blocked. All individuals function differently on the cycle and studying this gives a rough guide as to where interventions should concentrate and in what form. For example, some rarely deeply relax because there is never enough time given or there can be a fear of fully letting go; instead they may 'express' a lot with no resolution. Others find it difficult to rouse themselves sufficiently to get started with anything.

Information from the self-monitoring process can be used to construct a 'creative self-care and personal nurture plan designed to maximise vitality'.[36] Often, self-awareness derived from monitoring will effect change, even before the next stage, which is to plan interventions. Monitoring, however, should continue, but may be focused more specifically on emerging themes. For example, observing unassertive reactions to situations.

The range of interventions

An holistic plan of interventions should consider mind, body, emotions, spirit and the environment beyond the individual (see Box 20.1). Wilbur[39] has theorised on different levels of consciousness addressed by different psychotherapies and spiritual traditions. If these ideas are applied to stress management, light may be shed on why some strategies appeal to some and not others; and why they are effective for some and not others.

Physical

Physical interventions may lower or boost arousal. Keable[40,41] has reviewed relaxation techniques and their effectiveness. Exercise facilities installed in organisations have been shown to reduce absenteeism.[4] Massage comes in different forms with differing aims.[42,43] Diet changes are indicated in a number of diseases. Drugs can be helpful in the short term, but non-prescribed drugs, smoking, alcohol and caffeine all have deleterious effects on energy levels.

Box 20.1 A holistic view of individual interventions (adapted from Tubesing and Tubesing)[36]

Physical
Balance energising activity with relaxation
Exercise aerobic, anaerobic
Relaxation
Autogenics
Biofeedback
Breathwork
Massage
Yoga
T'ai Chi
Walking
Dance
Diet
Restrict drugs — prescribed, caffeine, alcohol, smoking

Emotional
Balance release of emotion with enjoyment of having done it
Emotional expression/discharge
Assertion/self-expression
Talking
Writing
Movement

Mental/intellectual
Balance mental strategies with recognition of external reality
Constructive self-talk
Reframing, restructuring
Thought-stopping
Reassess values and attitudes
Alter Type A behaviours
Recognise unchangeable
Withdrawal

Spiritual
Connect with deeper meaning of life – balance materialism with love
Meditation
Poetry
Art
Music
Nature
Caring as service

Social
Balance giving and receiving
Support groups
Networks
Interpersonal skills — giving and receiving:
social skills
Leisure

Environmental
Balance work with the rest of life
Time management
Problem-solving
Planning
Goal-setting
Conflict resolution
Lifestyle balance
Home/work interface

Emotional

These should enable self-expression, particularly of emotions that the individual cannot express, perhaps through lack of skill, a transferential component, or the inappropriateness of the emotion in the work context. Sometimes it is possible to transform the energy of the emotion into a social form. For example, anger can be sublimated in strenuous physical exercise or dance.

Intellectual

Matteson and Ivancevich[31] describe cognitive strategies to neutralise a stress-provoking situation or to develop resistance to one. Cognitive appraisal, i.e. getting the stressor in perspective; cognitive restructuring, i.e. looking at the individual's relationship between thoughts, feelings and behaviour, and replacing negative feelings with neutral ones; and cognitive rehearsal, considering events beforehand, are some possibilities.

Spiritual

The lack of connection with the spiritual dimension can underly malaise when all is apparently going well. Questions to consider are what is most important in life? What is the personal life meaning for me in doing this work and experiencing this crisis now? What nourishes the spirit in my life?

Social

Social support of various kinds will alleviate and prevent stress. Non-work supports are important, as well as sharing leisure activities with colleagues.

Environmental

This involves placing oneself harmoniously in the wider environment. Time management, for example, involves skills in how to use time efficiently, and self-awareness about the personal relationship with time. For example, how the individual compulsively fills up time with no spaces allowed for rest. It also includes balancing work, home life and leisure.

WORKPLACE INTERVENTIONS

Workplace interventions belong alongside individual ones.

Acknowledge job stress and burnout

The first step for an organisation is to acknowledge that job stress and burnout exist, and that the organisation can begin to deal with it.

Role characteristics

Management can reduce role stress by ensuring employees know clearly the core job requirements. This is more than giving the employee a job description. Employees will need help with job functions, i.e. clusters of duties. From this information, supervisor and supervisee can prioritise duties. The supervisor will need to consider how to communicate clearly. Role clarity will decrease anxiety from role confusion. Job overload and underload will also be alleviated by the above strategy, as long as there is a climate where the employee feels able to say 'No' to excessive demands, and managers appreciate overload and underload have an individual subjective component.[9]

Job characteristics

Ross and Altmaier[9] think that many managers need training to deal with jobs which are unhealthy. Strategies for dealing with stressful job characteristics include:

1. Job redesign — for example, reducing overload by the introduction of computerised systems or restructuring working periods to give pauses.

2. Job enrichment to make a job more meaningful and rewarding.[31]

3. Job enlargement to give an individual more responsibilities in role underload.

4. In role overload situations the job might involve more responsibility for fewer patients. Quantitative aspects will increase, but qualitative ones will decrease.

5. Examining and changing core job features to give more skill, variance or autonomy.

6. Allowing flexible work schedules. This might include a compressed working week, working more hours over fewer days; flexitime; and job sharing. Some health authorities enable working parents to have school holidays off. Within mental health some health authorities have mental health days, an agreed number of paid days, which the employee may take when they are emotionally depleted, or in need of a break.

7. Providing facilities such as on-site child-care and holiday play schemes may also help to ease job stress.

Interpersonal relationships

Skilled communication between employees will enhance relationships as well as provide the information needed to perform tasks. Staff meetings can be used to give information and provide opportunities to air feelings about policy changes. Team-building activities will develop group cohesion. Away days and review days can clarify goals and give perspective.

Organisations can encourage staff to support each other informally by recognising the importance of meal breaks and non-direct work time. Mental health has a history of formal support groups, also called supervision groups, sensitivity groups and awareness groups in recognition that people's work needs an institutionalised support structure.[15] However, their usefulness is not limited to mental health. Management can facilitate these groups by providing work time and funding for an outside consultant to run the group. Hawkins and Miller[44] point out the need for clear aims for such a group, particularly when it is open-ended: the facilitator being clear about what is being asked for; having a group contract and review process. Sometimes staff have the skills to run a self-help support group, using, for example, relaxation, massage, exercise.

Belfiore[45] described the use of 20 sessions of art therapy to prevent burnout. Art with its use of metaphor and symbol enabled the participants, who were working in the community with terminally ill cancer patients, to express profound personal experiences in their work. Support groups should look at the individual in terms of their experience in fulfilling their work role, and should not slip into group psychotherapy.[8]

Clinical supervision and consultation is an important aspect in caring work, and can be used to understand the counter-transference, the feelings that the therapist has towards the client. The supervisor can encourage the mobilisation of the therapist's internal resources.[8]

Organisational structures and climate

Management which is decentralised and where there is participation in decision-making is less stressful. Decentralisation involves giving departments and individuals more autonomy. It is important for managers to clarify what decisions can be made autonomously, what issues are for consultation and those that are not within the remit of an individual or department. Issues for discussion should not be too trivial, nor too complex nor irrelevant to the department or individual. After consulting individuals, it should be clear to them that their opinions have been heeded if they are not to see participation as a cosmetic exercise and thereby become cynical and demoralised.[9] Ashton[46] emphasises the importance of clear objectives within an overall strategic plan being clearly communicated to the workforce.

Human resource management

Within the remit of human resource management the following factors should be considered:

- recruitment
- selection
- induction
- goal-setting
- performance feedback
- career development and planning

- health promotion, health screening and health awareness
- employment assistance programmes
- physical factors.

Recruitment

Matteson and Ivancevich[31] recommend realistic job previews of negative and positive aspects in order to dispel illusions about the job and organisation which could later lead to distress.

Selection

Selection of a new member of staff should involve looking at the candidate's skills, knowledge, experience and abilities, but also the values and attitudes that the individual holds. The interview process should be a two-way one for maximum communication. This will enable a better person–environment fit.

Induction

After selection, the first stage of the socialisation process occurs, i.e. 'getting in' is followed by 'breaking in'.[31] Induction is the phase where the new employee and organisation get to know each other. Ideally there will be structured induction which introduces the employee to relevant information on jobs and duties, responsibilities, training and career opportunities and the prevailing management structure. Alongside this, there should be less formal induction. In caring work induction is likely to be an ongoing process over a lengthy period, particularly for basic grade staff.

Goal-setting

Goal-setting reduces role ambiguity and confusion, thereby reducing stress. Goals need to be mutually agreed, challenging, but obtainable. Management by objectives is a system of management based on goal-setting, but it should be noted that this approach can create pressures as well as alleviate them.[9]

Performance feedback

Performance appraisal can give the employee retrospective information on performance, as well as future development possibilities. For this to work well there needs to be some mutuality in the appraisal. The implementation of performance appraisal schemes often evokes anxiety and the performance appraisal process can be anxiety-provoking for supervisor and supervisee.[9] Problems can arise when unfairness is seen to operate, or when appraisal is linked with salary increase, but there is an inadequate budget actually to give the increase merited.

Career development and planning

Some organisations run career planning activities which involve self-assessment and guidance in career opportunities. Others provide a library of resources for employees to use. Such schemes demonstrate commitment to the employee by the organisation and enable both a pro-active and interactive approach to career progression that will maximise satisfaction.[31] However, Pelletier[29] found that many of his 'transcenders' did not plan their careers, but were able to adapt and use opportunities as they arose. Ross and Altmaier[9] also observed that the aspirations of employees have changed. Nowadays, employees look for opportunities 'to create new job situations and pursue non-traditional career paths'.

Health promotion, health screening and health awareness

Health promotion in the workplace includes stress management, weight control programmes, information on diet, cardiovascular fitness, programmes on reducing alcohol intake and ceasing smoking. Some run seminars on balancing work and home demands for working parents. Programmes are delivered via video, display stands, seminars and lectures, and regular group meetings. Health screening is done in some organisations on an individual basis, the results interpreted and suitable programmes jointly selected.

Employment assistance programmes

Employment assistance programmes (EAPs) enable individuals to explore personal responses to stress and have grown out of other health promotion activities. Some are run in-house, but many make use of outside psychotherapists and counsellors which provides more confidentiality. Many organisations have seen counselling as a last resort for those who have failed to cope with job stress. Depending on the model of psychotherapy being used, the employee can become pathologised, masking very real problems in the organisation which are not tackled and to which the employee is returned. Humanistic psychotherapy, as well as a growing number of other psychotherapies, would look both at intrapsychic phenomena as well as organisational ones. Some EAPs pick up patterns of stressors in organisations and are able to feed these back into the organisation confidentially where they can be addressed.[4]

Physical factors

Often employees will know what could be done in this area. Interventions might be relatively straightforward, but sometimes will involve those with specialist skills like architects and engineers for radical change. Basically the environment can be changed, the individual protected from the stressor or given periods of escape from the stressor.[9]

CONCLUSION

Health care professionals are valuable and in scarce supply. Strategies need to be developed to prevent and cope with the job stress they experience. Interventions need to be applied both at individual and organisational levels. Sociology, psychotherapy, organisational psychology and medicine all have contributions to make. However, it is important to bear in mind that job stress may ultimately be more than the individual and organisation can tackle alone, since governmental policy and trends in global economic structure also have a significant impact.

REFERENCES

1 Cambridge and District Chamber of Commerce 1995 Newsletter, November
2 Howard G 1995 Occupational stress and the law: some current issues for employers. Journal of Psychosomatic Research 39(6):707–719
3 Dearlove D 1996 The Times 29th February
4 Sutherland V, Cooper C 1990 Understanding stress. A psychological perspective for health professionals. Chapman & Hall, London
5 French J R P, Caplan R D, Van Harrison R 1982 The mechanisms of job stress and strain. John Wiley, Chichester
6 Lazarus R S 1995 Psychological stress in the workplace. In: Crandall R, Perrewe P L (eds) Occupational stress, a handbook. Taylor and Francis, London
7 Menzies Lyth I 1988 Containing anxiety in institutions. Selected essays. Volume 1. Free Association, London
8 Skynner R 1991 Institutes and how to survive them. Routledge, London
9 Ross R R, Altmaier E M 1994 Intervention in occupational stress. Sage, London
10 Maslach C 1982 Burnout — the cost of caring. Prentice-Hall, New Jersey
11 Boadella D 1982 Transference, resonance and interference. Journal of Biodynamic Psychology (3):73–93

12 Farber B A, Heifetz L J 1982 The process and dimension of burnout in psychotherapists. Professional Psychology 13:293–301
13 Koeske G F, Kelly T 1995 The impact of overinvolvement on burnout and job satisfaction. American Journal Orthopsychiatry 65(2)
14 Garden A-M 1995 The purpose of burnout: a Jungian interpretation. In: Crandall R, Perrewe P L (eds) Occupational stress, a handbook. Taylor and Francis, London
15 Clark D H 1981 Social therapy in psychiatry, 2nd edn. Churchill Livingstone, London
16 Margison F 1987 Stress in psychiatrists. In: Payne R, Firth-Cozens J (eds) Stress in health professionals. John Wiley, London
17 Carroll J F X, White W L 1982 Theory building integrating individual and environmental factors within an ecological framework. In: Stewart Paine W (ed) Job stress and burnout, research, theory, and intervention perspectives. Sage, London
18 Freudenberger H J 1975 The staff burn-out syndrome in alternative institutions. Psychotherapy Theory Research Practice 12:73–82
19 Friedman M, Rosenman R H 1974 Type A behaviour and your heart. Knopf, New York

20 Sinatra T S, Lowen A 1987 Heartbreak and heart disease: the origin and essence of coronary-prone behaviour. Holistic Medicine 2(3):169–172

21 Eysenck H J 1967 Biological basis of personality. Charles C. Thomas, Springfield, Illinois

22 Rotter J B 1966 Generalised expectancies for internal versus external control of reinforcement. Psychology Monograph 80, 1–28

23 Cooper C L, Cooper R, Eaker L H 1988 Living with stress. Penguin, Harmondsworth

24 Sweeney G M, Nichols K A, Kline P 1993 Job stress in occupational therapy: an examination of causative factors. British Journal of Occupational Therapy 56(3):89–93

25 Tyler P, Cushway D 1995 Stress in nurses: the effects of coping and social support. Stress Medicine 11:243–251

26 Constable J F, Russell D W 1986 The effect of social support and the work environment upon burnout among nurses. Journal of Human Stress 12:20–26

27 Lazarus R S, Folkman S 1984 Stress, appraisal, and coping. Springer, New York

28 Kobasa S C 1982 The hardy personality. In: Sanders G, Suls J (eds) Social psychology of health and illness. Lawrence Erlbaum, New Jersey

29 Pelletier K R 1994 Sound mind, sound body, a new model for lifelong health. Simon & Schuster, New York

30 Delbecq A L, Friedlander F 1995 Strategies for personal and family renewal. How a high-survivor group of executives cope with stress and avoid burnout. Journal of Management Inquiry 4(3):262–269

31 Matteson M T, Ivancevich J M 1987 Controlling work stress: effective resource management strategies. Jossey-Bass, San Francisco

32 Quick J C, Quick J D 1984 Organizational stress and preventive management. McGraw-Hill, New York

33 Ketz de Vries M F R 1984 Organizational stress management audit. In: Sethi A S, Schuler R S (eds) Handbook of organizational stress coping strategies. Ballinger, Cambridge, MA

34 Levinson H 1978 The abrasive personality. Harvard Business Review 56, May

35 Handy J 1990 Occupational stress in a caring profession: the social context of psychiatric nursing. Avebury, Aldershot

36 Tubesing N L, Tubesing D A 1982 The treatment of choice: selecting skills to suit the individual and the situation. In: Stewart Paine W (ed) Job stress and burnout, research, theory, and intervention perspectives. Sage, London

37 Gendlin E 1982 Focussing. Bantam, New York

38 Boyesen, M 1975 Psycho-peristalsis, part IV, Dynamics of the vasomotoric cycle: nuances of membrane pathology according to the mental condition (based on papers of Gerda Boyesen). Energy and Character 6(2)

39 Wilbur K 1993 The Spectrum of consciousness, 2nd edn. Quest, London

40 Keable D 1985a Relaxation training techniques — a review. Part one: What is relaxation? British Journal of Occupational Therapy 48(4):99–102

41 Keable D 1985b Relaxation training techniques — a review. Part two: How effective is relaxation training. British Journal of Occupational Therapy 48(7):201–204

42 Westland G 1993 Massage as a therapeutic tool. Part 1. British Journal of Occupational Therapy 56(4):129–134

43 Westland G 1993 Massage as a therapeutic tool, Part 2. British Journal of Occupational Therapy 56(5):177–180

44 Hawkins P, Miller E 1994 Psychotherapy in and with organisations. In: Clarkson P, Pokorny M (eds) The handbook of psychotherapy. Routledge, London

45 Belfiore M 1994 The group takes care of itself: art therapy to prevent burnout. The Arts in Psychotherapy 21(2):119–126

46 Ashton D 1989 The corporate healthcare revolution, strategies for preventive medicine at work. Kogan Page with the Institute of Personnel Management, London

USEFUL CONTACTS

British Association of Counselling
  1 Regent Place
  Rugby
  Warwicks
  CV21 2PJ
  01788 578328

UK Council for Psychotherapy
  167–169 Great Portland Street
  London
  WIN 5FB
  0171 436 3013

The anxiety management course client packs

This appendix contains the client training material to accompany each session of the anxiety management course described in Chapter 11. The packs are for the therapist's guidance in preparing sessions and contain detailed information on what each topic should cover.

Client Pack 1
Introduction: what is anxiety?

What is anxiety?

What do we really mean when we talk about suffering from 'tension', 'nerves' or 'stress'? What does it feel like? Anyone who suffers from severe anxiety will have no difficulty answering the last question. Anxiety is an extremely unpleasant feeling — it can make people feel frightened, uneasy, unhappy and sometimes desperate. There are many ways in which people describe anxious feelings, not always recognising that these feelings are associated with anxiety. This may happen all too easily since the range of anxiety symptoms is very wide, and some may mimic quite severe mental or physical illness. Anxiety can affect anyone, man or woman, at any age and from all social backgrounds. Different people suffer anxiety in different ways, as the following examples of common symptoms will show. These may affect the body, the thoughts and emotions, and the lifestyle of the individual.

Bodily feelings

The bodily feelings associated with anxiety (see Fig. 1) include:

- breathing difficulties
- feeling faint/dizzy
- dry mouth
- shakiness
- pounding heart
- headaches
- muscle aches and pains
- excess sweating
- bowel and urinary problems
- 'lumps' in the throat
- persistent tiredness.

Anxiety also shows in the way people hold themselves — stooped posture, clenched fists, furrowed brow, clenched jaw. An astonishingly wide variety of distressing physical symptoms

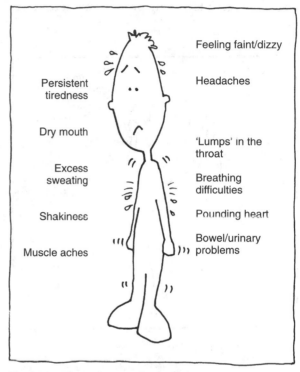

Persistent tiredness

Dry mouth

Excess sweating

Shakiness

Muscle aches

Feeling faint/dizzy

Headaches

'Lumps' in the throat

Breathing difficulties

Pounding heart

Bowel/urinary problems

Figure 1   The bodily symptoms of anxiety.

can occur as a result of anxiety. This can easily lead people to assume that they are seriously ill, when they are actually suffering from the symptoms of severe anxiety.

Thoughts and emotions

Fear of a variety of things, people or situations may develop as a result of anxiety:

- going out of doors
- meeting people
- travelling on buses or trains
- Ill-health.

Anxious people may also find themselves increasingly subject to episodes of crying, panicking, worrying, being irritable, unable to concentrate and feeling guilty. They may hold negative or unreasonable ideas about themselves or the feared situation, e.g. 'I can't cope', 'If I go out I might collapse/make a fool of myself/be sick/have an accident' (Fig. 2). Sometimes these fears may reach terrifying proportions and suffer-

ers may find themselves subject to panic attacks. It is easy to see how anxious people may lose their confidence so that even small stresses which are an ordinary part of life become huge obstacles.

Lifestyle

Lifestyle may be seriously curtailed by a tendency to avoid stressful situations or escaping them wherever possible. This might include:

- not going out
- not going to work
- not meeting people
- not using public transport
- not being able to do the shopping
- not being able to stand up for oneself.

This involves a great many 'NOTS' and 'CAN'TS' which reduce quality of life and make a happy and fulfilled existence impossible. We all need a certain amount of stimulation and stress in our lives in order to remain healthy. For others, anxiety might mean taking on too much work and responsibility, but the end result is the same — a poor quality of life.

Work performance and relationships can also suffer. The roles that we adopt in life — wife,

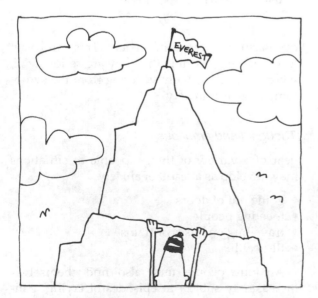

Figure 2 The anxiety trap.

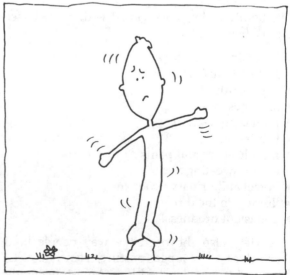

Figure 3 Goal-setting and 'setting yourself up' . . . for failure.

husband, employer, employee, mother, father — can become too difficult for us to carry out successfully when we are burdened with anxiety. It may be hard to trust others or, alternatively, our anxiety may make us ask too much of other people, thus becoming too dependent or demanding. Those who do attempt to tackle their difficulties may find that they set themselves unrealistic targets, attempting either too much or too little, again leading to a vicious circle of failure (see Fig. 3). So anxiety can get out of hand and seriously affect our mental, emotional and bodily reactions as well as our relationships and lifestyles.

Why do some people suffer so much with anxiety and not others?

Well, first of all, *everybody* feels some degree of anxiety — this is normal and useful. If you were unable to get anxious at all, it would be extremely dangerous. You need some anxiety to help you to cross the road safely, for example. You also need it to give you an extra spur to deal with difficult situations like exams and interviews. It may sound surprising, but moderate anxiety can improve your strength of purpose and also help you to perform better (Fig. 4). Psychologists' experiments have shown that people who are moderately anxious do better on a variety of tasks than people who have either very high or very low levels of anxiety.

Anxiety can become a problem when it rises beyond these normal limits, if it goes on for too long, or if it happens too often and in inappropriate situations like the supermarket. This may happen to some people because of painful feelings and experiences that they have not been able to come to terms with. It may be simply because they have not learnt how to cope with their anxiety or that they have learnt ways of coping which do not work very well — like avoiding stressful situations. Even if you could find out exactly why you're anxious, it probably wouldn't help very much. What counts is dealing with it.

So what causes the symptoms of anxiety?

The body

The symptoms that we call anxiety are the same as those that primitive man experienced when faced by life-threatening dangers such as ferocious animals. His reaction in such a situation would be either to fight the wild animal or to run

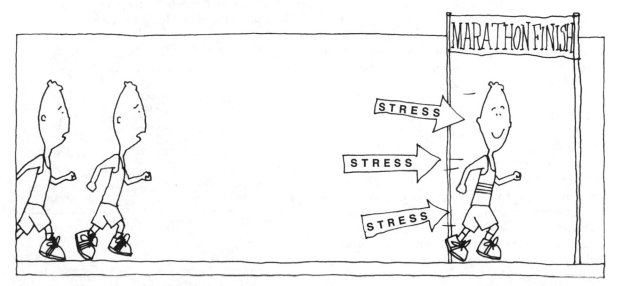

Figure 4   Stress can sometimes help you to be a winner.

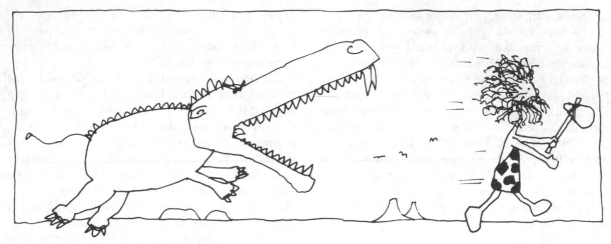

Figure 5   The primitive 'fight/flight' response.

away in order to survive, and that is why we call the bodily reactions that cause anxiety the 'fight or flight' response (Fig. 5). These responses are geared to prepare the body to deal with danger and cope with vigorous physical activity like fighting or running. When our primitive forefathers had dealt with danger in either of these ways, the anxiety feelings disappeared. Clearly we cannot relieve our anxieties in modern times in this way — often our worries are too subtle and deep-seated for this — and it would not be appropriate to run away from an interview or attack the interviewer, for example! Consequently, when we are anxious, the pent-up feelings tend to stay with us, causing some very uncomfortable symptoms like headache, muscular pain, nausea, palpitations. You may have noticed how physical exercise has the effect of draining off this tension and helps you feel better and think more clearly. Exercise has great benefits in stress control if carried out as a sensible and regular routine.

The autonomic nervous system There are two different branches to the autonomic nervous system which governs how anxious or relaxed you feel. One branch works to get you 'keyed-up' for 'fight or flight', and the other branch works to calm you down so that you can rest, recuperate and digest your food more efficiently.

The first branch of the autonomic system, let us call it the 'arousal' system, can be very useful

and even life-saving as has already been mentioned. It prepares you for immediate action when you are threatened by some danger, speeding up your heart and breathing, increasing muscle tone and releasing that familiar surge of adrenalin. However, if this arousal state continues for lengthy periods, unrelieved by exercise or relaxation, the result is distressing and persistent anxiety.

The second branch of the autonomic nervous system, we'll call it the 'relaxation' system, cannot act whilst the 'arousal' system is 'turned on'. This makes it difficult to sleep or calm down and also blunts the appetite. See Figure 6.

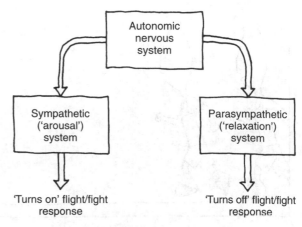

Figure 6   The autonomic nervous system.

This is why we need to learn relaxation skills in order to turn the 'arousal' system off, so that the 'relaxation' system can work properly. More of this in Pack 2.

And what are the mental causes of anxiety?

Two main reasons for persistent anxiety are avoidance of the feared situations and faulty thinking. Let's look at these two in turn.

Avoidance We may avoid situations which we know will cause us anxiety because the symptoms are so uncomfortable that we would rather not face up to them. Unfortunately, each time we avoid a situation, its power to cause an anxiety response in us increases. See Figure 7.

● ●

What would happen if you went into a situation that you find highly stressful and stayed there instead of leaving it as soon as possible? Which of the following results would you think the most likely?

1. My anxiety level would go on getting worse.
2. My anxiety level would stay the same.
3. My anxiety level would be high at first, then it would gradually die away.

Many people would automatically opt for the first result, but the third result is actually the correct one (Fig. 8). Experiments have shown that very high anxiety levels do drop after a while because they simply cannot be maintained for long periods. This fact highlights two very simple but important truths which apply to all those who find it hard to face the situations they fear:

● *If you keep avoiding the situation you fear, you will become more and more afraid of tackling it.*

● *If you always leave stressful situations quickly you will never find out that your anxiety will gradually die away of its own accord.*

● ●

Faulty thinking What is faulty thinking? Here are a few examples:

● 'I can't cope — I'm just a failure'
● 'nobody else seems to find things as difficult as I do — I'm sure everyone thinks I'm stupid'
● 'I should never let people down in any way'
● 'real men don't cry'
● 'it's a woman's job to do the housework'
● 'if the bus doesn't come along soon, I'm going to collapse/have a heart attack'.

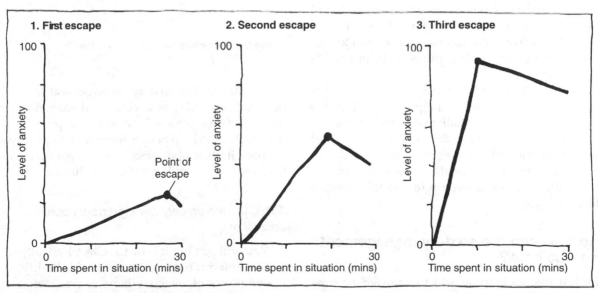

Figure 7   Avoidance/escape — the consequences.

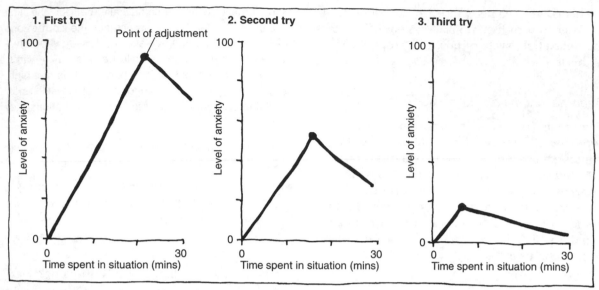

Figure 8 Facing the fear — the consequences.

Faulty-thinking patterns include the kind of thoughts and beliefs we have which are negative and irrational. Firstly, they make us expect the worst. Secondly, they are usually incorrect and unreasonable, often making us expect far too much from ourselves or others. This leaves us open to constant disappointment. These patterns of thought are often self-fulfilling prophecies — tell yourself you can't cope and you probably won't. Anxiety is related to what we think and believe, and the examples above show how our ways of thinking can sabotage our efforts to succeed and overcome difficulties — before we've even started.

We have to learn to replace negative thoughts with positive ones which help us cope. We also need to examine and challenge the truth of some of our irrational beliefs and assumptions about ourselves and others. Are they really realistic? Negative and unreasonable ways of thinking make life difficult to live up to and failure more likely (Fig. 9).

So how can the anxiety management course help?

By just that — helping you to 'manage' or cope with anxiety and reduce its distressing symp-

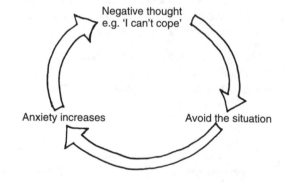

Figure 9 The vicious cycle of negative thinking.

toms and effects. Anxiety management training does not pretend to be a 'cure' — there is no such thing, because *anxiety is normal*. The purpose of the course is to help people learn how to put anxiety back in its proper place, under their own control, and keep it within acceptable limits.

'What will the anxiety management course consist of?'

1. You will be taught how to relax physically so that you can reduce uncomfortable bodily symptoms of anxiety wherever you are.
2. You will be taught how to challenge faulty

thinking and use a positive approach that will help you achieve more control over your fears.

3. The course will also cover problem-solving methods and help you to improve your confidence in using social skills, such as assertiveness. See Figure 10.

● ●

At the risk of putting you off, a few serious points must be mentioned right at the beginning so as not to waste your time:

1. If you want to succeed you must be committed to the course. This means attending punctually and regularly and completing all the self-help tasks set throughout the course. Otherwise, you are very unlikely to benefit from this kind of therapy.

Anxiety management is a self-help technique!

2. Please do your best to participate in the group work and discussion periods as much as you can. Of course, it is understood that you will need support initially, especially if you are anxious in a group situation. However, the more you put into the course, the more benefit you will get back.

3. Remember that if you do succeed in overcoming problems as a result of attending the course, it will have been entirely due to your own efforts, not the therapist's. You will then have the confidence of knowing that you have made the achievement by yourself — it is acknowledged that few people will find the course easy!

4. The general tone of the course may seem rather business-like, and even a little unsympathetic at times. This is intentional. Although it is certainly appreciated that anxiety is a miserable feeling, the priority is to help you put yourself back in charge of your life. In order to achieve this, the practical approach we will be using is usually the most effective.

5. If you really don't like the sound of the course so far or you feel it isn't right for you, it may be better not to start it at all, or at least, not at the present time. Your decision will be respected. If you are unsure about the course you will be unlikely to complete it and might end up feeling more discouraged. However, if you are willing to give the course a try, despite your doubts and fears, then go ahead — and good luck!

● ●

Supplement: 'Contrast muscle relaxation'

The purpose of this technique is to help you to improve your awareness of muscle tension so that you will be able to recognise and release it when you first become tense. This exercise also helps you to appreciate what the feeling of muscle relaxation is like, and how pleasant it can actually be.

The exercises cover each major muscle group and for each one you should perform the following sequence *twice, slowly*:

- tense / tighten the muscles
- relax / loosen the muscles
- concentrate hard on the sensations you can feel — notice the difference between tension and relaxation.

Either lie down or find a comfortable chair in which to practise.

Breathing

Repeat this exercise 2–3 times over the whole relaxation period:

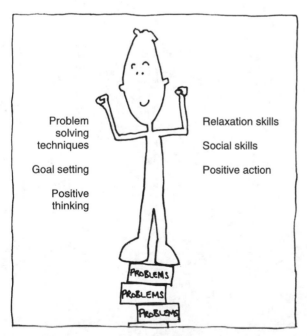

Problem solving techniques

Goal setting

Positive thinking

Relaxation skills

Social skills

Positive action

Figure 10   How to get on top of your problems.

Take a deep breath, hold for a count of three and very slowly breathe out. Continue breathing normally in between each deep breath.

Going round the body

Hands and forearm Clench your right fist and feel the tension spread around your knuckles and up your forearm. Hold this for a slow count of three and then let go, noticing as you do so the feeling of looseness and warmth in your hand and forearm — this is relaxation. After a few moments repeat once more using your right hand and then do the same exercise twice using your left hand.

Continue in the same way for the remaining muscle groups.

Upper arms Press your elbows into your sides and continue as for above. Release.

Forehead Raise your eyebrows and wrinkle your forehead with eyes closed. Release.

Face Screw up your eyes, wrinkle your nose and clench your jaw. Pull back the corners of your mouth. Release.

Neck Press your chin down onto your chest and thrust your head forward. Release.

Chest, shoulders and back Arch the lower part of your back and pull your shoulder blades together. Release.

Stomach Pull your tummy in hard. Release.

Legs Press the backs of your knees down, straightening your leg and point your toes towards your face. Release.

Now survey each body part again and make sure that it is as relaxed as possible. If it is not, repeat the exercise for that muscle group again.

It is suggested that you practise the relaxation exercises for 20 minutes at least twice a day.

Note that it is very important not to get up too quickly after relaxation, especially if you have been lying down, because the sudden change of position may make you feel dizzy. Of course it would also defeat the object of the exercise if you were to start rushing around after relaxation, so try to preserve the feeling of calm for the rest of the day.

Self-help assignments

Name ....

1. Complete your stress diary (p. CP 44) and relaxation practice (p. CP 45) sheets every day.

2. Practise contrast relaxation (see the supplement for instructions).

3. In the space below, make a list of any personal tension spots you experience when anxious and bring it in for the next session. For example, people can suffer from headaches, neck-aches, stomach-aches and even bowel problems as a result of anxiety.

Remember to bring all your completed homework in for the next session.

Client Pack 2
Physical tension control

Fight or flight

In the previous pack, we spoke of the body's reaction to stress — the 'fight or flight' response. This is a normal protective mechanism but can get out of hand in those who are excessively anxious, causing a variety of unpleasant feelings. Everyone tends to react in a different and highly individual way to stress, but some of the common responses include those described below. Also see Figure 11.

Pounding heart

This happens because the heart is beating stronger and faster in order to pump more blood to and from the muscles. This extra blood carries oxygen and glucose to the muscles which increases their efficiency should we have to run away from danger or turn to fight it. If we do not engage in such physical activity to drain off this extra energy, the resulting symptoms can sometimes feel quite alarming.

Breathlessness

This happens because the lungs are working harder in order to increase the oxygen levels in the blood. In threatening situations this helps us to think more clearly as well as increasing muscle efficiency. Again, if the muscles are not burning off the extra oxygen through physical activity, then we may develop a number of uncomfortable sensations because the gases in our blood become unbalanced. For example, we may feel dizzy or panicky, and even experience sensations of numbness or pain anywhere in the body.

Tense or shaky muscles

We automatically react by tensing our muscles when we are feeling anxious. This can result in pain, such as headache, backache or neck-ache. Feelings of shakiness are generally associated with the stress hormone, adrenalin, which is released into the bloodstream when we are threatened. This is supposed to help us to react more effectively to a threat, but when we remain sedentary it can have the opposite effect and make us feel weak and dizzy.

Nausea and digestive problems

When we are under stress our digestive system shuts down so that all our energy can be diverted to the 'fighting' muscles. In extreme conditions, we may respond by vomiting to clear the stomach of undigested food. Symptoms may be felt as 'butterflies' or feelings of churning in the

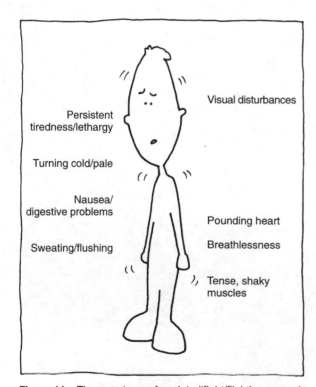

Figure 11   The symptoms of anxiety ('fight/flight' response).

stomach. Alternatively, we may react with diarrhoea or frequent urination when under stress. We may also experience a dry mouth as body fluids are diverted into the bloodstream in order to increase blood volume.

Increased sweating or flushing

As the blood flow to the muscles on the body surface increases, this brings with it a feeling of being hot, sweaty and flushed.

Turning cold and pale

This may occur in states of extreme fear or shock as the blood drains from the body surface. It may be accompanied by fainting in some cases if the blood pressure also drops dramatically. Some people seem to react with this kind of 'faint/freeze' response when under stress, rather than the more usual fight/flight reaction. Both phenomena may be seen in the animal kingdom in which some animals tend to fight or flee when in danger, whereas others feign death. Both reactions are nature's way of increasing the chance of survival.

Visual disturbances

While under stress our eyesight tends to become sharper in order to increase our ability to spot signs of danger. As this wears off, our vision may seem to have become blurred until we adjust. When first taking off a pair of spectacles, the wearer may notice a similar feeling.

Persistent tiredness and lethargy

This can occur as a result of long-standing unrelieved anxiety. The body literally becomes worn out from the constant demands made upon it by the continual pressure to maintain the accelerated bodily state associated with arousal. The chronic anxiety sufferer is subject to persistent sleeping difficulties, lowered resistance to infection and depression.

How relaxation works

As we mentioned in Pack 1, the stress responses are governed by the autonomic nervous system in combination with the stress hormones, notably adrenalin. Although this system is involuntary, there is a great deal that we can do to gain control over our responses to stress. You will remember that the autonomic nervous system has two branches:

- the 'arousal' (sympathetic) system: responsible for the 'fight/flight' response to stress
- the 'relaxation' (parasympathetic) system: responsible for helping us to sleep, digest our food and rest.

Only one of these systems can work at any one time. This means that if we find a way of 'turning on' the relaxation system when needed, then the arousal system will automatically 'switch off'. So, although we do not have direct control over the nervous system responsible for producing the stress reactions, by learning relaxation techniques we gain a very powerful influence over the mechanism. Of course you cannot tell your heart to stop pounding or your body to stop sweating at will in the same way that you can make your arms or legs move when you want them to. Nevertheless, the mind and body are so closely linked that once you have learned the skill of relaxing your muscles your mind and body will automatically feel calmer. It is impossible for the mind to be tense when the body is deeply relaxed — this is the key to mental relaxation. It is a tried and tested scientific principle. Experiments on relaxation have shown that people can even reduce their blood pressure with regular practice! Anxiety can be switched off by learning how to switch relaxation on.

Stress positions

Have a look at Figure 12. Can you recognise yourself here? When we are under stress, frightened or anxious the body tends to adopt a characteristic position:

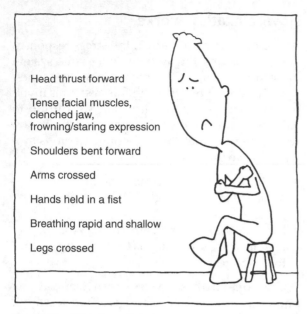

Figure 12   The stressed posture.

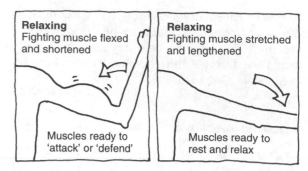

Figure 13   The principles of muscle tension and relaxation.

- head thrust forward
- shoulders held up towards the ears
- arms crossed or held tightly to the sides
- hands held in a fist
- legs crossed tightly, often the top foot pointing upwards
- body bent forward, held stiffly
- breathing shallow and rapid
- facial muscles tight, with clenched jaw, frowning forehead and eyes either open very wide or screwed up tightly
- standing and walking restlessly.

Maintaining our bodies in these positions not only communicates our anxiety to others, but also reinforces our own tension level. The more you hold onto a tense posture, the more your brain receives tension messages from your muscles and responds by causing you to feel more anxious — until you're exhausted. Eventually these positions will become painful as well as tiring. If you change to a relaxed position, you should notice the difference! From now on, keep a watchful eye on your posture. Try to identify what happens to your body when you are tense and change this for a relaxed position each time you catch yourself out.

How to relax

The relaxation technique which goes with this handout (see the supplement) was designed to move your body out of the tense positions and into relaxed ones. Certain muscle groups tend to place us into these tense positions and certain ones move us into relaxed positions. Both sets of muscle groups cannot work at the same time. This principle means that if we move the group that puts us into a relaxed position, the 'tensing' group has to stop and allow us to relax (see Fig. 13). The 'simple (physiological) relaxation' technique by Laura Mitchell shows how to make use of this natural law to help us deal with stress. Initially, we will concentrate on building up basic skills in relaxation as thoroughly as possible. Later we will look at how to apply them in stressful situations. Relaxation is good for you — everyone needs to relax — allow yourself to enjoy this pleasant interlude as a regular part of your daily life.

The benefits of regular exercise

Another way to relax is to take regular exercise. We mentioned this matter last time when we talked of how physical action relieves tension due to the 'fight/flight' principle. You can exploit this fact to your advantage and benefit in a number of ways. Firstly, before you start your relaxation practice it is advisable to do a few loosening up exercises to drain off tension before you start. People often find relaxing easier if they do this — especially if they feel restless. Secondly, as part of the anxiety management course, we recommend that you make exercise a regular part of your life. Even if you don't think of yourself as a 'sporty' person, you still need exercise to feel at your best. Of course it is possible to do many kinds of exercise indoors, but best of all, go to your library or local community centre and find out what fitness-related activities you can join outside the home. Decide on one, or even two, and go to it! You'll be very glad you did (see Fig. 14).

Through exercise you can:

- improve your health
- increase your energy, vitality and stamina
- improve your appearance
- meet people and develop your social life
- improve your confidence
- reduce anxiety, tension and depression
- enjoy yourself!

You need not feel that you'll make a fool of yourself — if you're a beginner at any sport you aren't expected to be an expert and you probably won't be the only one getting things wrong at first. If this worries you a lot, choose a non-competitive sport. Do take things easy at first, especially if the sport is very physically demanding like jogging or squash, and gradually build up your stamina within comfortable limits. Remember that it is vital to progress at a slow and sensible pace in any exercise regime. Almost everyone can take up some form of exercise even if they are disabled in some way or suffer from ill health.

However you should always check with your doctor first if:

- you have any doubts about whether a particular form of exercise is suitable for you
- you are unused to exercise
- you already have health problems which may indicate extra caution, e.g. asthma, high blood pressure, heart problems, painful/unstable joints.

But remember, taking no exercise at all is certainly bad for your health.

Tips for helping to make relaxation work for you

1. Tie up any loose ends. Make sure that you haven't left any simple, urgent chores undone before your relaxation practice. Do these first so you feel free to concentrate on the task in hand.
2. Choose a regular time to practise every day and keep to it.
3. Start learning in a comfortable position, lying down or sitting, as demonstrated in course sessions. This is very important to get right. In the initial stages choose a quiet place, free from interruptions. Pull the curtains or dim the lights if you wish.

There's something for everyone ...

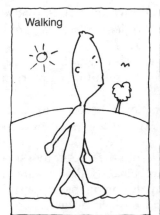
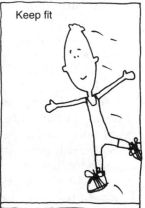
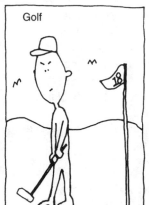
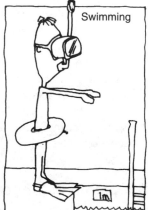

Figure 14   Beat stress with exercise.

4. Learn to breathe correctly — deeply and slowly.

• •

Try this:

Close your eyes and focus your attention on your breathing. Listen to the sound of your breathing. Take one deep breath and draw it right down into your abdomen, then let it go. Feel the tension escaping as you breathe out. Try to get the lower part of your chest to do the work of breathing, not your throat and upper chest. To ensure that you are breathing deeply enough, place your hands flat on your abdomen, at the bottom of your rib cage. You should feel movement as you breathe in and out. Continue breathing gently — don't force it — you don't have to *make* yourself breathe! Keep your shoulders down and relaxed. You can do this simple breathing routine at any time, in any place to help you relax. Check up on your breathing from time to time throughout the day until it comes naturally.

• •

5. Let relaxation happen — you can't hurry it, so don't get annoyed with yourself if you can't relax straightaway. Each time you practise it is doing you good so no effort is wasted. Allow thoughts to come and go but don't react to them, just passively let them go and gently bring your thoughts back to relaxation. You can deal with your problems after you've relaxed — you'll almost certainly find them easier to solve.

6. Observe your body, take notice when it tells you if it is tense or relaxed. You need to concentrate quite hard on your inner sensations, shutting out all external distractions, so that you eventually get really 'in tune' with yourself. This is necessary so that you can become expert at recognising and controlling your tension.

7. Enjoy relaxing. You deserve to relax, just like everyone else, so why not?

Supplement: 'Simple relaxation'

This exercise is based on: *Simple (physiological) Relaxation* by Laura Mitchell (1977 John Murray,

UK). Also see the 'How to relax' section above. For this technique you are not asked to tense your muscles — just to move the body part and then stop.

Positioning

Choose one of the following:

1. Lie flat with a small pillow under your head.
2. Sit in a comfortable chair with a high back on which to rest your head.
3. Sit on a chair with a table in front of you, with a pillow on top. Rest your head and upper body forward onto the pillow.

Orders

Shoulders Pull your shoulders towards your feet. STOP. Notice that your shoulders feel further away from your ears. Your neck may feel longer.

Elbows Slide your elbows away from your sides and open the angle so that they are slightly bent. STOP. Notice how your upper arms are now away from your sides and there is a wide angle at your elbows. The weight of both arms should be resting on a supportive surface, e.g. arm-rests.

Hands Keeping your wrists supported, stretch out your fingers and thumbs so they feel long. STOP. Notice that your fingers and thumbs are stretched out, separated and resting on the support surface.

Hips Turn your hips outwards. STOP. Notice how your thighs have rolled outwards. Your kneecaps are facing outwards.

Knees Move your knees slightly until they feel comfortable. STOP. Feel the resulting comfort in your knees.

Feet Push your toes away from your face, bending at the ankle. STOP. Feel your feet dangling and heavy.

Body Push your body into the supportive surface under/behind your back. STOP. Be aware of the weight of your body resting on the support.

Head Push your head back into the support. STOP. Be aware of the weight of your head on the support surface.

Breathing At your own pace, breathe in through the nose gently and slowly; then feel the lower ribs fall inwards and downwards as you breathe out.

Jaw Drag your jaw downwards. STOP. Notice your separated teeth, heavy jaw and loose lips.

Tongue Press your tongue downwards in your mouth. STOP. Let your tongue lie loosely in the middle of your mouth.

Eyes Close your eyes. STOP. Feel your lids resting gently over your eyes. Enjoy the darkness.

Forehead Smooth out your forehead from your eyebrows, up over your scalp and down to the back of your neck. STOP. Feel your hair move in the same direction.

Mind Either repeat the same sequence of movements around the body or choose some pleasant theme and let your thoughts wander upon this. Alternatively, choose something which has a sequence like a song, poem or a prayer. Don't be troubled if you get distracted by worrying thoughts, just dismiss them gently and return your mind to the pleasant ideas you have chosen.

Finishing routine Do this SLOWLY. Have a good stretch in all directions and yawn. Sit up for a few minutes before getting up and moving around again.

Self-help assignments 2

Name ....

1. Complete your daily stress diary and relaxation practice sheets as before.

2. Practise simple relaxation (see the Pack 2 supplement for instructions).

3. In the space below, make a list of the early-warning signs which occur just before your anxiety level rises. For example, many people notice that their breathing becomes faster, they start to perspire more or their muscles tremble or tighten. These must be the very first signs of anxiety you experience, not those of a full blown state of panic. We will be working on these in the next session.

Remember to bring all your completed homework in for the next session.

Client Pack 3
Relaxation in action

Now that you have begun to learn basic relaxation skills, it is time to start considering how to put them into practice when you most need them. It is all very well relaxing in a quiet, darkened room on a comfortable bed, but most of us need to be able to relax when life gets tough! Obviously, you won't be able to lie down on the supermarket floor, on the bus or at work whenever you feel tense! Because of this, the techniques discussed here concentrate firstly on helping you become more relaxed when you are going about your daily activities; and, secondly, on 'emergency' or quick relaxation methods that you can use to control anxiety in stressful situations. In previous sessions, you have been asked to recognise your own personal tension spots and early-warning signs of anxiety. It is important to be aware of these as you go about your daily activities so that you can intervene with a relaxed response before the tension and anxiety rise too high.

Differential (continuous) relaxation

This session deals with sitting, standing, walking and doing a task in a relaxed manner. It is important that you observe yourself carefully and retrain yourself to carry out activities using only the amount of tension that the task demands and no more.

This may take a lot of effort at first as you will have to keep correcting your posture and relaxing. With continued practice, though, you will lose the bad habits of tension that you have learned and find that you are more relaxed all the time without having to think about it. Also, you will need to speed up your ability to relax from 20 minutes down to one minute or less. Some people will be able to do this fairly quickly and others take longer. Note the length of time it takes you to relax completely and practise intensively until you can relax in one minute or less.

First practise differential relaxation sitting, then standing, walking, and then carrying out a simple, rhythmic task like peeling potatoes, painting or typing (Fig. 15).

Then, begin practising in a variety of different places — in different rooms, outdoors, at work, on public transport, etc.

Gradually work up to practising in more stressful situations.

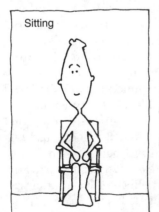 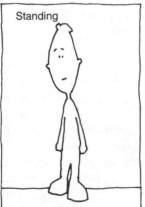 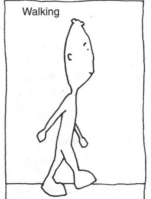 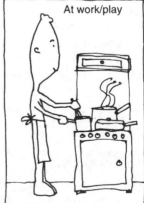

Figure 15   Differential relaxation — relaxation in action.

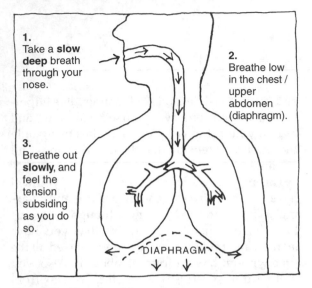

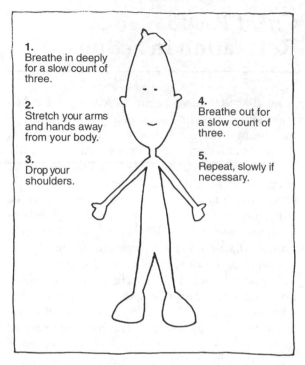

Figure 16 Deep breathing control.

• *Learn to recognise signs of tension*

• *Learn to relax quickly as soon as you notice signs of tension*

Figure 17 Mini relaxation.

Emergency (quick) relaxation methods

Deep breathing control

See the breathing exercise outlined in Pack 2. To adapt this for emergency use take a SLOW, DEEP BREATH. Make sure you are drawing your breath down as far as your lower chest/upper abdomen (Fig. 16). As you breathe out, slowly and fully, feel the tension dying away. You should notice that you feel more in control, steadier and calmer. Repeat this three times then continue breathing naturally, but still more deeply and slowly than usual. Quickly check your body for tension and let it go.

Mini relaxation

Make sure both feet are flat on the floor, whether you are sitting or standing. Take one deep breath in for a slow count of three while stretching out your arms and hands, slightly away from your sides. Pull your shoulders down and let your arms flop loosely by your sides. Breathe out for another slow count of three (Fig. 17). Lift your head up slowly. Finally, try a smile to relax your facial muscles.

We all feel tense in certain situations and you will find that what makes you tense might not affect another person and vice versa. Whether you feel at your most anxious on the bus, in a supermarket, at work or in social situations, the techniques we have recommended are similar. It is most important to tackle the difficult situations rather than stay on the easy ones — you won't achieve anything otherwise. So don't just talk about it — do it! You'll feel better when you've faced the problem. More help in facing up to anxiety and dealing with it effectively is on the way in the following sessions, so keep it up!

Self-help assignments 3

Name ....

1. Complete your daily stress diary and relaxation practice sheets as before.

2. Practise the 'everyday' and 'emergency' relaxation methods outlined in this pack and report on progress using the special relaxation application form attached (p. CP 46).

3. In the space below, make a list of ideas and thoughts that generally go through your mind when you are anxious, for example: 'I can't cope', 'I'm going to be ill' or 'I'm sure everyone is looking at me'. We will be working on this in the next session.

Remember to bring all your completed homework in for the next session.

Client Pack 4
Mental tension control

Negative thinking

As we have already made clear, anxiety can be useful and protect you from harmful situations. Unfortunately, it may also have the effect of making you think negatively. When you begin to have negative thoughts about situations, even if they are not really harmful, you will want to avoid them. Avoiding a situation causes even more negative thoughts, and in turn more anxiety, and so on.

This vicious circle starts to become a self-fulfilling prophecy: 'I *know* I'll feel ill if I go out'. The anxiety then increases so much that the person is bound to 'feel ill' when they go out, simply as a result of the uncomfortable symptoms of tension. After the trip they'll probably tell themselves: 'I *knew* I would feel ill if I went out'; and the damage will probably then be further reinforced by: 'I can't face going out again' (Fig. 18). This puts the person in the position either of having to get someone else to do all their errands for them, reducing their confidence, self-respect and independence still further — or of going without.

Another common example occurs when people misinterpret the physical sensations associated with anxiety. They may worry that they are seriously ill, perhaps even at risk of dying, and nothing the doctor says can dissuade them from this depressing view, despite numerous tests. This wastes precious time feeling really miserable, when the unpleasant bodily feelings associated with anxiety are rarely dangerous and can be overcome. Frequently, also, anxiety can complicate an existing physical condition, making it much more difficult to cope with.

Most of us probably fall into this trap from time to time when we're feeling worried and upset. So if you have recognised yourself in these descriptions, remember that you're not alone — the important thing is to question yourself as honestly as possible so that the problem can be solved. This takes real courage.

• •

Negative thoughts are very persuasive:

- they just 'appear' in your mind, out of nowhere

- they are not strictly true, and do not match the real facts

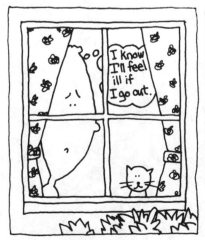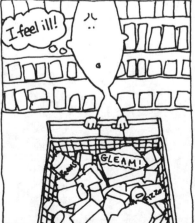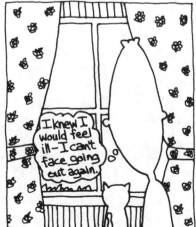

Figure 18   A self-fulfilling prophecy.

- they are unhelpful — they stop you fighting the anxiety

- they are seductive — it is easy to fall into the trap of believing them

- they seem overwhelming and very difficult to dismiss from your mind.

Irrational beliefs

Some of the beliefs we all develop about ourselves, our relationships and roles within society are irrational. They do not fit the true facts and may involve unreasonable expectations either of ourselves or others. Often, anxiety occurs as a result of a person putting pressure upon themselves to measure up to an ideal, or deeply held belief. We scarcely ever question out irrational beliefs and so never escape from the demands these place upon us.

A common example of an irrational belief:

'If I make a mistake, it means I'm stupid/everyone will think I'm stupid.'

Clearly, this is simply not justified, but so many of us cannot accept our own shortcomings in a realistic way.

Here's how this irrational belief can be challenged:

Of course *everybody* makes mistakes and it's best to be honest about it. This does not indicate stupidity — just ordinary human error which even the most skilled/intelligent people are subject to from time to time. Also, most mistakes can be corrected, and anyway, who's perfect? Who would want to be?

And here's a more realistic alternative:

'I'd rather not make too many mistakes — but I can't expect to be perfect — the odd slip doesn't mean I'm stupid.'

Let's look at some more examples of irrational beliefs.

Unreasonable expectations

These are the 'shoulds', 'musts' and 'oughts' that we live by. These are unreasonable when they are unrealistic and destructive either to others or to ourselves. Examples are:

- 'I *must always* be a good wife and mother'
- 'I *should never* allow myself to look foolish in front of others'
- 'I *ought* to show people that I'm *always* on top of things at work'.

Notice how the words 'always' and 'never' make the statements even more pressurised and anxiety-provoking. More irrational too, because in this world 'always' and 'never' hardly apply in personal matters such as these (Fig. 19).

Catastrophising

This simply describes how 'mountains can be made out of molehills'. Catastrophising is most unhelpful because it exaggerates and distorts the facts and also makes people miserable. Often we don't ask ourselves whether things really are as bad as all that — we just accept our own unrealistic assessment of the situation and expect those around us to see things the same way. The danger is that other people will probably find it difficult to understand why we are blowing things up out of all proportion and, understandably, may not give us the support we think we deserve. In this way, unreasonable expectations may lead to all kinds of conflict and disappointment.

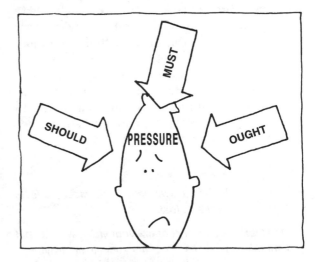

Figure 19 Unreasonable expectations.

Unreasonable assumptions

These are very similar to 'unreasonable expectations' but often involve some kind of social element. For example: 'caring mothers shouldn't go out to work'; 'strong men don't cry'; 'it's not polite to ask for second helpings' etc, etc. These assumptions keep us trapped in roles we may not want, or which make uncomfortable demands on us that we feel compelled to try and meet. These things can and must be questioned and challenged if it would lead to a happier and healthier way of life for you and those close to you! So what if the neighbours might not approve!

So what can you do about it?

There are three steps that you can carry out:

1. Learn to recognise your negative thoughts.
2. Challenge them! Are they really accurate, helpful and necessary?
3. Learn to replace them with positive thoughts.

Just as negative thinking can increase your anxiety, positive thinking can reduce it and put you in a more relaxed frame of mind. It also helps divert your attention from building up your anxiety level through focusing on the stressful situation and negative thoughts. When we have a difficult task ahead, we can choose to start thinking negatively about how we are bound to make a mess of it, (with the accompanying increase of anxiety we are more likely to make a mess of things!) or we could build up our resources with positive thinking. Perhaps we could take the attitude that this is a chance to show how well we can do, and our performance will improve as a result.

• •

- *Don't forget that the way you think directly affects the way you act and feel.*

- *Don't let your anxiety control your life — why not put yourself back in charge — it's your life anyway!*

• •

Guidelines on challenging faulty thinking

1. When you are worrying about something, try to isolate the underlying unreasonable belief you hold concerning the worry and re-evaluate it. You may be thinking, for example: 'it would be really unbearable if I made a fool of myself in front of people — I could never face anyone again'. Ask yourself whether it would really be so terrible as all that. After all, everyone is entitled to make mistakes.

    Often you'll find that it might be 'unfortunate' or 'inconvenient' if such and such happened, but rarely a complete disaster. Can you be sure that the worst is certain to occur in any case? Take a deep breath and get yourself thinking rationally.

2. Once you realise that you can be the author of your own anxiety, it puts you back in charge. It might be a bit hard to allow yourself to accept this at first. One reason might be that most of us prefer to blame other people or things and events outside ourselves for our difficulties. While we all suffer misfortunes that are out of our control, more often there is plenty that we can do to ease problem situations ourselves. Being in control of your anxiety is better than being at the mercy of it.

3. Use your new found control: *challenge* faulty thinking by being objective. Don't put things off — tackle problems quickly and with all your energy. Don't give yourself a chance to change your mind!

4. Tell yourself that you *can* handle the situations you worry about. When you find that your fears are not rational, be positive and face up to them. While you are in the feared situation, keep reminding yourself of the rational facts to help you cope, e.g. 'People are *not* looking at me/ I *won't* collapse'. Then PRACTISE, PRACTISE, PRACTISE over and over again until you've mastered your fear of the situation. You'll feel much more in control if you can achieve this. The alternative is for your anxieties to continue torturing you at the same pitch indefinitely.

5. Stop yourself briskly if you find yourself worrying about the same thing over and over again — actually say to yourself: 'STOP!' Then allow yourself some positive, rational thoughts — these are usually more comforting at the very least!

6. Don't worry about why you became anxious in the first place — you may never know. What really matters is dealing with the anxiety now.

7. Don't expect to master your anxiety in five minutes — a great deal of practice will be needed. Set backs must be expected too so don't let the odd slip make you so disheartened that you give up completely. After all, you may have had your anxieties for some time — they'll take time to conquer and you can't reasonably expect yourself to find things that easy.

8. Be kind to yourself. This is part of taking control over your own life too — it's not all hard work! Take responsibility to reward yourself when you've achieved something rather than expect others to do this. Give yourself a treat now and then. If you've tried to follow the guidelines given so far on this course, you certainly deserve it! How about now?

Supplement: mental tension control techniques — Part 1

The relaxation response

This exercise is based on *The Relaxation Response* (Benson H 1976 Collins).

For this technique you are advised to practise in a quiet environment, in a comfortable position and maintain a passive attitude. The latter means focusing on the exercise and just letting relaxation happen of its own accord. If you do find you get distracted by worries, just notice these thoughts calmly, let them pass, and then gently bring your thoughts back to the exercise. To help you keep your mind focused you are asked to repeat a word, any word you like, silently to yourself each time you breathe out. Carry out the exercise for ten to twenty minutes, twice daily.

Avoid practising if you've had a meal within the last two hours.

1. Sit quietly and comfortably.
2. Close your eyes.
3. Relax your muscles deeply, working up from feet to face, and stay relaxed throughout the exercise.
4. Breathing through the nose, focus your attention on this, and allow an easy natural rhythm.
5. Repeat the word 'one' (or any other word you prefer), silently to yourself each time you breathe out (see Fig. 20).

Visualisation

This technique involves using your imagination to help you relax and to overcome worries. While this technique is very simple, some people claim that it can help cure quite serious disease, so never underestimate the power of your own mind!

Here are some examples:

1. To aid muscle relaxation, imagine your muscles lying over your bones and under

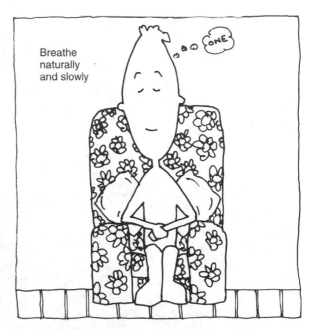

Breathe naturally and slowly

Figure 20   The relaxation response (Benson, 1976).

your skin; see the tension in them. Imagine them becoming softer and looser, lengthening out and relaxing. Take pleasure from the calming sensation and the feeling that just by thinking about it your muscles have relaxed.

2. To reduce the pain in a particularly tense spot, e.g. headache or backache, visualise the area that the pain is coming from in as much detail as you can. Paint a picture in your mind which seems near to the cause of the pain. For example, perhaps you feel that your stomach is 'tied up in knots'. Then slowly untie the knots in your imagination, focusing all the time on the painful area. Another example might be the feeling of tight bands around your head, as in tension headaches. In this case you could imagine the bands growing looser and slowly dropping away. You may notice the pain gradually reducing or dissolving away entirely.

3. To help you achieve mastery over situations you fear, imagine the situation in as much detail as possible. Where is it? Who is there? Set the scene in your mind, be it an approaching interview, confrontation, trip to the supermarket or bus trip. Then imagine yourself going into the situation and coping really well with the difficulties — just as you wish you could! Allow yourself time to linger over this and congratulate yourself.

You can probably think of some other ways of using visualisation to help you deal with problems or uncomfortable feelings. Do try them — it is best if you find your own way of adapting the method. Do be patient with yourself, though, and take all the time you need. Practise with your eyes closed, on your own, and in your most comfortable place. It also helps if you relax physically as much as possible first.

Self-help assignments 4

Name ....

1. Complete your daily stress diary and relaxation practice sheets as before.

2. Practise the mental relaxation techniques that have been described in this pack.

3. On the 'anxious thinking' form attached (p. CP 47) note examples of your own typical 'faulty thinking' patterns and challenge them, with a positive and rational thought. We will be working on these in the next session.

Remember to bring all your completed homework in for the next session.

Client Pack 5
Coping with life stress

Modern stresses

The sort of stresses we have to face these days are very different from those our forefathers had to deal with. Modern day stresses are often more subtle, complex, tending to wear us down gradually, sometimes without our being fully aware of it. Here are some examples:

1. Increased expectations of ourselves and those around us to live up to the impossibly ideal images portrayed through the media (Fig. 21).
2. Increased competitiveness leading to low self-esteem because our achievements, our homes, our appearance and social status often seem to compare unfavourably.
3. Reduced community and family support because it is no longer the norm for families to stay together in the same area. People frequently live alone, or in smaller family units. Support from the community is often lacking and many people do not even know their neighbours.
4. Linked to the above, loneliness is often a very real problem for many social groups, e.g. elderly and unemployed people.

5. Escalating work pressure, due to increasingly heavy demands / responsibilities and / or the threat of redundancy.
6. Increasing sense of threat to person, home and belongings associated with rising crime in many neighbourhoods.
7. Uncertainty or insecurity associated with the breakdown of former social norms such as regular church attendance and increased choices.
8. Unemployment, giving rise to loss of role and increased poverty.
9. Financial pressures — whether meeting mortgage demands or managing on meagre benefits.
10. Alienation and conflict in multicultural societies.
11. Continual bombardment by horrific news events from around the world through increasingly efficient media sources.

Life events

Many very ordinary events that occur as part of life can also be stressful — especially when they pile up on you! A test was designed by two researchers, Thomas Holmes and Richard Rahe, in 1967 to measure the 'stressfulness' of different life events. This test came up with 43 fairly common events including: pregnancy, retirement, Christmas, moving house, 'in-law' troubles, divorce, marriage and bereavement. Although you would expect such events as bereavement or divorce to be stressful, some of the events would normally be described as positive or happy ones. However, according to this famous research, any event which demands some kind of change or effort to readjust to a new situation is stressful, whether wanted or unwanted!

Incidentally, at the top of the 'stress table', by a long way, is the death of a spouse; next comes divorce and marital separation. If you are

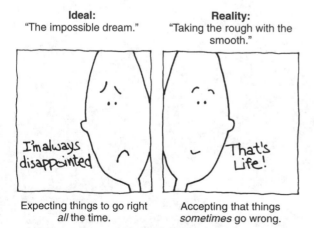

Ideal:	Reality:
"The impossible dream."	"Taking the rough with the smooth."
Expecting things to go right *all* the time.	Accepting that things *sometimes* go wrong.

Figure 21   Stress and the impossible ideal.

suffering from any of these stresses, it is very important to accept that you are going to feel desolate for a while. Such losses as these demand that you allow yourself to go through a period of grieving — this is normal and healthy. If you give yourself the space to express your pain and unhappiness, then things will improve all the sooner and you'll find life has some meaning again. Most of us have to suffer bereavement or the loss of an important relationship at some stage during our lifetime, so remember that you're not alone. It is helpful to find someone understanding to share your feelings with.

Of course we cannot avoid many of these life events, they simply are part of life! What we can do is to learn how to cope and adjust in a more healthy way to the demands life makes of us. Two ways of reducing stress stand out clearly. The first is to share your feelings, and accept the support of others (without leaning on them too heavily), as well as doing your share of giving. The second method is dealt with in this course — practical ways of coping with anxiety! (see Fig. 22)

Roles

Stress often results from difficulties in properly fulfilling the roles that we feel we *ought* to fulfil.

For example, we may demand of ourselves that we be a 'good mother/father/wife/husband/boss/employee'. Occasionally these roles conflict and we are torn between more than one demand. The working mother frequently experiences this kind of dilemma. Certain aspects of a role may also lead to stress. For example, you might be a good mother but not a particularly good cook, and feel a failure because you believe that your role as mother demands that you *should* be.

People sometimes place unnecessary burdens upon themselves trying to fulfil roles that they're not ideally suited to. There are often ways to reduce such stresses if people would only allow themselves to seek them. Alternatively, some people might prevent themselves from carrying out a role they would really like to take on because they believe it 'wouldn't be right'. For example, some mothers might be happier and healthier if they went out to work rather than staying at home, but deny themselves this opportunity because of guilt. Some men force themselves into competitive jobs with high salaries when they would rather do a more creative job, even if less highly paid (Fig. 23).

Relationships

Relationships cause a great deal of stress whether they are with our parents, our

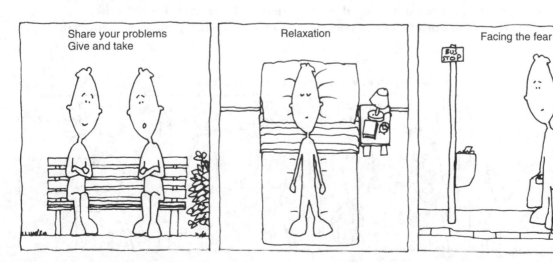

Figure 22   Coping strategies that work.

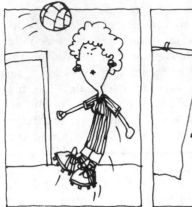
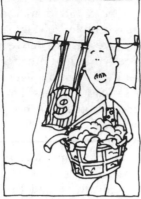

So what if the neighbours don't approve!

Figure 23 Roles: you can swap if you want to.

work-mates, our children or our partners. This is probably the most difficult area of all — few people find relationships easy all the time. Everyone's approach to relationships is unique and there are no clear 'wrongs' or 'rights'. However, there are things that seem generally helpful in easing the most common problems. We'll look at some of those now.

Communication

Talk over problems, no matter how painful and difficult this may seem. It is usually best to clear the air rather than just bottle things up; this can be really damaging to a relationship, so it is essential to keep the communication lines open (Fig. 24). Even arguments are usually better than cold silences which are especially destructive if they continue for any length of time. This doesn't mean to suggest that continually nagging at each other is a beneficial option though! One of the best ways of encouraging good communication is to listen. (Also see Pack 7). Communication problems, especially in a troubled relationship, can be extremely difficult to sort out. The situation may be helped by the intervention of a neutral third party that both people trust.

Understanding

This means thinking about what causes the problems between you so that you can deal with it. Understand your partner, but also yourself. There are rarely any totally innocent or guilty parties, but it helps to look at one's own contribution to the difficulties rather than to seek to apportion blame. The squabbles over issues like money, squeezing the toothpaste at the wrong end, leaving dirty socks around, etc. are frequently about much more important things in the relationship — like trust, sex, responsibility, sharing and caring (Fig. 25).

Give and take

In a partnership, making genuine efforts to understand and care for the other can help to keep the relationship alive. Showing affection is

Listening is the most important communication skill.

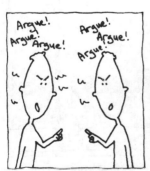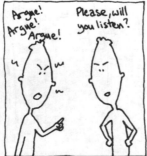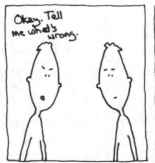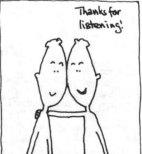

Figure 24 Communicate!

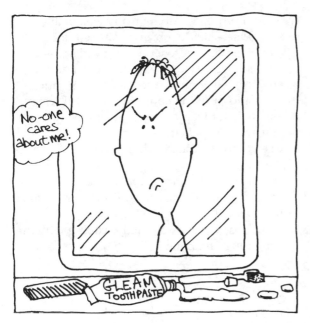

Figure 25 No-one cares about me!

also important in any close relationship.

Sadly, however, it is sometimes best to end a relationship and this is extremely gruelling for those concerned. A worse state of affairs occurs when people stay in mutually destructive relationships because they can't face parting. You may need to seek professional help to solve long-standing problems, or provide support during a separation process.

Indecision

When facing difficult choices, a great deal of stress results, especially when the decision-making period drags on. The only cure is to make the decision and accept the attendant problems — recognising that sometimes there is no ideal answer. Once this has been done, the stress is often reduced.

Time pressure

At no time before has there been greater time pressure than in the modern day; often our lives are run by the clock. Frustration mounts as time ticks inexorably onwards and we find we cannot meet the deadlines we set for ourselves. The principles of good time management include:

- planning ahead
- deciding on your priorities — tackle these first
- cutting out inessentials
- delegating more
- being realistic about the number of tasks you expect to complete within a certain time frame
- saying 'no' when demands get out of hand
- making good use of lists and diaries
- identifying time-wasting habits/practices and finding ways of controlling them
- getting away from it all as often as practicable.

Supplement: mental tension control techniques — Part 2

Putting it all together

By now you should have gained some mastery in the physical techniques of relaxation and have begun to practise some of the mental relaxation methods from the previous session. Exactly which techniques and which combinations of techniques is a personal matter at this stage, so select those which seem most suited to the occasion you require them for. Or choose one physical technique which you find works well for you, and one mental technique. You might, for example, use simple relaxation (Pack 2) to help you reduce physical tension and use 'visualisation' (Pack 4) to calm and focus your mind. The important thing is to find an effective combination which is convenient for the situation you are in, and which you feel comfortable using.

How to put your fears in order

In this session you were asked to think of three situations you found stressful and to practise controlling your anxiety level using relaxation. Continue practising these three until you can stay quite calm when you are thinking about them. Then put this achievement into practice by actually tackling the situation in real life.

1. Set yourself realistic targets that you can achieve and attempt them gradually. We will

be dealing with goal-setting in the next session.

2. Once you've done these three situations you may feel that there are more that you need to start tackling. Make a list of these and start the process again from the beginning.

3. Once you've conquered a situation, keep practising — *don't avoid it* — or you may end up back at square one!

Guidelines for imaginary rehearsal

1. Imagine the situation you are thinking of in as much detail as you can: Where is it happening? Who else is there, if anyone? What is happening? And so on.

2. Imagine yourself coping really well in the situation — closely observe yourself doing this, allowing yourself to feel strong and at ease.

3. If you begin to experience the first signs of anxiety — e.g. muscle tension, perspiration — then stop thinking about the stressful scene and switch to a pleasant, calm scene. Remind yourself that *you* are in control.

4. Use your relaxation techniques to reduce any anxiety.

5. When perfectly calm again, repeat the procedure until you can control your anxious reaction to it.

6. Now you're ready to practise coping with the situation in real life!

Self-help assignments 5

Name ....

1. Complete your daily stress diary and relaxation practice sheets as before.

2. Practise 'imaginary rehearsal' from this pack, using a combination of physical and mental relaxation techniques. Base your practice on a list of situations you find stressful and gradually work through the list from the easiest to the hardest situation.

Start putting these into practice in real-life situations as you progress.

3. In the space below, make a list of personal goals that you would like to achieve, in order of difficulty. For example: 'travel on buses alone', 'join an evening class or club', 'go on holiday', etc. It is very important to keep the goals practical and clear, like the examples given. We will be working on these in the next session.

Client Pack 6
Goal-setting and problem-solving techniques

Goal-setting

The first stage in solving a problem is to learn how to set realistic goals. Too often we aim either too high or too low and end up getting nowhere. This can make us feel even more defeated by our problems so that we are less likely to try again.

Each main goal should be broken down into smaller targets along the way. For example, suppose your main goal is to be able to join an evening class to pursue an interest, meet friends and get out and about. You want to do this because you are feeling lonely and cut off from the rest of the world due to fears of going out, especially alone, and at night! This might seem an impossible goal, but let's break it down into more digestible pieces.

Stages	Targets
0	Stay indoors alone each evening.
1	Ask someone round to spend the evening with.
2	Go out during the daytime with a friend.
3	Go out at night with a friend.
4	Go out alone during the daytime to practise the journey to the class.
5	Go out at night alone to practise the journey to the class.
6	Go out to class and if possible arrange for someone to meet you afterwards.
7	Go out to class and return independently.

Each of these targets could then be broken down even further where necessary, for example:

Target (stage 4): 'Go out alone during the daytime to practise the journey to the class':

1. Walk alone to the end of the road.
2. Walk alone to the end of the road and cross over.
3. Walk alone into town.
4. Walk into town and go into some shops.
5. Catch a bus and travel one stop.
6. Catch a bus and travel two stops.
   And so on . . . . . .

It helps a great deal to write down the targets and goals so that you know exactly what you are aiming for and how you are going to achieve it. It also helps to ask yourself how realistic your goals really are, and how long you should give yourself to achieve them.

Problem-solving

Everyone has problems — yes, *everyone*, no matter how successful they may seem to be on the surface! Regardless of what the problem is, the following technique can be applied to help you see new ways around a problem.

Ultimately, of course, the only way to solve problems is to take positive action. Negative thinking is also a way of making problems worse and keeping them 'alive and kicking'. Often, simply looking at the difficulty in a more positive and objective light makes an enormous difference. Here are some steps you can take.

1. Break the problem down into small parts as already described for goal-setting. What are your assumptions about it? Are they rational? What are the facts?
2. Ask yourself which parts of the problem are truly out of your control — just facts of life. Put these to one side.
3. Ask yourself which parts of the problem are under your control. List these.
4. Take each item on your list, and follow through this sequence:
   a. Brainstorming. Think of as many solutions to the problem as you can, using your imagination as wildly as you like. You do

not need to take the usual moral or social objections into account. Don't reject *any* ideas at this stage, no matter how bizarre they seem.

b. Assess all the solutions you've thought of in terms of:
- outcome
- feasibility
- likelihood of success.

c. Reject any solutions that do not score reasonably well on these three points. Don't forget that you are looking for a realistic solution.

d. You should be left with only two or three viable solutions. Choose the one you like the best.

e. Put this solution into practice, breaking it down into achievable goals. If it doesn't work, put the next solution on the list into practice.

5. This should work. If it doesn't then ask yourself:
a. Have I followed the method fully and correctly?
b. Have I identified the real problem?
c. Is my solution really practical/relevant?

Example: Peter's problem is that he doesn't have enough money to go out once he's paid all his bills. This makes him lonely, miserable and tense. He doesn't have a job although he has tried at his local job centre.

1. Break problem down:
- he hasn't got any training or special skills
- he doesn't know where/how to meet people
- unemployment is high in his area
- he spends too much money on drink in an attempt to 'drown his sorrows'
- his benefits aren't enough.

And so on ...

Table 1 Analysing possible solutions to Peter's problem

SOLUTION	OUTCOME	FEASIBILITY	SUCCESS RATING
1. Put up with it	Problem continues	Nil	Nil
2. Get unskilled job	Might increase funds but might not enjoy	Hard to find	Slight
3. Start own business	Good if successful	Difficult to borrow funds	Risky but worth a try
4. Get training/ apprenticeship	Good in long term	Fairly easy	Good
5. Get job using false qualifications	The sack	Slight	Unlikely

2. Identify parts of problem that are facts and out of personal control:
- high unemployment
- low benefits.
Ignore these.

3. Take the first part of the problem: 'No training/special skills', and brainstorm possible solutions, no matter how absurd.

And so on ...

See Table 1. Solution 4 is probably the best alternative. Having chosen a possible solution, Peter needs to set targets to achieve it:

1. Go to library/colleges and enquire about further education/training opportunities.
2. Study the literature and choose several of the best alternatives and apply to these in turn.
3. Apply for grant.

Think about how you can use this method to solve your own problems. You might be surprised at how objective and resourceful you can be when you try!

Self-help assignments 6

Name ....

1. Complete your daily stress diary and relaxation practice sheets as before.

2. List problems you would like to work on and set goals for tackling them using the special 'goal-setting' form attached (p. CP 48).

Carry out the problem-solving method for at least one problem using the special form attached (p. CP 49).

3. Commence the action decided upon to solve at least one problem and report on progress at the next session.

Client Pack 7
Improving your social life

Social skills and lifestyle

We all need people. That is a fact, so it is not surprising that people who are lonely, for whatever reason, are usually unhappy. However some people avoid situations that bring them into contact with others because of anxiety. Such people may feel shy, anxious about meeting people or convinced that they are uninteresting conversationalists. However, confidence can be increased by understanding how to improve your social skills.

Others might argue that being a loner is part of their character and cannot be changed. Often such people have never tried an alternative way of behaving and have just got stuck in an unrewarding pattern. Shy people may be ignored in company because of the 'don't come near me' signals that they unwittingly send out. In turn, being avoided makes them feel worse and less like going out. An outgoing person is rewarded for the interest and warmth they show towards others and so they continue to enjoy being with people. Actually it is perfectly possible to learn new ways of behaving in company, and the effort is nearly always well rewarded.

It is also important to have hobbies and interests that bring you into contact with other people. An empty life is usually a miserable, anxious one. Anxiety can make you lose interest in hobbies and social activities, leaving you more time to dwell on worries, leading to yet more anxiety. This vicious circle is not easy to break, but the alternative is to continue leading an anxious and lonely lifestyle.

Ask yourself what you'd really like to do, or where you'd like to go. Have you got an unfulfilled ambition? Perhaps you'd like to take up a sport, learn a new skill, study for an exam? Local libraries are usually full of information on local clubs and evening/day classes. Don't put it off — you could change your life for the better!

What are social skills?

These are our means of communicating effectively with others. Surprisingly, it is not so much what you say that makes you socially skilled, but what you do.

Posture

Someone who is anxious may sit huddled up on the edge of the chair, often looking away from people. They may walk with rounded shoulders and bent head. The confident person walks upright, looking around them (Fig. 26).

Hands

An anxious person's hands may often be seen twisting or fiddling. Confident people use their hands in a moderate way, just to emphasise their speech.

Personal space

An anxious person might stay too far away from

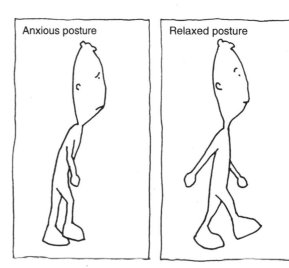

Figure 26   Body language.

others, making conversation and intimacy difficult. On the other hand, some people — you could call them 'space invaders' — come too close, which can be offensive. The confident person finds a comfortable distance, somewhere in between the two, depending on how well they know the other person (Fig. 27).

Touch

An anxious person might find it hard to make physical contact with people in an ordinary friendly way. However, an overbearing person might use too much physical contact. A confident person will use touch to help show warmth and friendship, without being intrusive.

Facial expression

Anxiety obviously shows on the face in a tense expression. Those who are anxious sometimes find it hard to show emotion on their face so that they may look rather rigid. Alternatively, they may look rather nervous and agitated. The facial expression of a confident person will be more animated, but calm at the same time.

Eye contact

An anxious person may find it hard to look at the person they are talking to. This might lead the other person to think they are not interested, and give up. An over-confident person might stare which can be a hostile gesture. A confident person will look at the person who is talking and look away briefly when replying.

Voice

Our feelings can show in our voices, by the tone, pitch and volume we employ. When anxious, this may be quiet and high-pitched. A confident person will speak clearly and emphasise certain points.

Check over these and ask yourself which of these are a problem for you. Then practise a more confident manner. You could practise first with people you don't know, like shop assistants or the bus conductor. A cheery good morning and a smile to a neighbour might be the start of a new friendship. You'll find people will respond to you much better if you only make the effort.

There are other things to consider regarding our interaction with people.

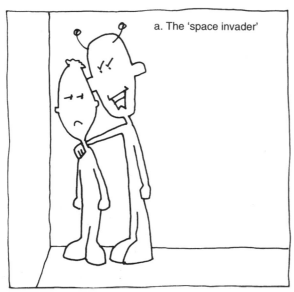
a. The 'space invader'

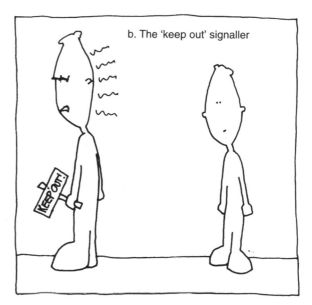
b. The 'keep out' signaller

Figure 27   Personal space.

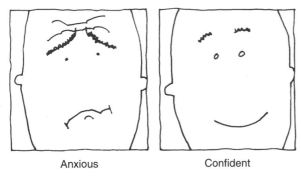

Anxious   Confident

Figure 28   Facial expression.

Appearance

How we dress and present ourselves to the world gives out a message about us. Consequently, it is important to make sure that you're giving out the kind of message you really want to convey. It goes without saying that good hygiene is obviously necessary if we don't want people to avoid us! Dress can give various impressions — attractive, eccentric, outrageous, stylish, shabby or nondescript. It can be an important way of expressing your unique personality and communicating to the world around you.

Conversation skills

The most important thing about conversation is listening! You may be surprised at this, but people tend to value a good listener more than a good conversationalist. So if you're shy, stop thinking that you have to offer a never-ending stream of sparkling witticisms, and learn how to listen!

Listening, however, is NOT a passive process. It means encouraging the other person to talk using all the social skills we've already mentioned such as looking at the other person. It means simple things like nodding, saying: 'Oh yes' or 'mm' now and then, to show that you're following what is being said, and responding with appropriate facial expressions. It also means responding verbally with a simple comment or another question to draw the other person out. For example, if you're talking to someone who is telling you about their hobby, you can respond with: 'That sounds interesting', 'What do you do when that happens?', or 'How long did it take you to learn that?' If you forget yourself and really listen to what the other person is saying, you'll soon forget your nerves.

It is also important to share your feelings and thoughts with others as openly as possible. It is extremely unlikely that they'll bite your head off or ridicule you — especially if you've listened to them! They'll probably want to know about you, in their turn. Don't say that you haven't got any thoughts/opinions/feelings — of course you have! — say them and people will respect you for it. Finally, never assume that what you've got to say is stupid or wrong. It frequently happens that the person who has the courage to state the seemingly obvious is greeted only with a sigh of relief and general agreement — especially in a group debate/discussion situation.

Assertiveness

This can be difficult if you're anxious, but if you can't be assertive, the drawbacks are many:

- bottling things up and feeling resentful and tense
- avoiding confrontation — this puts barriers between you and others, setting up dishonest forms of communication, e.g. loaded humour/sarcasm/cold politeness/excessive formality
- putting up with unfair treatment from others, e.g. being unable to return faulty goods
- losing one's temper because things have gone too far, with resulting strain on, or loss of, the relationship
- reducing your own self-respect.

And so on...

Assertion is not the same as aggression. Assertiveness is a way of protecting our own rights and needs without violating those of other people.

Assertiveness is:

- asking for help when you need it, not just suffering in silence

- saying 'no' to requests from others whenever you feel it is justified
- asking for more information when you don't understand something
- starting and finishing conversations on your own initiative
- giving and receiving compliments without being embarrassed
- stating openly and clearly when you feel irritated or disappointed
- listening to negative feelings that someone is expressing towards you while keeping a rational frame of mind.

Firstly, it's not until you have stated the problem to the person concerned that it can be dealt with. Avoid blaming, apologising or exaggerating — just say how *you* feel about the problem in a calm, rational manner. After all, you are not trying to hurt the other person, so decide on what you want to gain from the exchange, and ask for that. Secondly, it is hard to hear things we don't like about ourselves, but you'll find it pays to listen before you react. That way, nasty arguments are avoided, differences are more likely to be resolved, and such discussions often bring people closer.

Dos and Don'ts of assertiveness

Don't forget to use your social skills when you are being assertive, e.g. speak directly and honestly, make eye contact, speak loudly and clearly. Hold yourself upright and listen to what the other person is saying back to you.

Don't try to smile when you are really angry — it looks as if you don't mean what you're saying.

Choose an appropriate time to bring the issue up, e.g. not in front of others or during busy moments.

Facing up to things — coping with anxiety in social situations

Let us say you've decided to take an evening class, but you're dreading it. You are feeling very anxious and apprehensive that this will show. You're worried about how to cope with getting

there. The following is an example of what your negative thoughts might be and how to challenge them.

Before the event

Negative thoughts: This is going to be awful, I'm going to make a fool of myself, I know it. I won't go this week (avoidance!).

Challenge: STOP! Relax. What am I so worried about? Am I being reasonable about this? Going to an evening class won't hurt me, but it might help.

Negative thoughts: I know I'll make a fool of myself — everyone will see I'm nervous.

Challenge: So might the others — they'll all be beginners too. Anyway, what is really so bad about making a fool of myself — everyone does from time to time and life still goes on.

Negative thoughts: But I can't bear the idea — I'll feel terrible.

Challenge: That's an exaggeration. It's unlikely that I'll make a fool of myself. This wouldn't stop anyone else from going — am I going to let it stop me? No, I'm not going to waste all the effort I've made to make the arrangements. Anyway, I might meet someone who feels the same.

And keep it up . . .

Getting there

Negative thoughts: If the bus doesn't come soon I'll be sick!

Challenge: I'm feeling sick because I'm anxious, not because I'm ill. STOP. I'll take a deep breath and do my relaxation routine, then I'll feel better.

Negative thoughts: What am I doing on this horrible bus? Perhaps I'll get off and go home as fast as I can — I'm obviously not ready for this yet.

Challenge: This is something I want to do. I'm getting fed up with spending every evening indoors. Besides I'll never be ready unless I fight the anxiety.

At the event

Negative thoughts: I'll take a chair right at the

back so nobody will notice me. I feel as if everybody is looking at me.

Challenge: If I try to hide away people will think I don't want them to come near me and that will defeat the whole object of coming. Besides, no-one is looking at me — what's so special about me, anyway? If I see anyone looking my way they're probably being friendly, so I'll smile at them.

Actually, this is going quite well — I'm glad I came now. The class is really interesting so I've almost forgotten about my nerves. People seem friendly too. I bet the journey home won't be so bad — I'll have something to think about, besides my nerves!

The next day

I think I coped really well last night and that's the first time I've been out on my own for ages!

Negative thoughts: But what about the next time — things might not go so smoothly. How will I cope if I feel sick again?

Challenge: Well, I did cope and that is all that matters! The more I practise the easier it will be — I'm not likely to feel wonderful at first but its *action* that really counts!

This script shows how much effort is needed to counter anxious and negative thinking patterns. It also shows how easily anxiety could have sabotaged all your efforts to tackle the situation and damaged your self-confidence still further. It is important to keep up the positive challenges from the beginning to the end of a task like this, and evaluate your own coping performance realistically afterwards. Coping is very hard work at first, but it pays great rewards, giving you the freedom to live a happier and fuller life.

Self-help assignments 7

Name ....

1. Complete your daily stress diary and relaxation practice sheets as before.

2. Complete the 'revision checklist' attached.

3. Make a note of any aspects of the course you're not sure of that you would like covered again in the final revision session.

Also, decide on another problem for the final role-play session — don't forget this will be your last chance!

Revision checklist

Some of the statements below are false/incorrect. Please cross out any you disagree with:

1. Anxiety is abnormal and dangerous.
2. Anxiety can help improve your performance.
3. A tense posture goes with a tense mind.
4. When you are feeling anxious, you should avoid any physical exertion.
5. A relaxed body usually means a relaxed mind.
6. Negative thoughts automatically result in anxiety.
7. When you avoid a situation you dread, your fear of it increases.
8. If you stay in a situation you fear, your anxiety will get worse and worse.
9. Anxiety is just a feeling.
10. If you want to overcome fear you have to face up to it.
11. It's best not to plan ahead for difficult tasks — just plunge in without thinking about it too much.
12. Setting realistic, practical targets helps you succeed.
13. When you have a bad setback, you may as well give up trying.
14. Some people are 'loners' — they're happiest if they avoid social contacts wherever possible.
15. An empty, boring lifestyle is as stressful as a very busy one.
16. Learning better ways of communicating with others boosts confidence.
17. You have to be witty and extroverted to be popular — people who just sit and listen tend to be ignored.
18. If you assert yourself, people will turn against you.
19. Assertiveness means standing up for your rights without being aggressive.
20. Anxious people can't cope with life.

Client Pack 8
Keeping up the good work

This pack aims to help you revise the main points covered in the course but it is strongly suggested that you read over all the handouts from the beginning so that you are really well acquainted with the information. The following are only intended as memory joggers.

Physical tension control

1. Remember that anxiety is normal and useful — use yours as a cue for action.
2. The fight/flight system is the body's way of preparing you to deal with stress — keep yours in control to help you succeed.
3. Stress positions — watch your body language! This will help you feel better and more in control.
4. Relaxation — learn the difference between tension and relaxation.
5. It's difficult to be physically relaxed and mentally tense at the same time. This is how relaxation works, so use this scientific principle to your advantage, through relaxation techniques.
6. Early warning signs of anxiety — make sure you know what yours are and respond immediately by relaxing.
7. Use relaxation as often as you can — become really skilled at this and you'll be in control of your body rather than letting it be in control of you!
8. Apply relaxation to everyday activities — don't use more tension than necessary to perform daily tasks and activities.
9. Emergency relaxation techniques — remember that you can use them when you're in a tight spot.
10. Exercise — a healthy, beneficial way of releasing tension, improves your quality of life and helps you reduce anxiety and depression.

Mental tension control

1. Faulty thinking causes anxiety. This means thinking negatively, irrationally, catastrophising and allowing unreasonable expectations and assumptions to rule your life.
2. Beat faulty thinking by challenging it positively.
3. Invent your own little maxims to get you through difficult situations, e.g. 'I can, I ought, I will'.
4. Avoidance increases anxiety. This is very important to remember. Never avoid a situation because of anxiety, always face it. Anxiety will try to stop you doing things — don't let it. It is your life!
5. Concentrate on facts and the steps you can take, not your fears.
6. Don't let anxiety run away with you. When you're tackling a stressful situation resist the urge to rush and get it over with. Take a deep breath, go slowly and 'stay with' the anxiety. This way you'll find it will subside — give this a chance to happen.
7. Use mental relaxation to calm your mind and keep anxious thoughts at bay.
8. Use imaginary rehearsal before you tackle situations you're dreading. This will help you work through much of the anxiety even before you actually go into the situation.
9. Evaluate your performance after you've tackled something — be realistic and positive.
10. Reward yourself as you achieve your goals — even the small steps are important.
11. Don't give up just because you have a setback — some setbacks must be expected. After all, if it was going to be that easy, you wouldn't have needed to join the course. The important thing is to pick yourself up and keep trying — you will certainly succeed.

12. Life stresses — deal with these as positively as possible. Keep them to a realistic minimum, but remember that boredom is stressful, too!
13. Life events — these are difficult to predict or control at times but apply coping skills and get support from others.

Goal-setting and problem-solving

1. Break your main goals down into practical targets.
2. Set realistic goals for yourself so that you can succeed.
3. Practise on easier problems before you tackle bigger ones.
4. Use the problem solving technique in Client Pack 6 for a new way of looking at things.
5. Make sure you select realistic solutions and then *act* on them.

Social life

1. Don't avoid contact with others — we all need people.
2. Don't look for excuses to continue leading an empty life — get out and about, take up a hobby or join a club/class.
3. Loneliness and shyness — you don't need to put up with it, you can change.

4. Learn how to improve your social skills to boost your confidence.
5. Body language — this can speak volumes if you're anxious. Being aware of it helps you to change.
6. The most important ingredient in the art of conversation is *listening*. Improve your listening skills and it will pay off.
7. Image — are you really happy with the messages you are sending out?
8. Assert yourself — don't always be the 'victim' or 'wallflower'. You deserve better.
9. Assertiveness is not the same as aggression.
10. Assertiveness is standing up for your own rights and needs without violating those of others.

Lastly, if you've made it through the course you deserve CONGRATULATIONS! This has been a very intensive course but we hope that you have been able to enjoy as well as benefit from it. The vital thing to remember is that any achievements you have made were done through your own efforts.

Now you're on your own, *keep up the good work* and don't let things slide — you'll only have to go through all this hard work again — just think of that!

Name ....

Please use this form whenever you experience a marked increase of anxiety:

Date & time	Anxiety trigger situation or activity	Feelings and thoughts	Strength of anxiety 0 ——— 10	How did you try to cope?	Strength of anxiety after trying to cope 0 ——— 10

Client Pack Form 1. Daily stress diary.

Name ....

Date & time	Type of relaxation method used	Progress ratings	
		Before relaxing	After relaxing
		0 ————— 10	0 ————— 10
		0 ————— 10	0 ————— 10
		0 ————— 10	0 ————— 10
		0 ————— 10	0 ————— 10
		0 ————— 10	0 ————— 10
		0 ————— 10	0 ————— 10
		0 ————— 10	0 ————— 10
		0 ————— 10	0 ————— 10

Key: 0 = Completely relaxed
    5 = Moderately tense
  10 = Extremely tense

Client Pack Form 2. Daily relaxation practice form.

Name ....

Nature of activity or situation	First rating	Final rating
Sitting	0 —— 10	0 —— 10
Standing	0 —— 10	0 —— 10
Walking	0 —— 10	0 —— 10
Simple task	0 —— 10	0 —— 10
Stressful situation	0 —— 10	0 —— 10

Key: 0 = Completely relaxed
          5 = Moderately tense 10 = Extremely tense

Client Pack Form 3. Relaxation application form.

Name ....

Typical anxious/ faulty thoughts	Useful positive challenges

Client Pack Form 4. Anxious thinking form.

Name ....

Main problem	Main goal	Mini targets leading to main goal in order of difficulty

Client Pack Form 5. Goal-setting form.

Name ....

1. Describe basic problem

_____

2. Break problem down into smaller parts

_____

3. Select parts of problem under personal control

_____

4. Take each part of problem and "brainstorm" possible solutions on a piece of scrap paper.

_____

5. Write Solutions down under these headings:

Solution	Consequence	Practicality	Success rating

_____

6. Select the best alternatives and set targets using the "Goal-setting form".

_____

7. Carry them out!

Client Pack Form 6. Problem-solving form.

Index